Unlocking the Potential of AI and Big Data in Cancer Research: Advances and Applications

Unlocking the Potential of AI and Big Data in Cancer Research: Advances and Applications

Guest Editors

Federico Mastroleo
Giulia Marvaso

MDPI

Basel • Beijing • Wuhan • Barcelona • Belgrade • Novi Sad • Cluj • Manchester

Guest Editors
Federico Mastroleo
Division of Radiation Oncology
IEO, European Institute of Oncology, IRCCS,
Milan
Italy

Giulia Marvaso
Division of Radiation Oncology
IEO, European Institute of Oncology, IRCCS,
Milan
Italy

Editorial Office
MDPI AG
Grosspeteranlage 5
4052 Basel, Switzerland

This is a reprint of the Special Issue, published open access by the journal *Cancers* (ISSN 2072-6694), freely accessible at: https://www.mdpi.com/journal/cancers/special_issues/NJW5BNV213.

For citation purposes, cite each article independently as indicated on the article page online and as indicated below:

Lastname, A.A.; Lastname, B.B. Article Title. *Journal Name* **Year**, *Volume Number*, Page Range.

ISBN 978-3-7258-8197-0 (Hbk)
ISBN 978-3-7258-8198-7 (PDF)
https://doi.org/10.3390/books978-3-7258-8198-7

Contents

About the Editors . . . . **vii**

Federico Mastroleo and Giulia Marvaso
Unlocking the Potential of AI and Big Data in Cancer Research: Advances and Applications
Reprinted from: *Cancers* **2026**, *18*, 1234, https://doi.org/10.3390/cancers18081234 . . . . **1**

Nicholas Nicholson, Francesco Giusti and Carmen Martos
Ontology-Based AI Design Patterns and Constraints in Cancer Registry Data Validation
Reprinted from: *Cancers* **2023**, *15*, 5812, https://doi.org/10.3390/cancers15245812 . . . . **5**

Maria Giulia Vincini, Mattia Zaffaroni, Marco Schwarz, Giulia Marvaso, Federico Mastroleo, Stefania Volpe, et al.
More than Five Decades of Proton Therapy: A Bibliometric Overview of the Scientific Literature
Reprinted from: *Cancers* **2023**, *15*, 5545, https://doi.org/10.3390/cancers15235545 . . . . **25**

Ashlee J. Thomson, Jacqueline A. Rehn, Susan L. Heatley, Laura N. Eadie, Elyse C. Page, Caitlin Schutz, et al.
Reproducible Bioinformatics Analysis Workflows for Detecting *IGH* Gene Fusions in B-Cell Acute Lymphoblastic Leukaemia Patients
Reprinted from: *Cancers* **2023**, *15*, 4731, https://doi.org/10.3390/cancers15194731 . . . . **38**

Mi Jung Kwon, Ho Suk Kang, Min-Jeong Kim, Nan Young Kim, Hyo Geun Choi and Hyun Lim
Chronic Periodontitis and the Potential Likelihood of Gastric Cancer: A Nested Case-Control Study in the Korean Population Utilizing a National Health Sample Cohort
Reprinted from: *Cancers* **2023**, *15*, 3974, https://doi.org/10.3390/cancers15153974 . . . . **51**

Lukas Glänzer, Husam E. Masalkhi, Anjali A. Roeth, Thomas Schmitz-Rode and Ioana Slabu
Vessel Delineation Using U-Net: A Sparse Labeled Deep Learning Approach for Semantic Segmentation of Histological Images
Reprinted from: *Cancers* **2023**, *15*, 3773, https://doi.org/10.3390/cancers15153773 . . . . **63**

Rytis Maskeliūnas, Robertas Damaševičius, Audrius Kulikajevas, Kipras Pribuišis, Nora Ulozaitė-Stanienė and Virgilijus Uloza
Pareto-Optimized Non-Negative Matrix Factorization Approach to the Cleaning of Alaryngeal Speech Signals
Reprinted from: *Cancers* **2023**, *15*, 3644, https://doi.org/10.3390/cancers15143644 . . . . **86**

Jonas Wüster, Max Heiland, Susanne Nahles, Robert Preissner and Saskia Preissner
Statin Medication Improves Five-Year Survival Rates in Patients with Head and Neck Cancer: A Retrospective Case-Control Study of about 100,000 Patients
Reprinted from: *Cancers* **2023**, *15*, 3093, https://doi.org/10.3390/cancers15123093 . . . . **105**

Qingyuan Zheng, Jun Jian, Jingsong Wang, Kai Wang, Junjie Fan, Huazhen Xu, et al.
Predicting Lymph Node Metastasis Status from Primary Muscle-Invasive Bladder Cancer Histology Slides Using Deep Learning: A Retrospective Multicenter Study
Reprinted from: *Cancers* **2023**, *15*, 3000, https://doi.org/10.3390/cancers15113000 . . . . **115**

Vincent Bourbonne, Adrien Laville, Nicolas Wagneur, Youssef Ghannam and Audrey Larnaudie
Excitement and Concerns of Young Radiation Oncologists over Automatic Segmentation: A French Perspective
Reprinted from: *Cancers* **2023**, *15*, 2040, https://doi.org/10.3390/cancers15072040 . . . . **131**

Lars Johannes Isaksson, Paul Summers, Federico Mastroleo, Giulia Marvaso, Giulia Corrao, Maria Giulia Vincini, et al.
Automatic Segmentation with Deep Learning in Radiotherapy
Reprinted from: *Cancers* **2023**, *15*, 4389, https://doi.org/10.3390/cancers15174389 . . . . **144**

Ting-Wei Wang, Chih-Keng Wang, Jia-Sheng Hong, Heng-Sheng Chao, Yuh-Min Chen and Yu-Te Wu
Deep Learning in Thoracic Oncology: Meta-Analytical Insights into Lung Nodule Early-Detection Technologies
Reprinted from: *Cancers* **2025**, *17*, 621, https://doi.org/10.3390/cancers17040621 . . . . **158**

About the Editors

Federico Mastroleo

Federico Mastroleo is a Radiation Oncologist affiliated with the Division of Radiation Oncology at the European Institute of Oncology (IEO IRCCS), Milan, Italy, and a PhD student at the European School of Molecular Medicine—University of Milan. His research interests include radiation oncology, prostate cancer, medical imaging, artificial intelligence, big data applications in oncology, and translational cancer research. He has contributed to multidisciplinary projects aimed at improving precision medicine and integration of advanced technologies into clinical oncology practice. Dr. Mastroleo has authored and co-authored scientific publications on topics ranging from radiotherapy and imaging biomarkers to emerging applications of artificial intelligence in cancer research and care. His work combines clinical and technological innovation to support the development of data-driven strategies for cancer diagnosis, treatment optimization, and outcome prediction.

Giulia Marvaso

Giulia Marvaso is a Radiation Oncologist at the Division of Radiation Oncology, European Institute of Oncology (IEO IRCCS), Milan, Italy, and an assistant professor in the Department of Oncology and Hemato-Oncology at the University of Milan. Her research focuses on radiation oncology, oligometastatic disease, prostate cancer, stereotactic body radiotherapy (SBRT), translational oncology, imaging biomarkers, and personalized cancer treatment. She has led and contributed to several national and international clinical and translational research projects, including the RADIOSA phase II trial investigating SBRT with or without androgen-deprivation therapy in oligorecurrent prostate cancer. Dr. Marvaso is actively involved in multidisciplinary and cooperative research initiatives and has contributed to international consensus and guideline activities in radiation oncology. She has authored numerous peer-reviewed scientific publications and is recognized for her work advancing evidence-based and patient-centered approaches to cancer care.

cancers

Editorial

Unlocking the Potential of AI and Big Data in Cancer Research: Advances and Applications

Federico Mastroleo [1,2,*] and Giulia Marvaso [1,2,*]

1 Division of Radiation Oncology, IEO European Institute of Oncology IRCCS, 20141 Milan, Italy
2 Department of Oncology and Hemato-Oncology, University of Milan, 20122 Milan, Italy
* Correspondence: federico.mastroleo@ieo.it (F.M.); giulia.marvaso@ieo.it (G.M.)

Artificial intelligence (AI) and big data analytics have fundamentally reshaped the landscape of modern oncology. Over the past decade, the exponential growth of digitized clinical data (genomic sequencing, radiomics, digital pathology, electronic health records [EHRs]) has created unprecedented opportunities to apply machine learning (ML) and deep learning (DL) algorithms to problems that were previously intractable through conventional statistical approaches [1,2]. In radiation oncology, AI-driven autosegmentation of organs at risk and target volumes has emerged as one of the most mature clinical applications, with the potential to reduce inter-observer variability and planning time substantially [3]. Radiomics, the high-throughput extraction of quantitative imaging features, has gained traction as a non-invasive complement to tissue-based biomarkers, supporting outcome prediction models across multiple tumor sites [4]. In parallel, natural language processing (NLP) and large language models (LLMs) are beginning to unlock the vast unstructured textual information embedded in clinical notes, pathology reports, and the published literature, offering new avenues for automated data curation and clinical decision support [5,6].

1. Knowledge Gaps and How This Special Issue Addresses Them

Despite the rapid pace of methodological innovation, several critical knowledge gaps persist. First, the translational gap between proof-of-concept AI studies and clinically validated, prospectively tested tools remains substantial. Most published models have been developed and evaluated on retrospective, single-institution cohorts, with limited external validation and insufficient attention to generalizability across patient populations, imaging protocols, and institutional workflows [7].

Second, the interpretability and explainability of AI models continue to pose challenges for clinical adoption. While performance metrics such as area under the curve (AUC) are commonly reported, the mechanisms by which models arrive at their predictions are often opaque, limiting clinician trust and regulatory acceptance [8]. The recently published TRIPOD+AI statement [9] and the TRIPOD-LLM reporting guideline [10] represent important steps toward standardized, transparent reporting of prediction model studies, but their adoption in oncological research remains inconsistent.

Third, integrating AI tools into existing clinical information systems, including EHRs and treatment planning systems, presents substantial informatics and interoperability challenges. Real-time deployment of AI models requires not only technical infrastructure (e.g., FHIR-based interfaces, cloud or edge computing) but also robust governance frameworks to ensure data quality, patient privacy, and algorithmic fairness [11].

The contributions assembled in this Special Issue collectively address several of these gaps. The published articles span a wide thematic range, including deep learning for auto-

 https://doi.org/10.3390/cancers18081234

mated segmentation in radiotherapy planning, radiomics-based outcome prediction, bibliometric analyses of rapidly evolving oncological subfields, multi-omics data integration, and the application of AI to specific diagnostic and prognostic tasks. By bringing together original research and comprehensive reviews, this collection provides both methodological advances and critical evaluations of the state of the art, offering readers a cross-sectional view of how AI and big data are being translated into oncological practice.

2. Future Research Directions

Looking forward, several priority areas warrant focused investigation.

2.1. Prospective Validation and Clinical Implementation

The field must transition from retrospective model development to prospective, multi-institutional validation studies embedded within clinical trials or real-world deployment frameworks. Pragmatic trial designs, including stepped-wedge, cluster-randomized, and adaptive platform trials, are well-suited to evaluating AI-augmented workflows in oncology. Regulatory science for AI-based medical devices is evolving rapidly, and collaborative engagement between researchers, clinicians, and regulatory agencies will be essential [12,13].

2.2. Foundation Models and Large Language Models

The emergence of multimodal foundation models, pretrained on large-scale imaging, genomic, and textual corpora, represents a paradigm shift in how AI systems can be adapted to oncological tasks [14]. Transfer learning, few-shot learning, and prompt engineering may enable the development of high-performing models even in data-scarce clinical scenarios, such as rare tumor types or pediatric malignancies. The integration of LLMs with retrieval-augmented generation (RAG) architectures is particularly promising for clinical decision support systems that draw on institutional knowledge bases and current evidence.

2.3. Multi-Omics Integration and Digital Twins

The fusion of genomic, transcriptomic, proteomic, radiomic, and clinical data into unified predictive frameworks is an area of active development [15]. Longitudinal, multi-omics datasets that capture the evolution of disease biology and treatment response over time will be critical for building dynamic, patient-specific models, so-called digital twins, capable of informing adaptive treatment strategies. In silico clinical trials leveraging synthetic cohorts derived from such models may accelerate the evaluation of novel therapeutic approaches.

2.4. Federated Learning and Data Governance

Overcoming the barriers to multi-institutional data sharing without compromising patient privacy is a prerequisite for building generalizable AI models in oncology. Federated learning, differential privacy, and synthetic data generation are emerging as viable technical solutions [16], but their implementation at scale requires coordinated governance frameworks, standardized data models (e.g., OMOP-CDM, FHIR), and institutional commitment to interoperability.

2.5. Equity, Bias, and Ethical AI

As AI tools become increasingly embedded in clinical decision-making, ensuring that they perform equitably across diverse patient populations is paramount. Algorithmic auditing, fairness-aware model training, and the inclusion of underrepresented populations in training datasets are critical safeguards against perpetuating or amplifying existing health disparities [17].

https://doi.org/10.3390/cancers18081234

3. Conclusions

This Special Issue illustrates both the breadth and the depth of current research at the intersection of AI, big data, and cancer. The contributions highlight meaningful progress in autosegmentation, outcome modeling, bibliometric characterization of emerging fields, and the integration of multi-dimensional data for clinical decision support. At the same time, they underscore the work that remains: prospective validation, clinical implementation, regulatory alignment, and equitable deployment.

We are grateful to all the authors who contributed their work to this Special Issue, to the reviewers who ensured the rigor of the published articles, and to the editorial team at *Cancers* for their support throughout the process. We hope that this collection will serve as both a reference for the current state of the field and a stimulus for the next generation of studies that bring AI-driven cancer research closer to clinical impact.

Conflicts of Interest: The authors declare no conflicts of interest.

References

1. Rajpurkar, P.; Chen, E.; Banerjee, O.; Topol, E.J. AI in health and medicine. *Nat. Med.* **2022**, *28*, 31–38. [CrossRef]
2. Topol, E.J. High-performance medicine: The convergence of human and artificial intelligence. *Nat. Med.* **2019**, *25*, 44–56. [CrossRef] [PubMed]
3. Isaksson, L.J.; Mastroleo, F.; Vincini, M.G.; Marvaso, G.; Zaffaroni, M.; Gola, M.; Mazzola, G.C.; Bergamaschi, L.; Gaito, S.; Alongi, F.; et al. The emerging role of Artificial Intelligence in proton therapy: A review. *Crit. Rev. Oncol./Hematol.* **2024**, *204*, 104485. [CrossRef] [PubMed]
4. Lambin, P.; Leijenaar, R.T.H.; Deist, T.M.; Peerlings, J.; De Jong, E.E.C.; Van Timmeren, J.; Sanduleanu, S.; Larue, R.T.H.M.; Even, A.J.G.; Jochems, A.; et al. Radiomics: The bridge between medical imaging and personalized medicine. *Nat. Rev. Clin. Oncol.* **2017**, *14*, 749–762. [CrossRef] [PubMed]
5. Singhal, K.; Azizi, S.; Tu, T.; Mahdavi, S.S.; Wei, J.; Chung, H.W.; Scales, N.; Tanwani, A.; Cole-Lewis, H.; Pfohl, S.; et al. Large language models encode clinical knowledge. *Nature* **2023**, *620*, 172–180. [CrossRef] [PubMed]
6. Thirunavukarasu, A.J.; Ting, D.S.J.; Elangovan, K.; Gutierrez, L.; Tan, T.F.; Ting, D.S.W. Large language models in medicine. *Nat. Med.* **2023**, *29*, 1930–1940. [CrossRef] [PubMed]
7. Park, S.H.; Han, K. Methodologic Guide for Evaluating Clinical Performance and Effect of Artificial Intelligence Technology for Medical Diagnosis and Prediction. *Radiology* **2018**, *286*, 800–809. [CrossRef] [PubMed]
8. Papanastasopoulos, Z.; Samala, R.K.; Chan, H.P.; Hadjiiski, L.; Paramagul, C.; Helvie, M.A.; Neal, C.H. Explainable AI for medical imaging: Deep-learning CNN ensemble for classification of estrogen receptor status from breast MRI. In *Proceedings of the Medical Imaging 2020: Computer-Aided Diagnosis*; Hahn, H.K., Mazurowski, M.A., Eds.; SPIE: Houston, TX, USA, 2020; p. 52.
9. Collins, G.S.; Moons, K.G.M.; Dhiman, P.; Riley, R.D.; Beam, A.L.; Van Calster, B.; Ghassemi, M.; Liu, X.; Reitsma, J.B.; Van Smeden, M.; et al. TRIPOD+AI statement: Updated guidance for reporting clinical prediction models that use regression or machine learning methods. *BMJ* **2024**, *385*, e078378. [CrossRef] [PubMed]
10. Gallifant, J.; Afshar, M.; Ameen, S.; Aphinyanaphongs, Y.; Chen, S.; Cacciamani, G.; Demner-Fushman, D.; Dligach, D.; Daneshjou, R.; Fernandes, C.; et al. The TRIPOD-LLM reporting guideline for studies using large language models. *Nat. Med.* **2025**, *31*, 60–69. [CrossRef] [PubMed]
11. Char, D.S.; Shah, N.H.; Magnus, D. Implementing Machine Learning in Health Care—Addressing Ethical Challenges. *N. Engl. J. Med.* **2018**, *378*, 981–983. [CrossRef] [PubMed]
12. Muehlematter, U.J.; Daniore, P.; Vokinger, K.N. Approval of artificial intelligence and machine learning-based medical devices in the USA and Europe (2015–20): A comparative analysis. *Lancet Digit. Health* **2021**, *3*, e195–e203. [CrossRef] [PubMed]
13. Mastroleo, F.; Marvaso, G.; Jereczek-Fossa, B.A. Artificial intelligence in muscle-invasive bladder cancer: Opportunities, challenges, and clinical impact. *Curr. Opin. Urol.* **2025**, *35*, 543–548. [CrossRef] [PubMed]
14. Moor, M.; Banerjee, O.; Abad, Z.S.H.; Krumholz, H.M.; Leskovec, J.; Topol, E.J.; Rajpurkar, P. Foundation models for generalist medical artificial intelligence. *Nature* **2023**, *616*, 259–265. [CrossRef] [PubMed]
15. Acosta, J.N.; Falcone, G.J.; Rajpurkar, P.; Topol, E.J. Multimodal biomedical AI. *Nat. Med.* **2022**, *28*, 1773–1784. [CrossRef] [PubMed]

 https://doi.org/10.3390/cancers18081234

16. Rieke, N.; Hancox, J.; Li, W.; Milletarì, F.; Roth, H.R.; Albarqouni, S.; Bakas, S.; Galtier, M.N.; Landman, B.A.; Maier-Hein, K.; et al. The future of digital health with federated learning. *npj Digit. Med.* **2020**, *3*, 119. [CrossRef] [PubMed]
17. Obermeyer, Z.; Powers, B.; Vogeli, C.; Mullainathan, S. Dissecting racial bias in an algorithm used to manage the health of populations. *Science* **2019**, *366*, 447–453. [CrossRef] [PubMed]

https://doi.org/10.3390/cancers18081234

cancers

MDPI

Article

Ontology-Based AI Design Patterns and Constraints in Cancer Registry Data Validation

Nicholas Nicholson [1,*], Francesco Giusti [2] and Carmen Martos [3]

1 European Commission, Joint Research Centre (JRC), 21027 Ispra, Italy
2 Belgian Cancer Registry, 1210 Brussels, Belgium; francesco.giusti@registreducancer.org
3 Rare Diseases Research Unit, Foundation for the Promotion of Health and Biomedical Research in the Valencian Region (FISABIO), 46020 Valencia, Spain; carmen.martos@fisabio.es
* Correspondence: nicholas.nicholson@ec.europa.eu; Tel.: +39-0332-78-9365

Simple Summary: Ontology-based AI promises a more flexible and cost-effective approach to the validation of cancer registry data over traditional approaches and may allow a more straightforward means of federating centralised data-harmonisation processes. The advantage of using ontologies is that they unite the conceptual and logical aspects of a given domain and, therefore, provide an inherent means for expressing data validation rule sets. The idiosyncrasies of data validation, however, impose certain constraints on the ontology structure of AI-based reasoning and require design patterns that are not immediately obvious. The design patterns presented in this work are generic to other domains beyond cancer registries and serve to point out the types of issues that validation ontologies have to confront, with proposed solutions for tackling them.

Abstract: Data validation in cancer registration is a critical operation but is resource-intensive and has traditionally depended on proprietary software. Ontology-based AI is a novel approach utilising machine reasoning based on axioms formally described in description logic. This is a different approach from deep learning AI techniques but not exclusive of them. The advantage of the ontology approach lies in its ability to address a number of challenges concurrently. The disadvantages relate to computational costs, which increase with language expressivity and the size of data sets, and class containment restrictions imposed by description logics. Both these aspects would benefit from the availability of design patterns, which is the motivation behind this study. We modelled the European cancer registry data validation rules in description logic using a number of design patterns and showed the viability of the approach. Reasoning speeds are a limiting factor for large cancer registry data sets comprising many hundreds of thousands of records, but these can be offset to a certain extent by developing the ontology in a modular way. Data validation is also a highly parallelisable process. Important potential future work in this domain would be to identify and optimise reusable design patterns, paying particular attention to avoiding any unintended reasoning efficiency hotspots.

Keywords: data validation; knowledge representation; ontology-based AI; ontology design patterns; machine reasoning; cancer registries

1. Introduction

Population-based cancer registries collect data on cancers occurring in a defined population and are an essential element in cancer surveillance [1]. They are also a useful reference for cancer epidemiology. Data validation is an important process in the work of registries since statistical bias can lead to erroneous conclusions with potentially far-reaching implications. Apart from the more simple and generic types of validation checks, tailored data validation software is, however, often necessary and leads to costly and complex development and maintenance processes [2]. At a generic level, data validation requirements are similar and revolve around tasks that need: (a) to describe the validation rules in unambiguous terms; (b) to develop the associated validation software and test-data sets; (c) to manage the change control and maintenance processes; (d) to handle and coordinate the various version releases; and (e) to ensure the correct application of the data validation procedures.

1.1. Centralised Validation Process of Cancer Registry Data

These validation requirements underlie the centralised validation process of data collected from cancer registry members of the European Network of Cancer Registries (ENCR) for the purpose of providing accurate and comparable cancer indicators across Europe [3]. In this process, data are submitted to the central processing point from the individual European cancer registries. Owing to the fact that health services are regionally based in a number of EU Member States, there are over 150 cancer registries. The data are submitted in a common data template prescribing the data variables and their permissible ranges and formats. The data are thereafter checked against a predefined and agreed set of data rules using dedicated software [4] that outputs any errors found to a data log. The data logs are then returned to the associated cancer registries for correction/verification. Once this process is completed, the data are aggregated for public release on the European Cancer Information System (ECIS) data browser [3].

The centralised process has a number of drawbacks. One major issue is that it incurs time delays in the availability of data and compromises their usefulness in feeding back into health-policy initiatives. The delays are inherent in the process of coordinating data collection and validation across so many different entities and are compounded by administrative and bureaucratic processes relating to increasingly stricter EU data protection laws that are often implemented differently according to national/regional policies. Another issue relates to the centralised collection point itself. The ENCR is not a legal entity in its own right and receives no funding for its operation. The European Commission's Joint Research Centre currently provides a type of secretariat to handle the data-cleaning operation but relies on the knowledge and experience of staff who are often recruited on temporary contracts, resulting in potential risks of continuity. The difficulties and time delays associated with the ENCR centralised collection and validation of sensitive data could be alleviated by devolving these activities to the local cancer registry level. A process federation of this type, however, would require a straightforward and manageable mechanism for handling the individual steps of the data validation lifecycle. Ontologies provide a possible means of accomplishing this.

1.2. Role of Ontologies

The word ontology derives from two Greek words and, crudely interpreted, means the study of things that exist. In relation to this definition, computer ontologies express a knowledge domain via a set of representational primitives (such as classes, attributes, and relationships) [5]. Classes represent specific entities in the knowledge domain and are related to each other via a set of well-described relationships. For example, in the cancer registry domain, classes might represent such concepts as topography, morphology, grade, stage, etc. Relationships might then express the dependencies between such classes; for example, specifying which morphologies could be associated with which topographies, and which grades can be used with which morphologies, etc.

In contrast to databases, ontologies are able to integrate the conceptual aspect of the domain (describing the semantics of the domain and the scope of the model) and the logical aspect (describing the structure of the information) [6]. A particularly useful aspect is that the associated expressions can be represented in description logics (DLs) and, therefore, benefit from a formal representation as well as the predisposition to AI-based reasoning, giving rise to the term ontology-based AI.

The ENCR data validation rules [7] describe tumours according to the international classification of diseases for oncology (ICD-O-3) [8] and the internationally recognised

TNM classification for solid tumours (where "T" encodes the size and tissue invasion of the tumour; "N", the number of local lymph nodes involved; and "M" any distant metastases) [9]. ICD-O-3 describes the tumour in terms of: topography (associated with 330 codes specifying the site of the tumour); morphology (associated with just under 2000 codes specifying the type of tumour); and behaviour (associated with six codes describing the nature of the tumour). The TNM classification identifies the stage of the tumour; a further ICD-O-3 term describes the grade (associated with eight codes specifying the extent of the tumour); and the basis of diagnosis is an additional code set comprising eight codes describing how the tumour was diagnosed. The ENCR validation rules stipulate the permissible combination of the ICD-O-3 codes and their restrictions on other factors such as age, sex, and basis of diagnosis. While some ENCR rules apply internationally accepted rules (such as the TNM classification and the definition of multiple primary tumours), others are agreed within working groups comprising members with specific expertise from the European cancer registries. The outputs from the working groups result in a series of recommendations for adherence by the European cancer registry community. The ENCR rules form the basis of the data-cleaning checks, and divergences from the rules trigger error and warning messages in the resulting data logs that are sent back to the registries for verification.

1.3. Tabular Presentation of the ENCR Validation Rules

The ENCR data validation rules are generally presented in tabular form [7]. For reasons of clarity, a tabular representation is only able to show a limited number of dependencies at a time, and the whole set of dependencies therefore have to be displayed across a number of tables. As an example, morphology is related to practically all other variables (topography, behaviour, grade, stage, age, and basis of diagnosis). It becomes a laborious task to check each of these dependencies separately from each table and constructing a test-case data set for verifying the rule-checking software is particularly tedious. Any valid combination of variables can only be verified after cross-checking each of the tables in turn. An ontological representation of the rules has the advantage that all the dependencies are visible at the same time for any given class; it is, moreover, applicable to any data domain where dependencies between variables can be captured by a set of rules.

Initial work showed the viability of applying ontology-based AI to cancer registries' data validation requirements [10] but also highlighted the challenge of achieving good ontology designs that are serviceable to the needs of federating a relatively complex process. We present the design principles taken towards the realisation of this aim that may hopefully serve as a potential reference to other ontology developers facing similar issues. In the newly evolving field of ontology engineering, there is a sparsity of guidelines apart from some general recommendations [11–14]. Moreover, the information needs of an ontology may require justifiable compromises in the application of such recommendations. Whereas design patterns are becoming increasingly available [15], the needs of data validation applications tend to be quite specific.

2. Methodology

We used the web ontology language (OWL) and the Protégé ontology editor for designing the ontologies to validate the cancer registry data. OWL forms part of the semantic web architectural stack and can operate relatively seamlessly with other components in the stack, which is an advantage for semantic operability. With Protégé, it is a straightforward task to create classes and the relationships between them. The expression editor uses Manchester OWL syntax [16], which is more intuitive and easier to understand than DL-style syntax.

By creating class hierarchy trees, it becomes a manageable task to assign relationships for the 2000 plus morphology codes. A relationship can be assigned at a relevant super-class level that is inherited by all the corresponding subclasses. For example, by creating two separate morphology code trees associated with haematological-type morphologies and solid-tumour-type morphologies, one can treat each block of codes as a whole and still distinguish between any of the individual subclassed codes in the two trees.

Using Protégé, it is possible to choose from a selection of DL reasoners for verifying the logic of the axioms throughout the development process. Prior to running the reasoner, the ontology consists only of asserted axioms (including classes, class trees, and expressions); after running the reasoner, the ontology consists of the original asserted axioms as well as the results arising from logical inferences drawn from those axioms. The logical inferences made by the reasoner include further class hierarchies that are not defined a priori in the asserted ontology. The process of determining other classification trees in the reasoning process is called class subsumption (a class is subsumed by another class when it is inferred to be a subclass of that class). This automatic class subsumption is the means of determining whether a cancer case record or part of it is valid or not. However, in order to ensure class subsumption, a number of design constraints may need to be imposed on the ontology for reasons described in the following sub-section.

2.1. Expressivity of Description Logics

DLs are a family of languages based on first-order logic that are described by their expressivity (or types of operations they support) [17]. Higher expressivity languages have greater modelling power but also increase computational requirements. An important aspect of DLs concerns decidability (deriving a correct answer from the reasoning process), and most of the expressivities supported by the OWL ensure this. The basic language is AL (associative language), which has a limited set of operators that allow axioms to specify the negation and intersection of classes and to construct certain containment relationships between classes. It comprises the operators: atomic negation "not" (¬), concept intersection "and" (⊓), universal restrictions "only have relationships" (∀), and limited existential quantification "at-least-one relationships" (∃). The addition of complex concept negation (C), including concept disjunction "or" (U) and full existential qualification (ε), to provide the ALC (attributive language with complements) furnishes a relatively powerful modelling language. The label S is used as a substitution for ALC with transitive roles (allowing inferences of direct relationships between otherwise indirectly connected classes). Higher expressivities include inverse properties (I), role hierarchy (H), nominals (O), cardinality restrictions that allow an exact number of relationships with other entities (N), and qualified cardinality restrictions (Q) that allow cardinality restrictions on specific classes of objects. These additional features provide a richer modelling language.

Tools are available for machine reasoning on the basis of axioms written in DL. The result of the reasoning process is an expanded classification hierarchy of the ontology based on the class subsumption decisions logically inferred by the reasoner from the asserted axioms. In terms of algorithm complexity, most logic-reasoning processes are hard, and computational performance demands account for one of the main current drawbacks, requiring circumspection in how an ontology is designed. By limiting the expressivity to the εLH (existential language with role hierarchy, i.e., including concept intersection, existential restrictions, and sub-properties), classification of the ontology can be performed in polynomial time (PTIME) [18], which is advantageous for processing performance. The higher expressivity of SHIQ has a worst-case complexity of EXPTIME [19] and SROIQ of N2EXPTIME [20], which, in the worst-case scenarios, would make them unusable. While the introduction of highly optimised implementations of Tableau-based algorithms [21] has enabled the use of higher expressivities in practical applications, care nevertheless has to be exercised to limit the expressivity as far as possible, especially for ontologies involving tens of thousands of axioms. Reasoners have different strengths in relation to different types of ontology structures, but it is not immediately clear which structure is more amenable to a given reasoner [22–29].

Moreover, two particular properties of DL provide challenges for modelling validation rules; one is the open-world assumption and the other is logic monotonicity. The open-world assumption considers that any information not explicitly stated a priori can only be assumed to be unknown. While this view is necessary from the perspective of having to model incomplete knowledge, which is a requirement for knowledge derived from web resources, it has important consequence for how classes are subsumed by others. Data validation is a process better described by the closed-world assumption, where information not explicitly known to be true is considered to be false. Logic monotonicity is a consequence of semantic entailment and, in practical terms, prevents the overriding of default values—if a default value is asserted in DL, it cannot thereafter be modified independently of how much extra information is provided that may warrant its modification. This presents difficulties for scenarios commonly encountered in data validation rules, for example when a default condition is specified at a super-class level and one or more subclasses present exceptions to that condition; it is not possible in these cases to override the default condition with another condition for the exceptional subclasses.

2.2. ENCR Ontology Suite

The ENCR data validation process can be handled with a suite of three main ontologies. While these three ontologies may be integrated into one large ontology without difficulty, the reasoning performance would be unduly affected. Moreover, given that not all validation checks are required for all of the tumour records, it makes sense to use only those ontologies that are relevant to a given set of cancer cases.

One of these three main ontologies contains the axioms required for validating rules affecting all cancer case records; the other two ontologies are used for validating subsets of cases that either have TNM-stage associated information or are instances of cases with multiple primary tumours. Multiple primary tumours are defined as a diagnosis of two or more independent primary tumours in the case records of a person with cancer. The conditions for the independency of tumours for cancer registration are defined by a set of international rules [30] for the consistent recording and reporting of cancer cases for comparability purposes among population-based cancer registries. All three ontologies draw from a number of common base ontologies (OWL files), thereby facilitating maintenance aspects. Figure 1 shows the ontology import tree of the three ontologies. The TNMEd6 and TNMEd7 imports contain the axioms specific to the TNM classification editions 6 and 7, respectively. The ICDO3DefinedTNMSite import consists of axioms related to the TNM sites expressed in terms of the ICD-O-3 codes, and the ICCC3_O import contains the morphology categories defined in the third edition of the international classification of childhood cancer (ICCC). The ENCRTumourSignature import consists of the axioms defining permissible combinations of morphology and topography codes, and the two generic-named imports consist of common axioms used by the different TNM editions (TNMGeneric) and ICD-O-3 versions (ICDO3generic). Together, the three imports ICDO3generic, ICDO3_1, and ICDO3_2 (ICD-O versions 3.1 and 3.2, respectively), constitute the ICDO3 ontology (ICDO3_O).

2.3. Modelling the ENCR Data Validation Rules

With regard to the design constraints of the ontology modules, a critical aspect was how best to specify the associations between classes that had bi-directional interdependencies (e.g., topographies and morphologies) whilst ensuring their consistency across different modules and allowing the necessary class subsumption outcomes, especially in relation to the open-world assumption of DL. The answers to such questions must take also into account the different DL expressivities required by each ontology in the suite.

While most ENCR validation rules can be modelled in the TBox (terminology component of the knowledge base), some may also require an ABox (assertion component of the knowledge base). The TBox of a knowledge base can be considered similar to the schema of a database; it contains the classification trees of the classes and the relationships between them. The Abox, in contrast, contains specific instances of classes defined in the TBox. Working only with the TBox is generally less computationally expensive than working with an Abox as well.

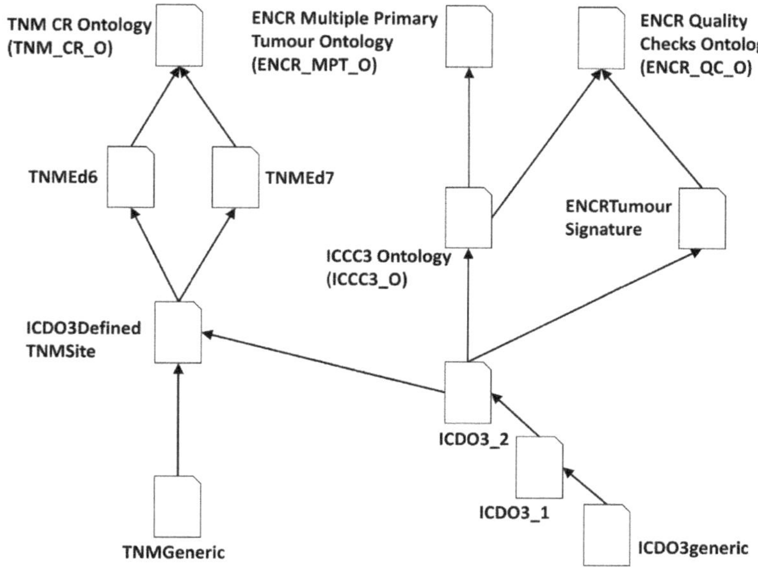

Figure 1. Ontology import tree for the three main ontologies—TNM_CR_O for validating TNM stage, ENCR_MPTO_O for validating multiple primary tumours, and ENCR_QC_O for validating all other rules.

Rules needing an ABox tend to require a higher expressivity DL and, consequently, may dictate the formulation of the properties used in the wider ontology space. As an example of this, a tumour may be expressed as a permissible combination of a morphology code and a topography code. In the multiple primary tumour ontology [31], for reasons related to the need for qualified cardinality restrictions (explicitly requiring an ABox), an appropriate axiom for a specific tumour defined by the ICD-O-3 morphology code 8082 and topography code C051 would be given by Equation (1):

$$\exists \text{hasMorphology.M\_8082} \sqcap \exists \text{hasTopography.C051} \sqsubseteq \text{Tumour} \quad (1)$$

The same axiom written in Manchester OWL syntax takes the more readable form:

(hasMorphology some M_8082) and
(hasTopography some C051) SubClassOf Tumour

This axiom loosely states that a hasMorphology relationship with the morphology code 8082, and a hasTopography relationship with the topography code C051together, constitute a tumour (the intersection of these existential relationships with the codes shown would, in the reasoning process, be subsumed by the tumour class).

2.3.1. Modelling Tumour Signature

The way in which axiom (1) is expressed influences how morphology and topography axioms are formulated in other parts of the ontology suite. Without the constraint of qualified cardinality restrictions, the way of associating the permissible set of topography and morphology codes could possibly be represented by the pattern of Equation (2):

$$\text{C051} \sqsubseteq \text{M\_8082} \quad (2)$$

which simply subclasses the topography code C051 under the morphology code 8082. While this expression makes it particularly easy in an ontology browser to see the whole set of topography and morphology associations from the asserted class hierarchy, it would insinuate that topography is a type of morphology, which is not the case. An alternative expression that breaks the direct class–subclass relationship would be:

$$\text{C051} \sqsubseteq \exists\text{hasMorphology.M\_8082} \quad (3)$$

which states that topography code C051 is a subclass of a hasMorphology relationship with morphology code 8082. This axiom would allow a user to derive both sets of associations, either by looking at the super-classes of the topography to see the corresponding morphologies or by running a DL query on the ∃hasMorphology existential relation of the morphology code to see the associated topography subclasses. There are two problems, however, with this formulation. The first problem is that it would require the topography code in a cancer case to be expressed in two different ways—first, as a simple or primitive class to derive the information from Equation (3) and, second, as an existential relation for the multiple primary tumour ontology in the formulation of Equation (1). The second problem is that it would encounter difficulties when specifying super-classes of morphologies (which is convenient for collectively referring to a large number of morphology subclasses). The morphology code M_8082 is subclassed from the set of morphology codes M_808 (which is itself subclassed from a further more general set). If one were to specify such a general morphology class in Equation (3) and execute a DL query to find the topography codes associated with the specific morphology code M_8082, the reasoner would not find the C051 association due to reasons of the open-world assumption of DL—there would not be enough information to warrant the subsumption of the topography class by the morphology class.

Reformulating Equation (3) as Equation (4) would circumvent the first problem (different formulations for the same concept) but not the second (class subsumption).

$$\exists\text{hasTopography.C051} \sqsubseteq \exists\text{hasMorphology.M\_8082} \quad (4)$$

Equation (4) subclasses a hasTopography relationship with the topography code C051 from a hasMorphology relationship with the morphology code 8082. This axiom would also make it more difficult to visualise the associations between topography classes and morphology classes since both sides of the expression consist of complex classes (classes within expressions). Moreover, neither of the patterns of Equation (3) or Equation (4) is able to model the validity of a combination of a specific topography and morphology without at least defining role compositions and incorporating inverse relationships to show their bilateral dependence. While role chain inclusions remain tractable in εL [32], inverse roles increase language complexity and generally lead to unsatisfactory performance using Tableau-based reasoners [33]. A more serious issue is that using inverse roles together with qualified cardinality restrictions leads to un-decidability [34], whereby the reasoner cannot return an answer.

A solution is not to define any relationship at all between the two class types but, instead, to decouple them via a duplicated or "surrogate" class hierarchy that mirrors the class hierarchy of one or other of the two class types. In this way, the morphology code classes could be subclassed from the surrogate topography classes according to the pattern of Equation (5):

$$\text{M\_8082} \sqsubseteq \text{C051Morph} \quad (5)$$

where, now, the morphology code is subclassed under the C051Morph class, which represents a surrogate topography class of C051. Using such a pattern still allows the associations in the visual terms of the class hierarchies to be made between the morphology and topography codes (via the similarly named surrogate topography codes). A further advantage is that the axiom in Equation (6) could then be used to expand the existential relationship ∃hasMorphology to the whole set of morphology codes subclassed from C051Morph (of which the morphology code 8082 in Equation (5) is just one example), thereby allowing the general formulation of a set of axioms specifying the valid combinations of topography and morphology codes, following the pattern of Equation (7).

$$\exists \text{hasMorphology.C051Morph} \quad (6)$$

$$\exists \text{hasMorphology.C051Morph} \sqcap \exists \text{hasTopography.C051} \sqsubseteq \text{VALID\_TumourSignature} \quad (7)$$

The intersection between a hasMorphology relation with any subclass of C051Morph and a hasTopography relation with any subclass of C051 would result in the subsumption of a valid tumour signature condition. An important point to notice from the first term of Equation (7) is that the surrogate topography codes are in fact morphology codes (unlike the situation in Equation (2)). The surrogate topography classification tree is, then, essentially a set of morphology codes organised following the structure of the topography classification tree (an example is shown in Figure A1 of the Appendix A). This would suggest a generic pattern in these types of problems where one needs first to create a duplicate set of surrogate classes of type B (but named and arranged according to the classification tree of type A) and, thereafter, to subclass the type-B classes under the surrogate code tree.

A drawback to this approach is the entanglement of the asserted ontology hierarchy (via multiple inheritance), which is not considered good practice owing to the fact that the trees cannot be split into disjoint branches to provide a more modular ontology [13]. While entanglement could be removed by subclassing existential relationships rather than primitive classes (c.f. the patterns of Equation (3) and Equation (2), respectively), the ease of visualising the associations—at least in an ontology editor such as Protégé—would then be lost.

2.3.2. Modelling Tumour Behaviour

A similar issue arises from the association of tumour behaviour with morphology. While some validation rules are only applicable to certain tumour behaviours, others are indifferent to them. It is, in any case, useful to know which morphologies are associated with any particular tumour behaviour. Given that a morphology may have more than one behaviour, it would seem appropriate to subclass the behaviours in some manner from the morphologies. Subclassing the behaviour codes directly under the morphology codes would confuse the meaning of tumour behaviour when using an existential relation ∃hasMorphology (at least without defining the associated role composition hasMorphology ∘ hasBehaviour), in much the same way as discussed in the previous section for the relationship between morphology and topography classes. Given the limited number of behaviour codes associated with each morphology code, we opted for creating a set of primitive classes under the morphology codes with the same names as the morphology code but appended with a number corresponding to the behaviour code, as in Equation (8) for behaviour code 3 (malignant behaviour). Although this increases the class structure both in size and depth, there is generally only a maximum of two or three behaviours per morphology code.

$$\text{M\_8082\_3} \sqsubseteq \text{M\_8082} \quad (8)$$

However, since the reasoner is unable to make inferences on the name of classes, an extra axiom, Equation (9), is needed to associate logically the behaviour code with the morphology:

$$\exists \text{hasMorphology.M\_8082\_3} \sqsubseteq \exists \text{hasBehaviour.BehaviorCode3} \quad (9)$$

The axiom in Equation (9) subsumes the class described on the left-hand side of the expression under the class of the right-hand side of the expression, which is relevant for axioms requiring knowledge of behaviour. Thus, whenever a hasMorphology relationship is used with a behaviour-appended morphology code, the expression will be subsumed by the reasoner under the associated hasBehaviour axiom.

This type of construct, which defines a complex subclass (left-hand side of Equation (9)), is termed by Protégé as a general concept inclusion (GCI). The approach in this case, however, costs an extra few thousand axioms (at least two axioms for each morphology code). Moreover, it requires axioms in all the other modules to specify the morphology code appended by the behaviour code, where knowledge of the behaviour is necessary (such that the class subsumption can be realised).

The important point to consider in a scalable ontology is how certain parts of the ontology might constrain the formulation of the axioms used in other parts of the ontology. ABox axioms in particular would form a good starting point from which to consider these constraints due to the greater restriction they place on class usage.

2.3.3. Overcoming Monotonicity Constraints

There are few ways around the limitations imposed by monotonicity on rules that are framed in terms of a default value for the majority of cases and another value for exceptional cases. Creating axioms that only flagged the exceptional cases would create ambiguities in knowing whether a non-flagged general case was valid or invalid. As a design decision, we opted to subclass a global axiom capturing all the conditions of the rule under a default value (for example, default valid or default invalid) and then to subclass the exceptions under a definitive exception flag. This would mean the user/application having to check not only the default condition class but also the presence or absence of the exception class before ascertaining whether the default condition was, in fact, correct or not. Equation (10) shows a global (invalid default value) rule applied to all cancer cases diagnosed from a clinical investigation (basis of diagnosis code 2), through a direct subclass relationship:

$$\exists \text{prevalidatedBoD.BoDcode2} \sqsubseteq \text{InvalidBoDDefaultCase} \tag{10}$$

This would mean that all basis of diagnosis codes of value 2 are, by default, subsumed under an invalid basis of diagnosis condition. In order to flag an exception to this default condition (for example, a basis of diagnosis code 2 is valid for a morphology code 8000 and behaviour code 1 in the case of tumours of the central nervous system), an axiom along the lines of Equation (11) can be used:

$$\begin{aligned}&\exists \text{prevalidatedBoD.BoDcode2} \sqcap \exists \text{hasMorphology.M\_8000\_1} \sqcap \\ &\exists \text{hasTopography.C751} \sqsubseteq \text{VALID\_BoD}\end{aligned} \tag{11}$$

The axioms modelling the various scenarios described in the preceding text are summarised, for convenience, in Table A1 of the Appendix A.

3. Results

The figures in this section show how the ontology suite is able to validate hypothetical cancer registry cases according to a selection of the validation rules. The yellow highlighted lines in the class description windows at the top of each figure relate to the inferences made by the reasoner. The non-highlighted lines relate to the information passed to the reasoner. The lines highlighted in green in the windows beneath the class description windows depict the traces provided by the reasoner for reaching the associated inference. The inferences illustrate some of the patterns referred to in Section 2.

3.1. Validation Results Using the General ENCR Quality Check Ontology (ENCR_QC_O)

Figure 2 shows the validation results for a hypothetical cancer case with the given class assertions. The reasoner has inferred that: (a) the tumour signature is a valid combination of morphology and topography codes; (b) the grade is incorrectly coded; and (c) the basis of diagnosis is valid. The first reasoner trace immediately below the class description window shows that the tumour signature instance c051_m8082 is defined by an existential relation with the morphology class M_8082 and an existential relation with the topography class

C051. The reasoner uses the fact that the M_8082 class is subclassed from the C051Morph surrogate topography class (c.f. Figure A1 of the Appendix A) to infer that the existential relation with M_8082 is subsumed by an existential relation with C051Morph. It then uses the axiom highlighted with the blue background to subsume the tumour signature instance c051_m8082 under the VALID_TumourSignature class, c.f. Equation (7).

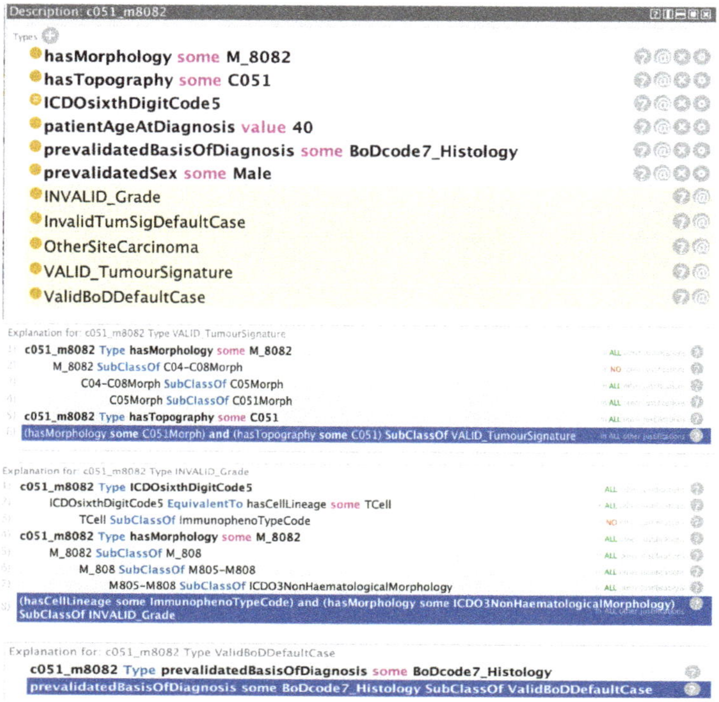

Figure 2. Inferences made by the reasoner (highlighted yellow text) on the basis of the asserted information provided (non-highlighted text) and the explanations provided by the reasoner (highlighted green text) for those inferences (valid tumour signature, invalid grade, and valid basis of diagnosis).

The second reasoner trace in Figure 2 provides the explanation for an invalid grade inference. From the predefined equivalence statement in the ontology, the reasoner recognises that the asserted value of grade is associated with a haematological morphology. The asserted morphology code is however subclassed from a non-haematological morphology. The axiom highlighted with the blue background is a rule that states a haematological-type grade with a non-haematological morphology is subsumed under an invalid grade condition.

The final reasoner trace relates to a valid basis for diagnosis inference. In this case, the inference is trivially determined since it is the default case for the basis of diagnosis involving a histological examination of an excised sample of the tumour (basis of diagnosis code 7). The reasoner infers the valid basis of diagnosis default case from the asserted basis of diagnosis code (7) and the associated default rule highlighted with a blue background in the window.

3.2. Validation Results Using the TNM-Specific Ontology (TNM_CR_O)

Figure 3 shows the validation results for a hypothetical cancer registry case with TNM data.

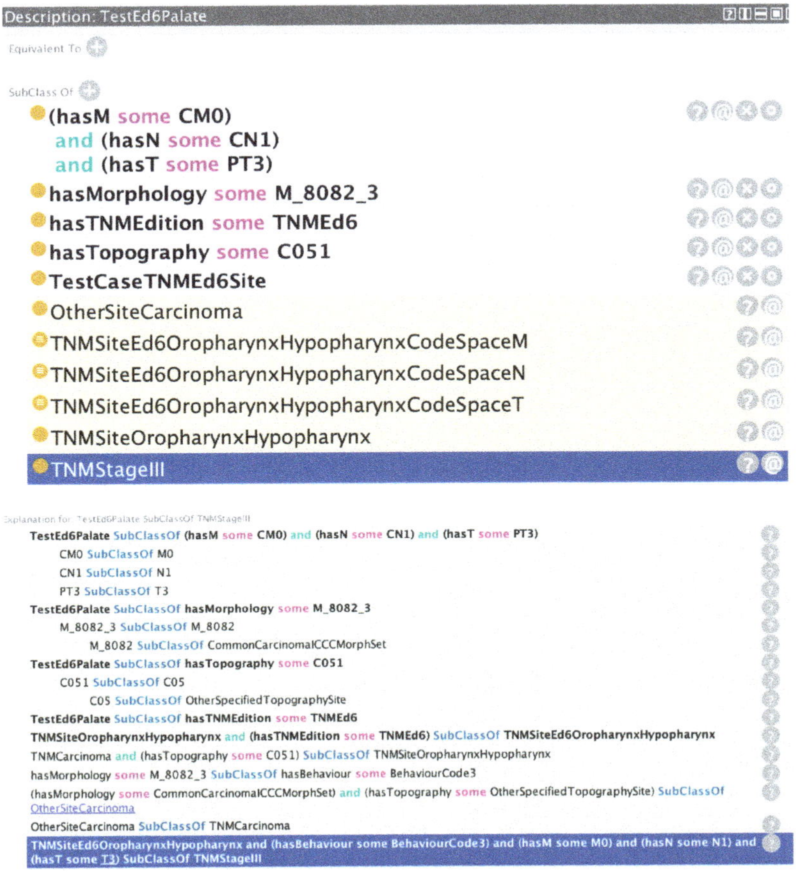

Figure 3. Validation results for a hypothetical cancer case with TNM data. The reasoner has correctly inferred stage group III (top window, bottom line highlighted with a blue background).

The reasoner has correctly inferred a stage group III based on the values asserted in the tumour case (morphology, topography, TNM edition, and T, N, and M parameters). The trace shows how the reasoner has determined a morphology group of common carcinomas from the asserted morphology and behaviour codes. Likewise, it has determined a topography site of "other specified site" from the asserted topography code. It then uses this information to find a subsumption under the class OtherSiteCarcinoma, which is itself a subclass of the TNMCarcinoma class, and this, together with the asserted topography class, results in a class subsumption under TNMSiteOropharynxHypopharynx—which for the asserted TNM edition results in a class subsumption under the TNMEd6 associated class. Finally, with the additional information of the asserted T, N, and M values, the reasoner infers a stage value of III from the rule highlighted with a blue background on the last line of the reasoner trace window.

3.3. Validation Results Using the Multiple Primary Tumour Ontology (ENCR_MPT_O)

Figure 4 is an example of a hypothetical multiple primary cancer case with three associated tumours, for which the reasoner has detected a violation of a condition for independent primary tumours. The asserted axioms are constructed using the three unique pairwise permutations (tumour couplets) of the three diagnosed tumours (tumours 1 and

2; tumours 1 and 3; and tumours 2 and 3, each corresponding to the three tumour couplet assertions shown in the figure).

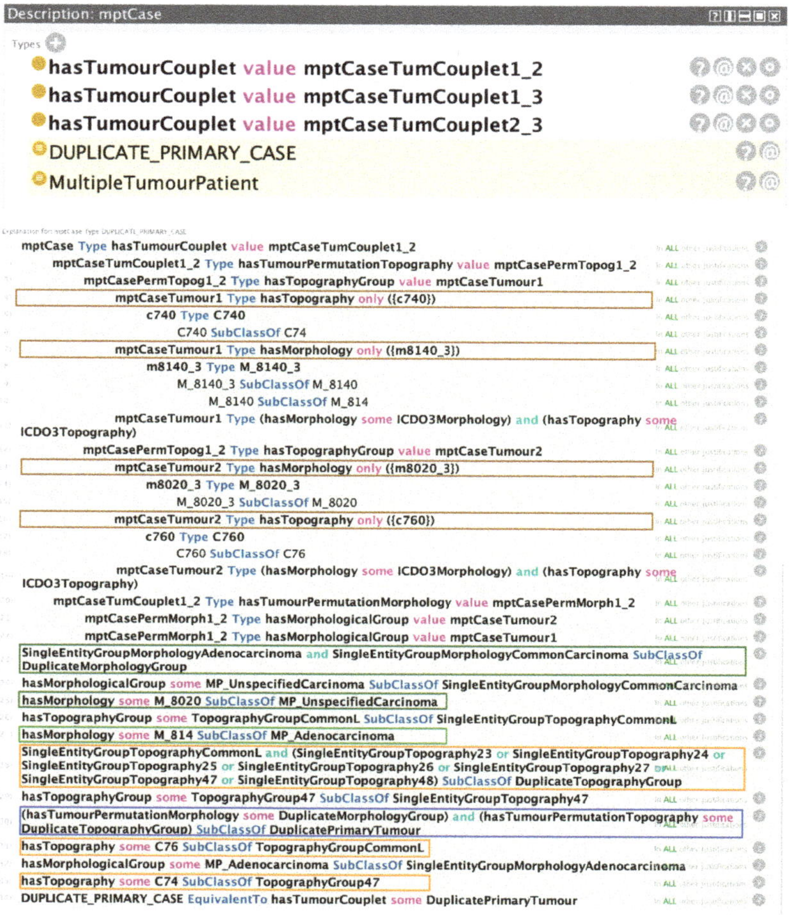

Figure 4. Example of a hypothetical multiple primary cancer case in which the reasoner has determined the occurrence of a duplicate primary tumour in one of the three tumour couplets.

The reasoner trace window provides the explanation for the rule violation inference with reference to the defaulting pair of tumours (the tumour couplet involving tumours 1 and 2). The first four boxed statements show the asserted topography and morphology values of the two tumours. The next three boxed statements show that the morphologies of the two tumours belong to a common morphology group. One of the morphologies belongs to the set of adenocarcinomas and the other belongs to the set of unspecified carcinomas; however, in combination, these two sets fall under a common morphology group, as shown. The three orange-boxed statements show that the topographies of the two tumours also belong to a common group. Tumours having morphologies and topographies both in common groups satisfy one of the conditions of a duplicate primary condition, as encapsulated in the axiom boxed by the blue rectangle. The equivalence statement on the last line leads the reasoner to infer a duplicate primary case, as indicated in the top window of Figure 4.

3.4. Metrics and Performance of the Ontology Modules

The main sets of metrics describing the ontology modules may be found in Table A2 of the Appendix A. The table includes the three main ontologies as well as a variety of composite ontologies incorporating other specific modules or main ontologies according to the modular design we used to allow such integration. The table also provides a comparison of reasoning performance between the four different reasoners we investigated (FaCT++, HemiT, Pellet, and ELK), all of which are freely distributed with Protégé.

4. Discussion

Ontologies are a powerful knowledge-organisation tool, and while data validation is not their primary function, they are able to support it via their foundation in description logics. The process of designing an ontology, however, is not an easy one, and ontology engineering is an emerging discipline; the ontology engineer must not only have an adequate understanding of the domain itself but be aware of the sorts of constraints that may influence the design of the axioms. Ontology development is seen as an iterative process [14] requiring frequent invocation of the reasoner; seemingly innocent changes can have major impacts on the speed of reasoning [35], and reasoning performance is also dependent on the reasoner used.

4.1. Main Findings

We have been able to show that ontology-based AI applications can successfully handle the majority of the ENCR validation rules for cancer registry data, even for quite complex inter-variable conditions. Using certain design patterns, we were able to overcome some of the DL restrictions that generally make DL reasoning challenging in applications more suited to the closed-world assumption. Other design patterns allowed us to limit the expressivity and reduce performance overheads. Regarding the reasoners we investigated, we found that FaCT++ and Pellet were more sensitive than HermiT to small changes in the axioms that disproportionately affected performance. Pellet performed consistently worst of all for reasons that appeared to be more associated with CPU load than memory space. While ELK performed consistently well, it is limited to a restricted set of operations and could not be used for validating the multiple primary tumour data. FaCT++ resulted in the best performance in the latter case.

4.2. Implications

Reasoning performance is an important factor to consider for any ontology-based AI application. Performance issues are, however, generally only noticeable for ontologies with more than several thousand classes, by which time it is more difficult to change the ontology structure. There are few guidelines available to help steer design choices, and the choice may, in any case, be constrained by the application domain. The requirements of data validation do impose certain restrictions on the design of the ontology, and we have highlighted a few issues and proposed some design patterns to help tackle them. One particular example is in relation to the open-world assumption of DLs; in order to force the necessary class subsumption requirements, we had to make extensive use of GCI constructs. GCIs can be expensive operations [36], but it is not otherwise possible to achieve the necessary containment. Moreover, the GCI construct is not so well supported in the Protégé editor (either in terms of text searching or visualisation of the asserted rules) and the value of the tool could be considerably enhanced were this functionality to be further developed. Reasoning performance is also an issue for ontologies with large ABoxes, and cancer registry data sets can run up to hundreds of thousands and even millions of records.

Designing an ontology using an appropriate modular architecture allows some performance gains on the basis of reasoner performance. For example, FaCT++ performed better for the multiple primary tumour ontology (ENCR_MPT_O) than the other reasoners we used, while HermiT was faster for the TNM ontology (TNM_CR_O), c.f. Table A2. Limiting expressivity to εL allows reasoning to be performed in polynomial time [35] (ELK is able to classify the 300,000 classes of SNOMED in the space of a few seconds [37]). The limitations of εL expressivity are not unduly restrictive for many types of validation checks, and ontologies can be designed carefully to respect the constraints. Only two particular types of checks in the ENCR validation process (age checks and multiple primary tumour checks) require greater expressivity and could be handled separately using other reasoners. Optimisation of reasoning algorithms remains an active field of research.

Other performance gains could be achieved via parallelisation. Validation is generally performed on a record-by-record basis, and the task is therefore highly parallelisable, serving to overcome performance bottlenecks on a single processor. The validation tests could themselves also be serialised and passed to the relevant ontology suite, c.f. Table A2, thus providing further motivation for a modular-based ontology design.

4.3. Motivations for the Ontology Approach to Data Validation

A major advantage of using ontologies for data validation is that of being able to maintain both the validation rules and the intelligence of the validation checks within the ontology itself. One need only invoke the reasoner on the basis of those axioms to validate any particular data. While this can be performed on a case-by-case basis using an ontology editor such as Protégé, complete data sets can be tested via the OWL application programming interface (OWL-API) [38]. The interface programme needs only to read in the individual records of a data set, translate them to the DL statements required by the ontology, and then invoke the reasoner. The application programme thus becomes more of a data-housekeeping task. The OWL-API can nevertheless also be used to perform the logic operations in the software and transfer the intelligence from the ontology to the application programme where necessary. Although this does have an impact on development and maintenance costs, it provides a means for overcoming limitations due to reasoning performance whilst still benefiting from the logical axioms defined in the ontology.

The unification of these aspects within a single application is attractive for the eventual devolution of centralised data-cleaning processes to the local cancer registry level. Application of a consistent and standard approach has been one of the hurdles in the past since it is critical that no biases are introduced from an inconsistent application of the validation rules. A further advantage of the ontological approach is that it allows some quantifiable and reproducible means of measuring several quality metrics of data sets, affording users greater assurance in the comparability/integration of data sets from different sources [39].

Ontologies are a useful tool allowing quick comparison and reference across multiple classification schemes, which can also serve to highlight where code hierarchies could be arranged more efficiently. For example, we had to define many different classification trees for the morphology codes (dependent on the specific validation checks). This resulted in considerable entanglement in the asserted classification trees due to multiple inheritance and conveys the need for greater rationalisation in morphology classification.

4.4. Limitations

In addition to reasoning performance issues, it must also be admitted that ontologies are not necessarily able to handle all types of validation checks; some notable exceptions are those that require the comparison of dates and the tracking of frequencies of variables. Such checks within the ENCR data, however, can be handled without undue difficulty in a pre-processing stage. The latter is, in any case, necessary for transcribing the raw data files into RDF prior to insertion into the ontology. Alternatively, there are other useful tools within the semantic web stack that can perform checks less suited to ontologies. The shape language ShEx is able to trap range and format errors and SPARQL scripts provides a versatile means for determining, amongst other things, the frequencies of variables in a given data set. The interesting aspect from the perspectives of maintenance and process harmonisation is that the tools all work on RDF data, which is one of the default representational formats of OWL ontologies.

4.5. Other AI-Based Approaches and Future Directions

Deep learning techniques could undoubtedly be used to validate data, and a commercial product along these lines is available for validating the accuracy of clinical trial results [40]. Such an approach has advantages in terms of reasoning speeds but requires a specific set of skills for developing and maintaining the associated application. Our reason for considering an ontological approach was to provide a range of functionalities, including: (a) a knowledge base allowing the integration of all the semantic relationships defined over a number of different classification schemes (ICD-O, TNM, and ICCC); (b) a means of formalising the data rules; (c) a means of defining and linking the metadata; and (d) a single application suite with a standard interface.

There is, however, no reason why the two approaches could not be used together, and a powerful symbiosis exists between extract, transform, and load (ETL) approaches and semantic representations of ontologies. The semantic relations, and even the rule base itself, could be derived and transformed using ETL into DL axioms from the whole of the European cancer registry data and stored in an ontology. The ontology could, thereafter, be used by any machine-learning process for data validation purposes.

More immediate aims to help consolidate ontology-based AI in the data validation domain would be to identify and optimise a full range of generic design patterns. It would be useful also to understand the underlying reasons for the formation of reasoning performance hotspots [35] and to find approaches/design patterns for avoiding them, as well as to deploy advanced reasoning tools as and when they become available.

5. Conclusions

Ontology-based AI can provide a number of advantages over traditional approaches to validating cancer registry data. Ontologies are able to describe the necessary conceptual and relational information associated with a given domain and express the dependencies in formal logic. The subsequent integration of the validation checks within the knowledge base means that any modifications to the rules base can be kept in synchronisation with the data model itself. This, in turn, simplifies maintenance issues and facilitates the federation of the validation process, thereby overcoming many of the hurdles associated with centralised data collection. Data validation is, however, not the primary purpose of ontologies, and the associated idiosyncrasies impose certain design constraints and patterns on the ontology structure for AI-based reasoning that are not immediately obvious. The design patterns and constraints presented here are generic to other domains beyond cancer registries and serve to point out the types of issues validation ontologies have to confront, with proposed solutions for tackling them. Discovery and optimisation (especially in overcoming reasoning hotspot issues) of other such patterns would provide an important and valuable contribution to the advancement of ontology-based AI for data validation purposes. It is hoped that this study may give impetus to further work in this area, which is relevant for all data domains.

Author Contributions: Conceptualization, N.N.; data curation, F.G. and C.M.; formal analysis, F.G. and C.M.; investigation, N.N.; methodology, N.N.; project administration, N.N.; resources, N.N.; software, N.N.; supervision, N.N. and C.M.; validation, F.G. and C.M.; writing—original draft, N.N.; writing—review and editing, N.N., F.G. and C.M. All authors have read and agreed to the published version of the manuscript.

Funding: This research received no external funding.

Institutional Review Board Statement: Not applicable.

Informed Consent Statement: Not applicable.

Data Availability Statement: The ontologies are available as follows: ENCR core-validation ontology: http://data.europa.eu/89h/efd6acd1-2cfd-401b-b5ea-d05f8efbb123 (accessed on 8 December 2023); stage-validation ontology: http://data.europa.eu/89h/9fa603ff-a118-41f3-82a2-bf8d4f0d7ea3 (accessed on 8 December 2023); ICD-O-3 ontology: http://data.europa.eu/89h/88ff4ec5-1832-40

3e-abe1-64928592568f (accessed on 8 December 2023); ICCC-3 ontology: http://data.europa.eu/89h/6f69e886-e5bc-4cd8-9b2d-8aaccf836789 (accessed on 8 December 2023); and multiple primary tumour-validation ontology: http://data.europa.eu/89h/2a110a2e-d1e2-439d-9b9f-7e2e5436cc49 (accessed on 8 December 2023).

Acknowledgments: This work was conducted using Protégé.

Conflicts of Interest: The authors declare no conflict of interest.

Abbreviations

AI	artificial intelligence
DL	description logic
ECIS	European cancer information system
ENCR	European Network of Cancer Registries
ENCR_QC_O	ENCR quality checks ontology
ETL	extract, transform, and load
GCI	general concept inclusion
ICCC	International classification of childhood cancer
ICCC3_O	ICCC3 ontology
ICD-O	International classification of diseases for oncology
ICDO3_O	ICD-O-3 ontology
OWL	web ontology language
OWL-API	OWL application programming interface
TNM	classification standard of malignant tumours
TNM_CR_O	TNM cancer registry ontology

Appendix A

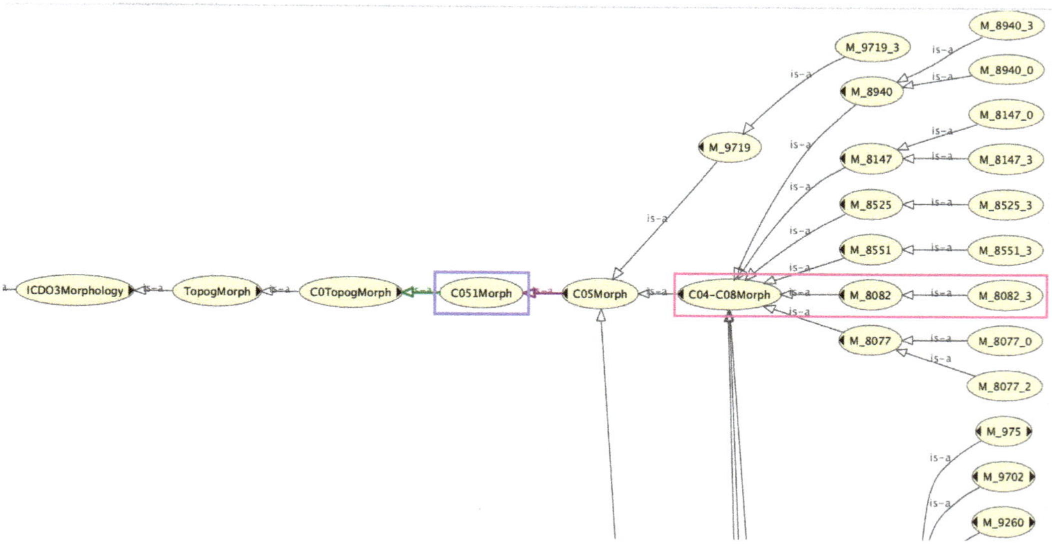

Figure A1. Part of the classification tree of the surrogate topography class C051Morph, showing its subsumption of the morphology class M_8082_3 (highlighted in the boxed sections).

Table A1. Summary of mechanisms described in Section 2.3 that can be employed to ensure the desired class subsumption results and that overcome some of the inherent constraints of DLs in closed-world reasoning.

DL Constraint	Mechanism to Circumvent Constraint Whilst Limiting Expressivity	Example	Axiom(s)
open-world assumption	GCI (to force the required class subsumption by subclassing the axiom under the desired outcome class)	behaviour	∃hasMorphology.M_8082_3 ⊑ ∃hasBehaviour.BehaviorCode3 (the existential relation ∃hasMorphology.M_8082_3 is automatically subsumed under the existential relation ∃hasBehaviour.BehaviorCode3, allowing other axioms to deduce that the existential relation with the class M_8082_3 is associated with the malignant behaviour code 3)
open-world assumption and inverse roles	GCI and "surrogate" classes	tumour signature	M_8082 ⊑ C051Morph (subclassing of morphology class under the associated "surrogate" topography class) ∃hasMorphology.C051Morph ⊓ ∃hasTopography.C051 ⊑ VALID_TumourSignature (subsumption by a valid condition class of the intersection of the real topography class and the surrogate topography class, which links in all the subclassed morphology codes)
role chaining	subclassing a class with a name qualifier under a class of the same name without the qualifier, and using a GCI to force the qualified relation	behaviour	M_8082_3 ⊑ M_8082 (subclassing of behaviour-flagged morphology class under the corresponding morphology class) ∃hasMorphology.M_8082_3 ⊑ ∃hasBehaviour.BehaviorCode3 (c.f. axiom in the first row of the table. The axioms avoid having to define a chain role such as hasMorphology ∘ hasBehaviour ⊑ hasBehaviour)
monotonicity	default condition and secondary override condition	basis of diagnosis	∃prevalidatedBoD.BoDcode2 ⊑ InvalidBoDDefaultCase (subclassing a prevalidated class under a default class) ∃prevalidatedBoD.BoDcode2 ⊓ ∃hasMorphology.M_8000_1 ⊓ ∃hasTopography.C751 ⊑ VALID_BoD (subsuming the intersection, under a class with the opposing validity to the default value, of the prevalidated class with the set of conditions that serve to invalidate the default condition)

Table A2. Summary of the metrics for the ontologies and their various integrations into larger containing ontologies. The attribute $^{(D)}$ in the language expressivity refers to the use of datatype properties. An asterisk against the reasoning time in the last column indicates that any datatype expressions in the associated ontologies are ignored by the ELK reasoner.

Ontology	Expressivity	Logical Axioms	Class Count	Object Properties	Data Properties	SubclassOf	Defined Class	GCI Count	Reasoning Times (Seconds)			
									FaCT++	HermiT	Pellet	ELK
ICDO3_O	ALC	3971	2753	9	0	3948	11	1202	<1	<1	<1	<1
ICCC_O	ALC	6651	2891	5	0	6646	1	3465	<1	<1	7	<1
Tumour Signature (TS)	ALC	7661	3157	3	0	7654	1	1533	2	8	11	<1
ENCR_QC_O without TS	ALC$^{(D)}$	8428	2964	12	4	8349	11	5013	2	2	57	1 *
ENCR_QC_O	ALC$^{(D)}$	12,155	3392	12	4	12,074	11	5344	3	14	175	2 *
ENCR_MPT_ O	ALCOIQ$^{(D)}$	7966	3129	9	1	7399	15	3891	2	23	>900	N/A
TNM Ed6	ALCI$^{(D)}$	8926	3410	21	1	8682	141	4688	4	2	10	1 *
TNM Ed7	ALCI$^{(D)}$	9409	3501	21	1	9100	204	4939	5	2	20	1 *
TNM_CR_O	ALCI$^{(D)}$	10,740	3684	21	1	10,302	332	5777	15	3	53	1 *
CCS_TGL_O	ALC$^{(D)}$	7536	3358	23	0	7409	22	3544	2	2	12	<1 *
ENCR_QC_O without TS + TNMEd7	ALCI$^{(D)}$	10,956	3619	24	4	10,588	204	6269	6	4	90	1 *
ENCR_QC_O + TNMEd7	ALCI$^{(D)}$	14,683	4002	24	4	14,313	204	6600	9	10	450	1 *
ENCR_QC_O without TS + TNM_CR_O	ALCI$^{(D)}$	12,287	3757	24	4	11,790	332	7107	17	5	240	1 *
ENCR_QC_O + TNM_CR_O	ALCI$^{(D)}$	16,014	4185	24	4	15,515	332	7438	19	14	540	2 *
ENCR_QC_O + CCS_TGL_O	ALC$^{(D)}$	13,386	3834	24	4	13,201	22	5807	3	11	165	1 *

References

1. Izquierdo, J.N.; Schoenbach, V.J. The potential and limitations of data from population-based State cancer registries. *Am. J. Public Health* **2000**, *90*, 695–698. [PubMed]
2. Metwalli, S. What Is Data Validation. 2003. Available online: https://builtin.com/data-science/data-validation (accessed on 22 April 2023).
3. European Commission, European Cancer Information System (ECIS). Available online: https://ecis.jrc.ec.europa.eu/ (accessed on 22 April 2023).
4. Giusti, F.; Martos, C.; Adriani, S.; Flego, M.; Carvalho, R.N.; Bettio, M.; Ben, E. The Joint Research Centre-European Network of Cancer Registries quality check software (JRC-ENCR QCS). *Front. Oncol.* **2023**, *13*, 1250195. [CrossRef] [PubMed]
5. Gruber, T.; Liu, L.; Özsu, M. Ontology. In *Encyclopedia of Database Systems*; Springer: New York, NY, USA, 2016. [CrossRef]
6. TopQuadrant, Ontologies and Data Models—Are They the Same? 2011. Available online: https://topquadrantblog.blogspot.com/2011/09/ontologies-and-data-models-are-they.html (accessed on 22 April 2023).
7. Martos, C.; Giusti, F.; Van Eycken, E.; Visser, O. A Common Data Quality Check Procedure for European Cancer Registries, JRC132486, European Commission, Ispra, Italy. 2023. Available online: https://encr.eu/sites/default/files/Recommendations/JRC132486_cancer_data_quality_checks_procedure_report_2.0.pdf (accessed on 8 June 2023).
8. WHO. International Classification of Diseases for Oncology (ICD-O). Available online: https://www.who.int/standards/classifications/other-classifications/international-classification-of-diseases-for-oncology (accessed on 19 June 2023).
9. UICC, TNM Classification of Malignant Tumours. Available online: https://www.uicc.org/resources/tnm-classification-malignant-tumours-8th-edition (accessed on 19 June 2023).
10. Nicholson, N.C.; Giusti, F.; Bettio, M.; Carvalho, R.N.; Dimitrova, N.; Dyba, T.; Flego, M.; Neamtiu, L.; Randi, G.; Martos, C. An ontology-based approach for developing a harmonised data-validation tool for European cancer registration. *J. Biomed. Semant.* **2021**, *12*, 1. [CrossRef] [PubMed]
11. University of Manchester, Protégé OWL Tutorial. Available online: http://owl.cs.manchester.ac.uk/publications/talks-and-tutorials/protg-owl-tutorial/ (accessed on 19 June 2023).
12. DeBellis, M. New Protégé Pizza Tutorial. Available online: https://www.michaeldebellis.com/post/new-protege-pizza-tutorial (accessed on 19 June 2023).

13. Rector, A.; Drummond, N.; Horridge, M.; Rogers, J.; Knublauch, H.; Stevens, R.; Wang, H.; Wroe, C. OWL pizzas: Practical experience of teaching OWL-DL: Common errors & common patterns. In *Engineering Knowledge in the Age of the Semantic Web, EKAW 2004*; Lecture Notes in Computer Science; Motta, E., Shadbolt, N.R., Stutt, A., Gibbins, N., Eds.; Springer: Berlin/Heidelberg, Germany, 2004; Volume 3257. [CrossRef]
14. Noy, N.F.; McGuinness, D.L. Ontology Development 101: A Guide to Creating Your First Ontology. Available online: https://protege.stanford.edu/publications/ontology_development/ontology101.pdf (accessed on 19 June 2023).
15. ODPA, Ontology Design Patterns. Available online: http://ontologydesignpatterns.org/wiki/Ontology_Design_Patterns__org_(ODP) (accessed on 21 June 2023).
16. Horridge, M.; Drummond, N.; Goodwin, J.; Rector, A.; Stevens, R.; Wang, H.H. The Manchester OWL Syntax. In *CEUR Workshop Proceedings*; 2006; Volume 216. Available online: https://research.manchester.ac.uk/en/publications/the-manchester-owl-syntax (accessed on 1 December 2023).
17. Krötzsch, M.; Simančík, F.; Horrocks, I. A description logic primer. *arXiv* **2013**, arXiv:1201.4089v3. [CrossRef]
18. Tongphu, S.; Suntisrivaraporn, B. Algorithms for measuring similarity between ELH concept descriptions: A case study on SNOMED CT. *Comput. Inform.* **2017**, *36*, 733–764. [CrossRef]
19. Baader, F.; Horrocks, I.; Sattler, U. Description logic. In *Handbook on Ontologies, International Handbooks on Information Systems*; Staab, S., Studer, R., Eds.; Springer: Berlin/Heidelberg, Germany, 2009. [CrossRef]
20. Kazakov, Y. RIQ and SROIQ Are Harder than SHOIQ. In Proceedings of the Principles of Knowledge Representation and Reasoning: Proceedings of the 11th International Conference, (KR 2008), 353. 2008. Available online: https://aaai.org/papers/027-riq-and-sroiq-are-harder-than-shoiq/ (accessed on 18 April 2023).
21. Möller, R.; Haarslev, V. Tableau-based reasoning. In *Handbook on Ontologies. International Handbooks on Information Systems*; Staab, S., Studer, R., Eds.; Springer: Berlin/Heidelberg, Germany, 2009. [CrossRef]
22. Weithöner, T.; Liebig, T.; Luther, M.; Böhm, S. What's wrong with OWL benchmarks? In Proceedings of the Second International Workshop on Scalable Semantic Web Knowledgebase Systems (SSWS 2006), 101–114. Citeseer. 2006. Available online: https://citeseerx.ist.psu.edu/doc/10.1.1.139.6934 (accessed on 18 April 2023).
23. Gardiner, T.; Horrocks, I.; Tsarkov, D. Automated Benchmarking of Description Logic Reasoners. In Proceedings of the International Workshop on Description Logics (06) CEUR. 189. 2006. Available online: http://sunsite.informatik.rwth-aachen.de/Publications/CEUR-WS/Vol-189/submission_23.pdf (accessed on 18 April 2023).
24. Bock, J.; Haase, P.; Qiu, J.; Raphael, V. Benchmarking OWL Reasoners. In *CEUR Workshop Proceedings*; 2008; Volume 350. Available online: https://citeseerx.ist.psu.edu/viewdoc/download?doi=10.1.1.143.1363&rep=rep1&type=pdf (accessed on 18 April 2023).
25. Dentler, K.; Cornet, R.; Teije, A.T.; de Keizer, N. Comparison of reasoners for large ontologies in the OWL 2 EL profile. *Semant. Web* **2011**, *2*, 71–87. [CrossRef]
26. Abburu, S. A Survey on ontology reasoners and comparison. *Int. J. Comput. Appl.* **2012**, *57*, 17.
27. Kang, Y.-B.; Li, Y.-F.; Krishnaswamy, S. Predicting reasoning performance using ontology metrics. In *The Semantic Web—ISWC 2012, Lecture Notes in Computer Science*; Cudré-Mauroux, P., Heflin, J., Sirin, E., Tudorache, T., Euzenat, J., Hauswirth, M., Parreira, J.X., Hendler, J., Schreiber, G., Bernstein, A., et al., Eds.; Springer: Berlin/Heidelberg, Germany, 2012; Volume 7649. [CrossRef]
28. Khamparia, A.; Pandey, B. Comprehensive analysis of semantic web reasoners and tools: A survey. *Educ. Inf. Technol.* **2017**, *22*, 3121–3145. [CrossRef]
29. Singh, G.; Bhatia, S.; Mutharaju, R. OWL2Bench: A benchmark for OWL 2 reasoners. In *The Semantic Web—ISWC 2020. ISWC 2020*; Lecture Notes in Computer Science; Springer: Cham, Switzerland, 2020; Volume 12507. [CrossRef]
30. International Association of Cancer Registries. International rules for multiple primary cancers. *Asian Pac. J. Cancer Prev.* **2005**, *6*, 104–106.
31. Nicholson, N.C.; Giusti, F.; Bettio, M.; Carvalho, R.N.; Dimitrova, N.; Dyba, T.; Flego, M.; Neamtiu, L.; Randi, G.; Martos, C. An Ontology to model the international rules for multiple primary malignant tumours in cancer registration. *Appl. Sci.* **2021**, *11*, 7233. [CrossRef]
32. Meier, A.; Schneider, T. The Complexity of Satisfiability for Sub-Boolean Fragments of ALC. *arXiv* **2010**, arXiv:1001.4255v6. [CrossRef]
33. Ding, Y.; Haarslev, V. Towards efficient reasoning for description logics with inverse roles. In Proceedings of the 2005 International Workshop on Description Logics (DL-2005), Edinburgh, UK, 26–28 July 2005; pp. 208–215.
34. Grandi, F. On decidability of expressive description logics with composition of roles in number restrictions. *arXiv* **2003**, arXiv:cs/0308029. [CrossRef]
35. Gonçalves, R.S.; Parsia, B.; Sattler, U. Performance heterogeneity and approximate reasoning in description logic ontologies. In *The Semantic Web—ISWC 2012. ISWC 2012*; Lecture Notes in Computer Science; Springer: Berlin/Heidelberg, Germany, 2012; Volume 7649. [CrossRef]
36. Kang, Y.-B.; Krishnaswamy, S.; Sawangphol, W.; Gao, L.; Li, Y.-F. Understanding and improving ontology reasoning efficiency through learning and ranking. *Inf. Syst.* **2020**, *87*, 101412. [CrossRef]
37. W3C, ELK. Available online: https://www.w3.org/2001/sw/wiki/ELK (accessed on 19 June 2023).
38. W3C, OWL API. Available online: https://www.w3.org/2001/sw/wiki/OWLAPI (accessed on 19 June 2023).

39. Nicholson, N.; Giusti, F.; Neamtiu, L.; Randi, G.; Dyba, T.; Bettio, M.; Carvalho, R.N.; Dimitrova, N.; Flego, M.; Martos, C. Dotting the "i" of interoperability in FAIR cancer-registry data sets. In *Cancer Bioinformatics [Internet]*; Kais, G., Hamdi, Y., Eds.; IntechOpen: London, UK, 2021; pp. 131–156. [CrossRef]
40. Care2Data, Kwalify. Available online: https://care2data.com/product.php (accessed on 20 October 2023).

cancers

MDPI

Article

More than Five Decades of Proton Therapy: A Bibliometric Overview of the Scientific Literature

Maria Giulia Vincini [1], Mattia Zaffaroni [1,*], Marco Schwarz [2], Giulia Marvaso [1,*], Federico Mastroleo [1,3], Stefania Volpe [1], Luca Bergamaschi [1], Giovanni Carlo Mazzola [1], Giulia Corrao [1], Roberto Orecchia [4], Barbara Alicja Jereczek-Fossa [1,5] and Daniela Alterio [1]

1 Division of Radiation Oncology, IEO European Institute of Oncology IRCCS, 20141 Milan, Italy; mariagiulia.vincini@ieo.it (M.G.V.); federico.mastroleo@ieo.it (F.M.); stefania.volpe@ieo.it (S.V.); giulia.corrao@ieo.it (G.C.); barbara.jereczek@ieo.it (B.A.J.-F.)

2 Radiation Oncology Department, University of Washington, Seattle, WA 98109, USA; marcosch@uw.edu

3 Department of Translational Medicine, University of Piemonte Orientale, 28100 Novara, Italy

4 Scientific Directorate, IEO European Institute of Oncology IRCCS, 20141 Milan, Italy; roberto.orecchia@ieo.it

5 Department of Oncology and Hemato-Oncology, University of Milan, 20122 Milan, Italy

* Correspondence: mattia.zaffaroni@ieo.it (M.Z.); giulia.marvaso@ieo.it (G.M.)

Simple Summary: The therapeutic potential of proton therapy (PT) was first recognized in 1946 by Robert Wilson, and nowadays, over 100 proton centers are in operation worldwide, and more than 60 are under construction or planned. Bibliometrics allows us to assess the growth and development of the field and provides an overview of the most relevant sources, authors, and institutions in the chosen field. Additionally, keyword analysis can be performed to provide details that could aid in identifying research trends and hot topics. Indeed, bibliometrics allows for identifying the basic and dominant themes and trends, as well as those emerging or declining. The aim of this study is to provide a comprehensive bibliometric analysis of the current status and trends in scientific literature in the PT field. The analysis will give an overview of past scientific production and, most importantly, provide a useful point of view on the future directions of the research activities.

Abstract: Background: The therapeutic potential of proton therapy (PT) was first recognized in 1946 by Robert Wilson, and nowadays, over 100 proton centers are in operation worldwide, and more than 60 are under construction or planned. Bibliometric data can be used to perform a structured analysis of large amounts of scientific data to provide new insights, e.g., to assess the growth and development of the field and to identify research trends and hot topics. The aim of this study is to provide a comprehensive bibliometric analysis of the current status and trends in scientific literature in the PT field. Methods: The literature on PT until the 31st December 2022 in the Scopus database was searched, including the following keywords: *proton* AND *radiotherapy* AND *cancer/tumor* in title, abstract, and/or keywords. The open-source R Studio's Bibliometrix package and Biblioshiny software (version 2.0) were used to perform the analysis. Results: A total of 7335 documents, mainly articles (n = 4794, 65%) and reviews (n = 1527, 21%), were collected from 1946 to 2022 from 1054 sources and 21,696 authors. Of these, roughly 84% (n = 6167) were produced in the last 15 years (2008–2022), in which the mean annual growth rate was 13%. Considering the corresponding author's country, 79 countries contributed to the literature; the USA was the top contributor, with 2765 (38%) documents, of whom 84% were single-country publications (SCP), followed by Germany and Japan, with 535 and 531 documents of whom 66% and 93% were SCP. Considering the themes subanalysis (2002–2022), a total of 7192 documents were analyzed; among all keywords used by authors, the top three were radiotherapy (n = 1394, 21% of documents), intensity-modulated radiotherapy (n = 301, 5%), and prostate cancer (n = 301, 5%). Among disease types, prostate cancer is followed by chordoma, head and neck, and breast cancer. The change in trend themes demonstrated the fast evolution of hotspots in PT; among the most recent trends, the appearance of flash, radiomics, *relative biological effectiveness (RBE)*, and *linear energy transfer (LET)* deserve to be highlighted. Conclusions: The results of the present bibliometric analysis showed that PT is an active and rapidly increasing field of research. Themes of the published works encompass the main aspects of its application in clinical practice, such as the comparison with the actual photon-based standard of care technique and the continuing technological advances. This analysis gives an overview of past scientific production and, most importantly, provides a useful point of view on the future directions of the research activities.

Keywords: proton therapy; bibliometric analysis; bibliometrics

1. Introduction

The therapeutic potential of proton beams was first recognized in 1946 by Robert Wilson, with the idea that a proton beam can provide a higher energy deposit in tumors by minimizing radiation exposure to surrounding healthy organs [1]. This hypothesis was developed by the Lawrence Berkeley Laboratory, which initiated research related to proton irradiation in the clinical setting of patients with malignant tumors. The first patient was treated in 1954 [2] with a synchrocyclotron at the University of California, Berkley. The first hospital-based proton therapy (PT) facility was established in 1990 at the Loma Linda University Medical Center (CA), and since then, PT experienced exponential growth in both facilities available for clinical use and the number of treated patients [3]. Nowadays, over 100 proton centers are in operation worldwide, and more than 60 are under construction or planned for a total of more than 311,000 patients treated with protons by the end of 2022 [4].

PT is associated with several clinical, physical, and translational aspects. For instance, the peculiar dose distribution of protons leads to a significant reduction in the low "dose bath" absorbed by surrounding healthy tissues that are typically seen in photon-based techniques like intensity-modulated radiotherapy (IMRT). This could result in several advantages, like reducing (1) acute and late treatment-related side effects, (2) radiation-induced secondary-cancer risk (mainly in young patients), and (3) immune system depression (thanks to the lower exposure of circulating lymphocytes and immune organs like lymph nodes) [5–12]. Moreover, technological advances have allowed the transition from passive scattering to pencil-beam scanning (PBS), with even higher conformity of the dose distribution—a technique routinely introduced by the Paul Scherrer Institute (Villigen, Switzerland) in the late 1990s. Whether this improvement could translate into a better cost/benefit ratio in clinical results is still a matter of investigation [13,14]. To date, a number of issues remain to be addressed in PT, such as the dosimetric impact of uncertainties on the delivered dose distributions versus the desired one and the criteria to define clinical indications in a scenario of limited resources. Therefore, there is consensus on the need to improve scientific evidence about PT from the bench to the bedside [15].

Bibliometric data can be used to perform a structured analysis for large amounts of scientific data using various metrics, which comprise, for instance, the number of publications over time, citation counts, institutional affiliations, authors, and countries' contributions. Bibliometrics allows us to assess the growth and development of the field and provides an overview of the most relevant sources, authors, and institutions in the chosen field. Additionally, keyword analysis can be performed to provide details that could aid in identifying research trends and hot topics. Indeed, bibliometrics allows for identifying the basic and dominant themes and trends, as well as those emerging or declining. In the past, several bibliometric analyses have been carried out in various areas and, recently, also in the radiation oncology field [16–21].

Up to today, no bibliometric analysis regarding PT has been performed yet; therefore, in this study, we aim to provide a comprehensive analysis of the status of the available scientific documents in the field of PT. This will allow us to have a snapshot of current topics and developing trends from 1947, the year of the first publication on the matter, to 2022.

2. Material and Methods

All English language documents available in the Scopus database were considered eligible for the analysis.

The search string used was the following: (TITLE-ABS-KEY ((proton) AND radiotherapy) AND (TITLE-ABS-KEY (cancer OR tumor)) AND NOT (TITLE-ABS-KEY (pump))) AND PUBYEAR < 2023. All documents up to the date of the research (16 June 2023) were considered.

Data were exported in BibTex format, comprehensive of all the metadata regarding the title, abstract, citation information, corresponding author's country, bibliographical information, authors' keywords, and cited references in the manuscript. The Bibliometrix R package in the R environment (R-Studio 0.98.1091 software) and the Biblioshiny (version 2.0) [22] interface were used for the analysis.

The entire sample of documents was used for analyses regarding scientific production over the years. Based on the assumption of a uniform contribution of all co-authors to each document and neglecting the different types of documents, top relevant sources and authors were assessed based on the number of documents. Affiliations of all authors were considered to assess the top relevant institutions, and the corresponding author's country was considered to assess the top productive countries and network collaboration regarding countries. Country production was also evaluated through a productivity index, defined as the number of documents divided by the number of PT centers in operation at the time of the study. Moreover, single-country publications (SCP) and multiple-country publications (MCP), namely documents with authors from one country and documents in which at least one of the co-authors had a different country affiliation compared to the corresponding author, respectively, were considered as another index of collaborations among nations.

Given the wide time span involving scientific production and the fast pace of development, analyses of keywords and trends focused on the 2002–2022 period only to obtain a glimpse of the major driving themes of the last two decades. The authors' keywords analysis included frequent PT-associated keywords and a keywords co-occurrence network. A list of synonyms was loaded and is provided in the Supplementary Materials Table S1. In addition, to see the evolution of trend topics over time, the top three keywords for each year were considered. Lastly, the thematic map [23] was produced to provide the relevant lines of research.

3. Results

3.1. Overview

A total of 7335 documents were collected from 1947, the year of the first paper on the clinical application of PT in Scopus, to 2023, from 1054 sources. Roughly 84% (n = 6167) of the documents were produced during the last 15 years (2008–2022), and the mean annual growth rate in this period was 13%. The retrieved documents were mainly articles (n = 4794, 65%) and reviews (n = 1527, 21%).

3.2. Sources and Authors

A total of 21,696 authors contributed to the literature, and on average, each document was written by seven co-authors. The majority of contributors (n = 14,436, 70%) were occasional authors who contributed with one document only, while the top 10 authors contributed to 985 documents, 13% of the total. The last three completed years (years 2020–2021–2022) were the most productive, with 657, 749, and 693 documents, respectively (Figure 1). The top ten relevant sources and affiliations are provided in the Supplementary Materials Table S2. The top sources were the *International Journal of Radiation Oncology, Biology and Physics* (n = 727 documents), *Radiotherapy and Oncology (n = 375 documents),* and *Physics In Medicine and Biology* (n = 298 documents).

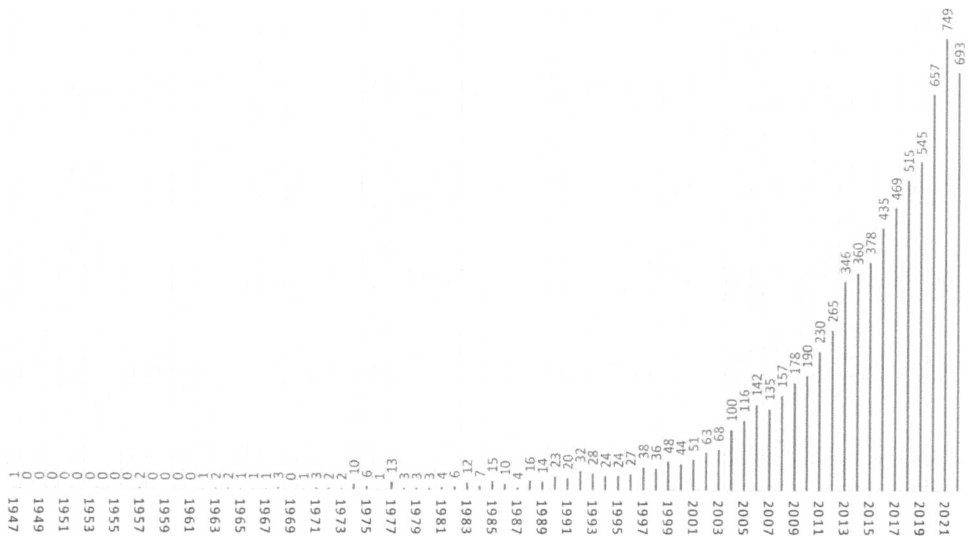

Figure 1. Annual scientific production in terms of documents produced.

The top three affiliations in terms of publication volume were the Massachusetts General Hospital—Harvard Medical School (Boston, MA, USA, n = 1050), the University Of Texas MD Anderson Cancer Center (Houston, Texas, USA, n = 646), and the Mayo Clinic (Rochester, MN, USA, n = 391 documents).

3.3. Countries

A total of 79 countries contributed to the literature (Figure 2, top). Among all considered documents, 21.1% were publications with authors from at least two countries.

Considering the corresponding author's country, the USA was the top contributor, with 2765 (38%) documents, of whom 84% were SCP, followed by Germany and Japan, with 535 and 531 documents, of whom 66% and 93% were SCP (Figure 2, bottom). Switzerland, France, and Germany were the countries with the greater productivity indexes. The country collaboration network (Figure 3) showed the main node, the USA, on its own, was strongly linked to two clusters: the blue one with European countries, with the strongest links with Germany and the United Kingdom, and the red one, with the strongest links with Canada and China.

3.4. Themes and Trends

Considering the themes' subanalysis (2002–2022), a total of 7192 documents were analyzed. Table 1 shows the top 20 PT-associated keywords, with the top 3 being *radiotherapy* (n = 1394, 21% of documents), *intensity-modulated radiotherapy* (n = 301, 5%), and *prostate cancer* (n = 301, 5%). Among the disease types, prostate cancer is followed by chordoma, head and neck, and breast cancer.

The co-occurrence network among the 25 top PT-associated keywords (Figure 4a) showed four different clusters. Among them, the wider cluster (blue), within *intensity-modulated radiotherapy, intensity-modulated PT*, and *prostate cancer* stand out; then, this is followed by the *pediatric/intracranic tumor* cluster (red), the stereotactic body radiation therapy (SBRT) cluster (green), and lastly, a cluster constituted by *particle therapy, relative biological effectiveness*, and *carbon-ion radiotherapy*. Among different cancer subsites in adults, prostate, head and neck, and base of the skull were the most frequently cited tumors. Moreover, the field of pediatrics was well-represented.

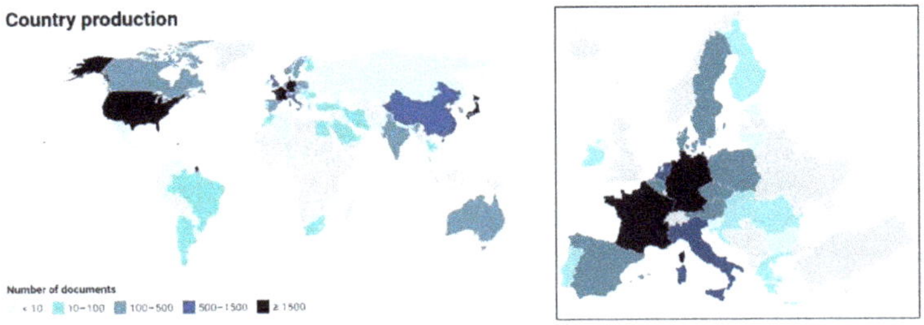

Country	Articles	centers in operation	Productivity index	SCP	SCP (blue)/MCP(red)*
USA	2765	44	63	2331	84%
GERMANY	535	5	107	352	66%
JAPAN	531	19	28	496	93%
FRANCE	360	3	120	292	81%
UNITED KINGDOM	317	6	53	240	76%
ITALY	309	3	103	203	66%
CHINA	208	4	52	176	85%
SWITZERLAND	202	1	202	103	51%
NETHERLANDS	190	3	63	101	53%

Figure 2. (**Top**): Country-specific production worldwide (left) and a focus on Europe (right) considering the corresponding author's country; (**Bottom**): top fifteen most productive countries considering the corresponding author's country and proportion between single-country publications (SCP) and multiple-country publications (MCP). * Publications with authors from more than one country.

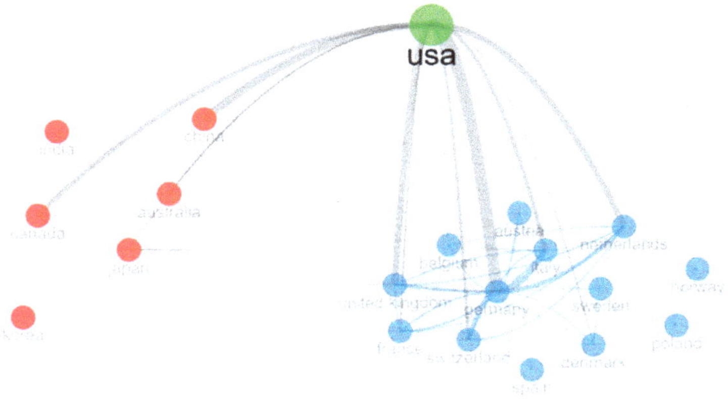

Figure 3. Countries collaboration network.

Figure 4b shows the change in trend themes over the period 2002–2022, with the three most frequent keywords for each year. The most recent topics were flash therapy and radiomics, which appeared in 2021 and 2020 and were in the top three keywords in 2022. From a clinical point of view, several tumors have been represented in the literature during the last twenty years and were mainly prostate, brain, and head and neck tumors in pediatric and lung settings.

The thematic map can be seen in Figure 5. This graph allows the identification of the hot topics (higher values of centrality and density) in the upper-right quadrant, the basic topics (higher values of centrality and lower values of density) in the lower-right quadrant, the peripheral topics (lower values of centrality and density) in the lower-left quadrant, and the niche topics (lower values of centrality and higher values of density).

The map highlights *RBE* and linear energy transfer (*LET)* as niche themes, isolated topics at a very high degree of development (upper-left side); less isolated and at a relevant degree of development were topics related to eye disease (*uveal melanoma, choroidal melanoma, eye*). *IMPT* and treatment planning-related themes (*treatment planning, PBS, Monte Carlo*) were central topics, and keywords, such as *chordoma, surgery, skull-base, condrosarcoma, chemotherapy, glioma, pediatric,* and *medulloblastoma* represent basic and transversal themes, and a low degree of development. Lastly, *prostate cancer, particle therapy, toxicity, breast cancer, and head and neck cancer* were basic themes at an average degree of development.

Table 1. Top 20 PT-associated keywords.

Words	Occurrences
Radiotherapy	1394
Intensity-modulated radiotherapy	301
Prostate cancer	301
Stereotactic body radiation therapy	255
Intensity-modulated proton therapy	219
Chordoma	182
Pediatric	175
Head and neck	174
Particle therapy	157
Chemotherapy	145
Cancer	137
Toxicity	131
Breast cancer	124
Carbon-ion radiotherapy	122
Surgery	120
Lung cancer	119
Brain tumor	110
Pencil-beam scanning	110
Hepatocellular carcinoma	105
Relative biological effectiveness	97

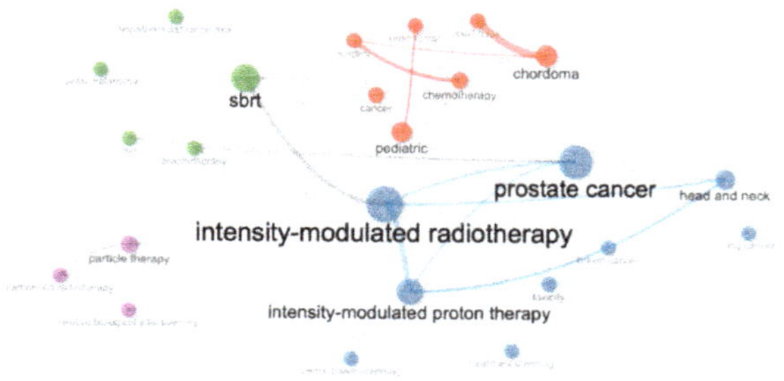

(a)

Figure 4. *Cont.*

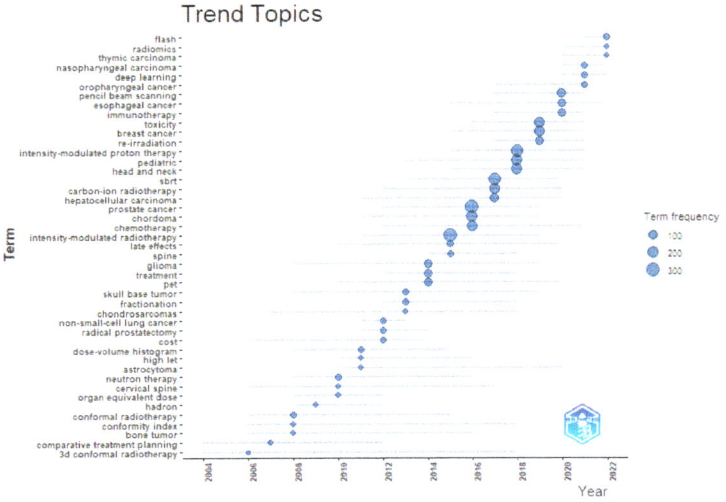

(**b**)

Figure 4. (**a**) Keywords co-occurrence network. Each vertex represents a keyword, and its size is proportional to the occurrence. Each cluster (colors) can be considered as a topic macro-area. The proximity among keywords in the network indicates a large proportion of articles addressing them together. "Radiotherapy" was excluded from the figure because it would have covered the other keywords. List of abbreviations: SBRT (stereotactic body radiation therapy). (**b**) Thematic evolution of keywords (2002–2022); blue dots: top three proton therapy-associated keywords for each year; the line-span indicates the interquartile range of the keyword distribution over years.

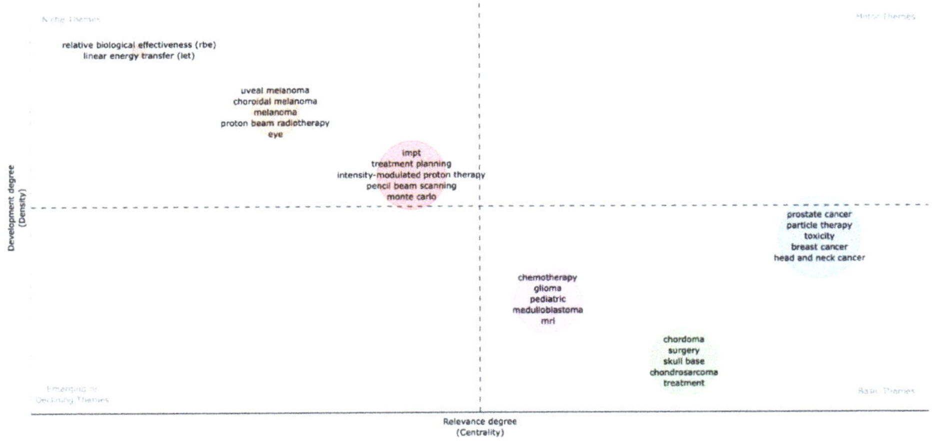

Figure 5. Thematic map [23] highlights the significant modifications in authors' keywords (2002–2022). Research themes are divided into four categories: (1) "Motor themes", with a high degree of centrality and density, refer to topics within the field that have a high level of importance and are continually developing; (2) "Niche themes", highly developed but isolated, refer to topics that are strongly developed but still marginal for the domain under investigation; (3) "Emerging or declining themes", with a low level of centrality and density, refer to themes that are not fully developed or marginally interesting for the domain; (4) "Basic themes", with high centrality but low development, refer to transversal themes that are considered to be fundamental and cross-cutting but have a lower level of development.

4. Discussion

Our bibliometric analysis included more than 7300 documents and allowed us to assess the state-of-the-art and the evolution of the current literature in the field of PT [24]. PT has undergone exponential growth in terms of treating facilities and treated patients. Such growth is also reflected by the number of scientific publications. Not surprisingly, we can observe that the scientific output has been increasing steadily, reaching more than 600 articles in each of the last three years (2020, 2021, and 2022).

4.1. Sources and Authors

The majority of top-contributor journals were addressed to the radiation oncologists and medical physics scientific communities. The two top sources, known in the field as the *Red Journal* and the *Green Journal*, are official journals of international organizations in the field of radiation oncology, namely the American Society for Radiation Oncology (ASTRO) and European Society for Radiotherapy and Oncology (ESTRO), respectively. They cover almost all areas of interest relating to the clinical application of radiation oncology. The finding that the majority of papers have been published in these journals represents a guarantee of the robustness of the methodology and reliability of the results reported in the published works. Moreover, it also reflects the high interest in the radiation oncology scientific community on the topic.

The third journal, *Physics in Medicine and Biology*, refers to the Institute of Physics and Engineering in Medicine (IPEM), whose mission is to improve health through physics and engineering in medicine, pointing at the inescapable link between PT and the development of technological and physical knowledge. Indeed, technical aspects are of paramount importance for translating the more favorable physical characteristics of protons into safe and effective treatments. In the last decades, several aspects of PT technological assets have been investigated, such as the implementation of the pencil-beam scanning (PBS) technique, the refinement of image guidance, set-up strategy techniques, as well as the development of compact systems [25–28]. Indeed, PBS and intensity-modulated PT (IMPT) were present as the top-associated keywords in the period of 2017–2021 [15,27]. The authors' indexing is naturally related to the publication type, and we found an equal distribution of physicians and physicists among the top four contributors.

4.2. Countries

Regarding the countries and affiliations analysis, the USA was found to be the top country contributor in terms of volume of publications, and eight out of the ten top affiliations are from facilities in the USA.

Particularly, the first top affiliation was the Massachusetts General Hospital (MGH)—Harvard Medical School (Boston, MA, USA), one of the leading hospitals in the USA. Indeed, one of the pioneers of PT was the research facility at the Harvard Cyclotron Laboratory (HCL) in Cambridge, Massachusetts, operating in conjunction with the MGH. Patient treatment lasted from 1961 to 2002, which was when the clinical program was transferred to the Northeast Proton Therapy Center (NPTC) at MGH [29]. MGH was thus one of the first hospitals in the world to establish its own proton therapy for cancer and, by now, has treated more than 10,000 patients [30].

Despite the huge production of documents, the USA productivity index is among the lowest. Indeed, the USA is the country with the highest number of PT facilities, with a total of 44 in operation and more than 10 under construction/planning stages [31]. It is followed by Japan, with 19 PT facilities in operation and 2 under construction, which, in turn, resulted in being second in terms of article production. Moreover, the USA, up to December 2021, has treated approximately 143,000 patients—51% of all patients treated worldwide at that date—and is, by de facto, the leading country in PT [4]. Moreover, the country collaboration network (Figure 3) highlighted the USA as an important node and showed a tendency for European countries to collaborate between them (blue cluster).

Scientific production in the United States is certainly also favored by the presence of many PT registries. A total of ten monocentric and multicentric PT registries are actively recruiting patients, and among them, the Proton Collaborative Group (PCG) registry (NCT01255748) is currently collecting data from 25 proton facilities [32].

Similarly, collaboration among European countries is boosted by initiatives promoted by Scientific Societies. A collaboration between the European Organization for Research and Treatment of Cancer (EORTC) and the ESTRO resulted in the creation of ParticleCare (EORTC 1833-RP), a common research platform to collect real-world data of patients treated with protons and C-ions in European centers [33].

Another project currently developing an infrastructure for automatic data registration is the PROTRAIT (PROton Therapy ReseArch regIsTry) [34] initiative in the Netherlands. The specific aim of the project is to establish an infrastructure for automatic data registration related to novel PT in the Netherlands to validate and strengthen the model-based approach used in this Country.

It should be noted that Switzerland is the country with the highest productivity index. This is not surprising, given its central role in the history of proton delivery, which can explain why such a small country with a small population and only one PT center is the eighth most productive country in terms of publications and the one with the highest productivity index.

In this scenario, low and middle-income countries (LMIC) remain very poorly represented. A study by Xia et al. [35] assessed extremely high inequality in the availability of PT centers throughout the world. Particularly in LMIC, cancer patients often have no access to PT despite the fact that these nations have a higher population and more cancer patients [35]. Undoubtedly, the scarce production of literature is another index of disparities affecting these nations.

4.3. Themes and Trend

The keywords subanalysis over the last twenty years reveals significant heterogeneity in the clinical keywords. This finding may be due to different clinical indications of PT among different countries. Zientara et al. [36] carried out a scoping review to explore various national and international clinical decision-making tools and dose comparison methods used for selecting cancer patients for proton versus X-ray radiation therapy. Great variability in indications emerged across different countries, especially for adult patients. With the exception of pediatric patients and adult patients with base of skull and chondrosarcomas [36], which were basic and transversal themes in the thematic map, there is uncertainty regarding patient cohorts that may benefit most from PT.

IMRT emerges from the associated keywords. Nowadays, IMRT and VMAT represent the standard of care for the vast majority of oncologic disease candidates for radiation treatment [37]. The methodology used does not allow us to assess the number of dosimetric studies emerging from the search. However, the strict association of IMRT with PT detected in the present analysis might reflect the high production of treatment planning studies in the last few years.

Among the technological advances in PT, FLASH therapy was found to be among the most recent and active fields of research in 2022. FLASH therapy allows treatment to be delivered at very high dose rates, and this approach has been proposed as a possible new frontier for radiation treatment, stimulating interest in preclinical, clinical, and technological studies [38–40]. Thus far, 10 patients have been treated within the FAST-01 non-randomized trial, the first and only trial on flash with protons. This trial was carried out at Cincinnati Children's/UC Health Therapy Center for patients with bone metastases in arms and legs, receiving a single palliative treatment fraction of 8 Gy [41,42].

Radiomics refers to the extraction of quantitative mineable data (*features*) from medical images and has been applied within oncology to enhance diagnosis, prognosis, and clinical decision support to provide increasingly tailored treatment [43–45]. The presence of radiomics, together with *deep learning*, found within the top keywords in 2021 and as a theme with a high degree of development, is not surprising; radiomics has experienced strong growth in recent years in the field of oncology, thanks to the ever-rising availability of images and technological advances in machine learning and artificial intelligence.

RBE and LET were also found to be topics at a high development rate in the thematic map. Currently, an RBE value of 1.1 is used to determine the clinical proton doses, which is thus 10% reduced due to the expected enhanced effectiveness [46]. However, this value represents only an approximation in the mid-part of the spread-out Bragg peak (SOBP). The use of a constant is currently under investigation, as RBE, in principle, may change as a function of both the proton LET and the specific clinical endpoint under consideration [47,48]. Radiobiological research on RBE is ongoing so as to fully comprehend how to model the complex relationship between RBE and LET in the SOBP; for example, the work package number six of the European Particle Therapy Network (EPTN) is fully centered on radiobiology and RBE [48,49].

The analysis performed in this work can be easily reproduced thanks to the Bibliometrix package [22], which is freely available to anyone and can be easily used in the R studio environment. The main limitation is that the literature search included only the Scopus database, which may have excluded other published work and citations. Moreover, the package used does not allow the documents collected to be divided into, e.g., mainly clinical papers, papers reporting trial results, methodological papers, or mainly physical papers. Lastly, the lack of bibliometric analysis regarding RT approaches comparable to PT (e.g., SBRT, FLASH) prevents the eventual comparison of results that could better highlight the specificities of PT.

For instance, assessing the number of papers reporting trial results by site of disease could be an interesting feature to add and would provide extra information. Although the theoretical benefit of protons over photons is high, to date, clinical shreds of evidence supporting its use are still conflicting [50]. As a matter of fact, PT can be considered an established treatment approach, with more than 100 facilities worldwide treating approximately 400 patients per year [31]. Promising results have been reported for several types of cancers, mainly in terms of toxicity reduction. Nonetheless, the majority of the reported data were retrieved from small, non-randomized studies, and widespread discussion regarding the lack of evidence of superior benefits makes PT a technique that still needs to find a role in radiation oncology [15].

Despite the limitations, we believe that the present analysis represents a reliable snapshot of the literature concerning PT.

5. Conclusions

PT is an active and rapidly increasing field of research and clinical application. Themes of the published works encompass the main aspects of its application in clinical practice, such as the comparison with the actual photon-based standard of care technique and the continuing technological advances. This analysis gives an overview of past scientific productions and, most importantly, provides a useful point of view on the future directions of research activities.

Supplementary Materials: The following supporting information can be downloaded at: https://www.mdpi.com/article/10.3390/cancers15235545/s1, Table S1: Considered synonyms in the present analysis. Table S2: Top ten sources and affiliations.

Author Contributions: Conceptualization, M.G.V., D.A.; methodology, M.G.V., D.A., M.S., M.Z., S.V. and F.M.; formal analysis, M.G.V. and M.Z.; investigation, M.G.V., D.A. and M.S.; data curation, M.G.V. and D.A.; writing—original draft preparation, M.G.V., D.A. and M.S.; visualization, M.G.V. and M.Z.; writing—review and editing, all authors; supervision, R.O., D.A. and B.A.J.-F. All authors have read and agreed to the published version of the manuscript.

Funding: This research received no external funding.

Institutional Review Board Statement: Not applicable.

Informed Consent Statement: Not applicable.

Data Availability Statement: Data supporting the results of this study are available from the corresponding authors upon reasonable request.

Acknowledgments: M.G.V. was supported by a research fellowship from the Associazione Italiana per la Ricerca sul Cancro (AIRC), entitled "Radioablation ± hormonotherapy for prostate cancer oligorecurrences (RADIOSA trial): potential of imaging and biology", registered at ClinicalTrials.gov NCT03940235 and approved by the Ethics Committee of IRCCS Istituto Europeo di Oncologia and Centro Cardiologico Monzino (IEO-997). S.V. is a Ph.D. student at the European School of Molecular Medicine (SEMM) in Milan, Italy. S.V. was partially supported by a research fellowship from Accuray Inc. L.B. received a grant from the European Institute of Oncology—Cardiologic Center Monzino Foundation (FIEO-CCM). The IEO, European Institute of Oncology, IRCCS, is partially supported by the Italian Ministry of Health (with "Ricerca Corrente" and "5 × 1000" funds). All described funds were outside the current study.

Conflicts of Interest: The division of Radiotherapy IEO received research funding from AIRC (the Italian Association for Cancer Research), Fondazione IEO-CCM (the Istituto Europeo di Oncologia-Centro Cardiologico Monzino), all of which were outside the current project. BAJF received speakers fees from Roche, Bayer, Janssen, Carl Zeiss, Ipsen, Accuray, Astellas, Elekta, and IBA Astra Zeneca, all outside the current project. MS received speakers fees from IBA, also outside of the current project. The remaining authors declare no conflicts of interest that are relevant to the content of this article.

References

1. Wilson, R.R. Radiological Use of Fast Protons. *Radiology* **1946**, *47*, 487–491. [CrossRef] [PubMed]
2. Lawrence, J.H.; Tobias, C.A.; Born, J.L.; McCombs, R.K.; Roberts, J.E.; Anger, H.O.; Low-Beer, B.V.; Huggins, C.B. Pituitary Irradiation with High-Energy Proton Beams: A Preliminary Report. *Cancer Res.* **1958**, *18*, 121–134. [PubMed]
3. Durante, M.; Paganetti, H. Nuclear Physics in Particle Therapy: A Review. *Rep. Prog. Phys.* **2016**, *79*, 096702. [CrossRef] [PubMed]
4. PTCOG—Home. Available online: https://www.ptcog.site/ (accessed on 20 April 2023).
5. Yahya, N.; Mohamad Salleh, S.A.; Mohd Nasir, N.F.; Abdul Manan, H. Toxicity Profile of Patients Treated with Proton and Carbon-Ion Therapy for Primary Nasopharyngeal Carcinoma: A Systematic Review and Meta-Analysis. *Asia-Pac. J. Clin. Oncol.* 2023; *ahead of print*. [CrossRef]
6. Fok, M.; Toh, S.; Easow, J.; Fowler, H.; Clifford, R.; Parsons, J.; Vimalachandran, D. Proton Beam Therapy in Rectal Cancer: A Systematic Review and Meta-Analysis. *Surg. Oncol.* **2021**, *38*, 101638. [CrossRef] [PubMed]
7. Ng, W.T.; But, B.; Wong, C.H.L.; Choi, C.-W.; Chua, M.L.K.; Blanchard, P.; Lee, A.W.M. Particle Beam Therapy for Nasopharyngeal Cancer: A Systematic Review and Meta-Analysis. *Clin. Transl. Radiat. Oncol.* **2022**, *37*, 41–56. [CrossRef] [PubMed]
8. Nie, M.; Chen, L.; Zhang, J.; Qiu, X. Pure Proton Therapy for Skull Base Chordomas and Chondrosarcomas: A Systematic Review of Clinical Experience. *Front. Oncol.* **2022**, *12*, 1016857. [CrossRef]
9. Qi, W.-X.; Fu, S.; Zhang, Q.; Guo, X.-M. Charged Particle Therapy versus Photon Therapy for Patients with Hepatocellular Carcinoma: A Systematic Review and Meta-Analysis. *Radiother. Oncol.* **2015**, *114*, 289–295. [CrossRef]
10. Ellsworth, S.G. Field Size Effects on the Risk and Severity of Treatment-Induced Lymphopenia in Patients Undergoing Radiation Therapy for Solid Tumors. *Adv. Radiat. Oncol.* **2018**, *3*, 512–519. [CrossRef]
11. Eaton, B.R.; MacDonald, S.M.; Yock, T.I.; Tarbell, N.J. Secondary Malignancy Risk Following Proton Radiation Therapy. *Front. Oncol.* **2015**, *5*, 261. [CrossRef]
12. Köthe, A.; Bizzocchi, N.; Safai, S.; Lomax, A.J.; Weber, D.C.; Fattori, G. Investigating the Potential of Proton Therapy for Hypoxia-Targeted Dose Escalation in Non-Small Cell Lung Cancer. *Radiat. Oncol.* **2021**, *16*, 199. [CrossRef]
13. Mishra, M.V.; Khairnar, R.; Bentzen, S.M.; Larson, G.; Tsai, H.; Sinesi, C.; Vargas, C.; Laramore, G.; Rossi, C.; Rosen, L.; et al. Patient Reported Outcomes Following Proton Pencil Beam Scanning vs. Passive Scatter/Uniform Scanning for Localized Prostate Cancer: Secondary Analysis of PCG 001-09. *Clin. Transl. Radiat. Oncol.* **2020**, *22*, 50–54. [CrossRef] [PubMed]
14. Yoo, G.S.; Yu, J.I.; Cho, S.; Jung, S.H.; Han, Y.; Park, S.; Oh, Y.; Lee, B.; Park, H.C.; Lim, D.H.; et al. Comparison of Clinical Outcomes between Passive Scattering versus Pencil-Beam Scanning Proton Beam Therapy for Hepatocellular Carcinoma. *Radiother. Oncol.* **2020**, *146*, 187–193. [CrossRef] [PubMed]
15. Mohan, R. A Review of Proton Therapy—Current Status and Future Directions. *Precis. Radiat. Oncol.* **2022**, *6*, 164–176. [CrossRef] [PubMed]
16. Franco, P.; De Felice, F.; Jagsi, R.; Nader Marta, G.; Kaidar-Person, O.; Gabrys, D.; Kim, K.; Ramiah, D.; Meattini, I.; Poortmans, P. Breast Cancer Radiation Therapy: A Bibliometric Analysis of the Scientific Literature. *Clin. Transl. Radiat. Oncol.* **2023**, *39*, 100556. [CrossRef]
17. Franco, P.; Segelov, E.; Johnsson, A.; Riechelmann, R.; Guren, M.G.; Das, P.; Rao, S.; Arnold, D.; Spindler, K.-L.G.; Deutsch, E.; et al. A Machine-Learning-Based Bibliometric Analysis of the Scientific Literature on Anal Cancer. *Cancers* **2022**, *14*, 1697. [CrossRef]

18. Zhang, J.; Zhu, H.; Wang, J.; Chen, Y.; Li, Y.; Chen, X.; Chen, M.; Cai, Z.; Liu, W. Machine Learning in Non-Small Cell Lung Cancer Radiotherapy: A Bibliometric Analysis. *Front. Oncol.* **2023**, *13*, 1082423. [CrossRef]
19. Liu, Y.; Li, J.; Cheng, X.; Zhang, X. Bibliometric Analysis of the Top-Cited Publications and Research Trends for Stereotactic Body Radiotherapy. *Front. Oncol.* **2021**, *11*, 795568. [CrossRef]
20. De Felice, F.; Crocetti, D.; Petrucciani, N.; Belgioia, L.; Sapienza, P.; Bulzonetti, N.; Marampon, F.; Musio, D.; Tombolini, V. Treatment in Locally Advanced Rectal Cancer: A Machine Learning Bibliometric Analysis. *Ther. Adv. Gastroenterol.* **2021**, *14*, 175628482110421. [CrossRef]
21. Wang, D.; Li, Z.; Zhang, Y.; Li, Y.; Wang, X.; Wang, S.; Gui, Y.; Dong, J.; Hou, W. Bibliometric Analysis of Research Relating to Radiation-Induced Lung Injury (2001–2020). *Ann. Palliat. Med.* **2021**, *10*, 11166–11176. [CrossRef]
22. Aria, M.; Cuccurullo, C. Bibliometrix: An R-Tool for Comprehensive Science Mapping Analysis. *J. Informetr.* **2017**, *11*, 959–975. [CrossRef]
23. Aria, M.; Cuccurullo, C.; D'Aniello, L.; Misuraca, M.; Spano, M. Thematic Analysis as a New Culturomic Tool: The Social Media Coverage on COVID-19 Pandemic in Italy. *Sustainability* **2022**, *14*, 3643. [CrossRef]
24. Koehler, A.M.; Dickinson, J.G.; Preston, W.M. The Range of Protons in Human Skullbone. *Radiat. Res.* **1965**, *26*, 334. [CrossRef] [PubMed]
25. Vilches-Freixas, G.; Unipan, M.; Rinaldi, I.; Martens, J.; Roijen, E.; Almeida, I.P.; Decabooter, E.; Bosmans, G. Beam Commissioning of the First Compact Proton Therapy System with Spot Scanning and Dynamic Field Collimation. *Br. J. Radiol.* **2020**, *93*, 20190598. [CrossRef] [PubMed]
26. Azcona, J.-D.; Aguilar, B.; Perales, Á.; Polo, R.; Zucca, D.; Irazola, L.; Viñals, A.; Cabello, P.; Delgado, J.-M.; Pedrero, D.; et al. Commissioning of a Synchrotron-Based Proton Beam Therapy System for Use with a Monte Carlo Treatment Planning System. *Radiat. Phys. Chem.* **2023**, *204*, 110708. [CrossRef]
27. Paganetti, H.; Beltran, C.; Both, S.; Dong, L.; Flanz, J.; Furutani, K.; Grassberger, C.; Grosshans, D.R.; Knopf, A.-C.; Langendijk, J.A.; et al. Roadmap: Proton Therapy Physics and Biology. *Phys. Med. Biol.* **2021**, *66*, 05RM01. [CrossRef] [PubMed]
28. Depuydt, T. Proton Therapy Technology Evolution in the Clinic: Impact on Radiation Protection. *Ann. ICRP* **2018**, *47*, 177–186. [CrossRef]
29. Levin, W.P.; Kooy, H.; Loeffler, J.S.; DeLaney, T.F. Proton Beam Therapy. *Br. J. Cancer* **2005**, *93*, 849–854. [CrossRef]
30. Proton Therapy for Cancer Treatment. Available online: https://www.massgeneral.org/cancer-center/radiation-oncology/treatments-and-services/proton-therapy (accessed on 25 September 2023).
31. PTCOG—Facilities in Operation. Available online: https://www.ptcog.ch/index.php/facilities-in-operation-restricted (accessed on 3 January 2023).
32. Home—ClinicalTrials.Gov. Available online: https://clinicaltrials.gov/ (accessed on 5 May 2023).
33. European Organisation for Research and Treatment of Cancer—EORTC. E^2-RADIatE: EORTC-ESTRO RADiotherapy InfrAstrucTure for Europe. 2019. Available online: https://project.eortc.org/e2-radiate/ (accessed on 17 October 2023).
34. Use Case: PROTRAIT, National Registration of Proton Therapy Data | The Personal Health Train. Available online: https://pht.health-ri.nl/use-cases/health-research/use-case-protrait-national-registration-proton-therapy-data (accessed on 2 February 2023).
35. Xia, Z.; Wang, J.; Xia, J.; Wang, M.; Cheng, Z. Inequality in Accessibility of Proton Therapy for Cancers and Its Economic Determinants: A Cross-Sectional Study. *Front. Oncol.* **2022**, *12*, 876368. [CrossRef]
36. Zientara, N.; Giles, E.; Le, H.; Short, M. A Scoping Review of Patient Selection Methods for Proton Therapy. *J. Med. Radiat. Sci.* **2022**, *69*, 108–121. [CrossRef]
37. Treatment by Cancer Type. Available online: https://www.nccn.org/guidelines/category_1 (accessed on 8 May 2023).
38. Hughes, J.R.; Parsons, J.L. FLASH Radiotherapy: Current Knowledge and Future Insights Using Proton-Beam Therapy. *Int. J. Mol. Sci.* **2020**, *21*, 6492. [CrossRef]
39. Lin, B.; Gao, F.; Yang, Y.; Wu, D.; Zhang, Y.; Feng, G.; Dai, T.; Du, X. FLASH Radiotherapy: History and Future. *Front. Oncol.* **2021**, *11*, 1890. [CrossRef] [PubMed]
40. Vozenin, M.-C.; Bourhis, J.; Durante, M. Towards Clinical Translation of FLASH Radiotherapy. *Nat. Rev. Clin. Oncol.* **2022**, *19*, 791–803. [CrossRef] [PubMed]
41. Daugherty, E.C.; Mascia, A.; Zhang, Y.; Lee, E.; Xiao, Z.; Sertorio, M.; Woo, J.; McCann, C.; Russell, K.; Levine, L.; et al. FLASH Radiotherapy for the Treatment of Symptomatic Bone Metastases (FAST-01): Protocol for the First Prospective Feasibility Study. *JMIR Res. Protoc.* **2023**, *12*, e41812. [CrossRef] [PubMed]
42. Proton FLASH Radiotherapy for the Treatment of Symptomatic Bone Metastases: The FAST-01 Nonrandomized Trial | Oncology | JAMA Oncology | JAMA Network. Available online: https://jamanetwork.com/journals/jamaoncology/fullarticle/2797843 (accessed on 25 April 2023).
43. Volpe, S.; Mastroleo, F.; Krengli, M.; Jereczek-Fossa, B.A. Quo Vadis Radiomics? Bibliometric Analysis of 10-Year Radiomics Journey. *Eur. Radiol.* **2023**, *33*, 6736–6745. [CrossRef] [PubMed]
44. Radiomics: Images Are More than Pictures, They Are Data | Radiology. Available online: https://pubs.rsna.org/doi/full/10.1148/radiol.2015151169 (accessed on 25 April 2023).
45. Rogers, W.; Thulasi Seetha, S.; Refaee, T.A.G.; Lieverse, R.I.Y.; Granzier, R.W.Y.; Ibrahim, A.; Keek, S.A.; Sanduleanu, S.; Primakov, S.P.; Beuque, M.P.L.; et al. Radiomics: From Qualitative to Quantitative Imaging. *BJR* **2020**, *93*, 20190948. [CrossRef]

46. Jones, B. Proton Radiobiology and Its Clinical Implications. *Ecancermedicalscience* **2017**, *11*, 777. [CrossRef]
47. Jones, B. Why RBE Must Be a Variable and Not a Constant in Proton Therapy. *Br. J. Radiol.* **2016**, *89*, 20160116. [CrossRef]
48. Sørensen, B.S.; Pawelke, J.; Bauer, J.; Burnet, N.G.; Dasu, A.; Høyer, M.; Karger, C.P.; Krause, M.; Schwarz, M.; Underwood, T.S.A.; et al. Does the Uncertainty in Relative Biological Effectiveness Affect Patient Treatment in Proton Therapy? *Radiother. Oncol.* **2021**, *163*, 177–184. [CrossRef] [PubMed]
49. EPTN. Available online: https://www.estro.org/Science/EPTN (accessed on 19 May 2023).
50. Mazzola, G.C.; Bergamaschi, L.; Pedone, C.; Vincini, M.G.; Pepa, M.; Zaffaroni, M.; Volpe, S.; Rombi, B.; Doyen, J.; Fossati, P.; et al. Patients' Needs in Proton Therapy: A Survey among Ten European Facilities. *Clin. Transl. Radiat. Oncol.* **2023**, *43*, 100670. [CrossRef]

cancers

MDPI

Article

Reproducible Bioinformatics Analysis Workflows for Detecting *IGH* Gene Fusions in B-Cell Acute Lymphoblastic Leukaemia Patients

Ashlee J. Thomson [1,2,*], Jacqueline A. Rehn [1,2], Susan L. Heatley [1,2,3], Laura N. Eadie [1,2], Elyse C. Page [1,2], Caitlin Schutz [2], Barbara J. McClure [1,2], Rosemary Sutton [4], Luciano Dalla-Pozza [5], Andrew S. Moore [6,7], Matthew Greenwood [8,9], Rishi S. Kotecha [10,11,12], Chun Y. Fong [13], Agnes S. M. Yong [1,14,15,16], David T. Yeung [1,2,17], James Breen [18,19,*] and Deborah L. White [1,2,3,20]

1 Faculty of Health and Medical Sciences, University of Adelaide, Adelaide, SA 5005, Australia; jacqueline.rehn@sahmri.com (J.A.R.); sue.heatley@sahmri.com (S.L.H.); laura.eadie@sahmri.com (L.N.E.); elyse.page@sahmri.com (E.C.P.); barb.mcclure@unisa.edu.au (B.J.M.); agnes.yong@health.wa.gov.au (A.S.M.Y.); david.yeung@adelaide.edu.au (D.T.Y.); deborah.white@sahmri.com (D.L.W.)
2 Blood Cancer Program, Precision Cancer Medicine Theme, South Australian Health & Medical Research Institute (SAHMRI), Adelaide, SA 5000, Australia; caitlin.schutz@sahmri.com
3 Australian and New Zealand Children's Oncology Group (ANZCHOG), Clayton, VIC 3168, Australia
4 Molecular Diagnostics, Children's Cancer Institute, Kensington, NSW 2750, Australia; rsutton@ccia.org.au
5 The Cancer Centre for Children, The Children's Hospital at Westmead, Westmead, NSW 2145, Australia; luciano.dallapozza@health.nsw.gov.au
6 Oncology Service, Children's Health Queensland Hospital and Health Service, Brisbane, QLD 4101, Australia; andy.moore@health.qld.gov.au
7 Child Health Research Centre, The University of Queensland, Brisbane, QLD 4000, Australia
8 Department of Haematology and Transfusion Services, Royal North Shore Hospital, Sydney, NSW 2065, Australia; matthew.greenwood@health.nsw.gov.au
9 Faculty of Health and Medicine, University of Sydney, Sydney, NSW 2006, Australia
10 Department of Clinical Haematology, Oncology, Blood and Marrow Transplantation, Perth Children's Hospital, Perth, WA 6009, Australia; rishi.kotecha@health.wa.gov.au
11 Leukaemia Translational Research Laboratory, Telethon Kids Cancer Centre, Telethon Kids Institute, University of Western Australia, Perth, WA 6009, Australia
12 Curtin Medical School, Curtin University, Perth, WA 6845, Australia
13 Department of Clinical Haematology, Austin Health, Heidelberg, VIC 3083, Australia; chun.fong@austin.org.au
14 South Australian Health & Medical Research Institute (SAHMRI), Adelaide, SA 5000, Australia
15 Division of Pathology & Laboratory, University of Western Australia Medical School, Perth, WA 6009, Australia
16 Department of Haematology, Royal Perth Hospital, Perth, WA 6000, Australia
17 Haematology Department, Royal Adelaide Hospital and SA Pathology, Adelaide, SA 5000, Australia
18 Black Ochre Data Labs, Indigenous Genomics, Telethon Kids Institute, Adelaide, SA 5000, Australia
19 James Curtin School of Medical Research, Australian National University, Canberra, ACT 2601, Australia
20 Australian Genomics Health Alliance (AGHA), The Murdoch Children's Research Institute, Parkville, VIC 3052, Australia
* Correspondence: ashlee.thomson@sahmri.com (A.J.T.); jimmy.breen@telethonkids.org.au (J.B.)

Simple Summary: B-cell acute lymphoblastic leukaemia (B-ALL) is a haematological malignancy driven by diverse genomic alterations, the most common being gene fusions, which can be detected via transcriptomic analysis. However, detecting gene fusions involving the Immunoglobulin Heavy Chain (*IGH*) region can be challenging due to its hyper variability. Our aim was to develop a workflow containing the algorithms FusionCatcher, Arriba, and STAR-Fusion, to achieve best-case sensitivity for *IGH* gene fusion detection. We analysed 35 patient samples harbouring *IGH* gene fusions and assessed the detection rates for each caller, before optimising the parameters to enhance sensitivity for *IGH* fusions. FusionCatcher and Arriba outperformed STAR-Fusion; however, by adjusting specific filtering parameters, we were able to improve STAR-Fusion's performance. This analysis highlights the importance of filtering optimization for *IGH* gene fusion events, offering alternative workflows for difficult-to-detect high-risk B-ALL alterations.

Abstract: B-cell acute lymphoblastic leukaemia (B-ALL) is characterised by diverse genomic alterations, the most frequent being gene fusions detected via transcriptomic analysis (mRNA-seq). Due to its hypervariable nature, gene fusions involving the Immunoglobulin Heavy Chain (*IGH*) locus can be difficult to detect with standard gene fusion calling algorithms and significant computational resources and analysis times are required. We aimed to optimize a gene fusion calling workflow to achieve best-case sensitivity for *IGH* gene fusion detection. Using Nextflow, we developed a simplified workflow containing the algorithms FusionCatcher, Arriba, and STAR-Fusion. We analysed samples from 35 patients harbouring *IGH* fusions (*IGH::CRLF2* n = 17, *IGH::DUX4* n = 15, *IGH::EPOR* n = 3) and assessed the detection rates for each caller, before optimizing the parameters to enhance sensitivity for *IGH* fusions. Initial results showed that FusionCatcher and Arriba outperformed STAR-Fusion (85–89% vs. 29% of *IGH* fusions reported). We found that extensive filtering in STAR-Fusion hindered *IGH* reporting. By adjusting specific filtering steps (e.g., read support, fusion fragments per million total reads), we achieved a 94% reporting rate for *IGH* fusions with STAR-Fusion. This analysis highlights the importance of filtering optimization for *IGH* gene fusion events, offering alternative workflows for difficult-to-detect high-risk B-ALL subtypes.

Keywords: B-cell acute lymphoblastic leukaemia; *IGH*; gene fusion; workflow

1. Introduction

B-cell acute lymphoblastic leukaemia (B-ALL) is a haematological malignancy that results in the over-proliferation of lymphoblasts [1]. While it is primarily diagnosed in children <5 years, younger patients tend to have a better prognosis than adolescents and adults diagnosed with the disease [2–4]. A number of genomic alterations have been identified as drivers of this disease, the most frequent being gene fusions secondary to chromosomal rearrangements [5,6], making them potential targets for therapeutic intervention and personalised medicine [6]. The accurate and rapid identification of these genomic alterations is therefore a crucial aspect of B-ALL diagnosis and treatment [7].

Prior to the introduction of Next-Generation Sequencing (NGS) and transcriptomic analysis, the detection of prognostically significant gene fusions with well-characterised breakpoints was performed using diagnostic analysis, such as fluorescence in situ hybridisation (FISH), reverse transcriptase polymerase chain reaction (RT-PCR) and G-banded karyotyping [7–9]; however, these processes are time-intensive, expensive, and inadequate for detecting novel and cytogenetically cryptic rearrangements [10,11]. With the implementation of transcriptome sequencing (mRNA-seq) and advanced bioinformatic analysis techniques, it is now possible to identify most fusion transcripts, including cytogenetically cryptic transcripts known to confer prognostic significance in a more time- and cost-effective manner [12,13].

Gene fusion detection via mRNA-seq involves identifying instances in which sequences from two distinct genes or genomic regions are combined, typically through structural variations, such as chromosomal rearrangements or translocations (Figure 1A). When sequencing reads are mapped to the reference genome, gene fusions are indicated by the presence of spanning and chimeric junction reads, which extend across the breakpoints in which the fusion occurs [8] (Figure 1B). To identify these transcripts, fusion calling algorithms analyse the sequencing data to detect and characterise events. Once potential fusion transcripts are identified, custom filters are applied to minimize the number of false positives caused by read alignment errors or technical artifacts. The filtering criteria implemented by fusion calling algorithms play a crucial role in reducing false positives. These criteria are often tailored to the specific characteristics of fusion events, such as read coverage, breakpoint sequence patterns, and the presence of discordant mate pairs. Some of these strict filtering guidelines, however, can result in important driver mutations not being reported. Additionally, evaluating highly repetitive and hypervariable regions of the genome, such as the immunoglobulin heavy (*IGH*) chain, remains a challenge for these algorithms [14,15].

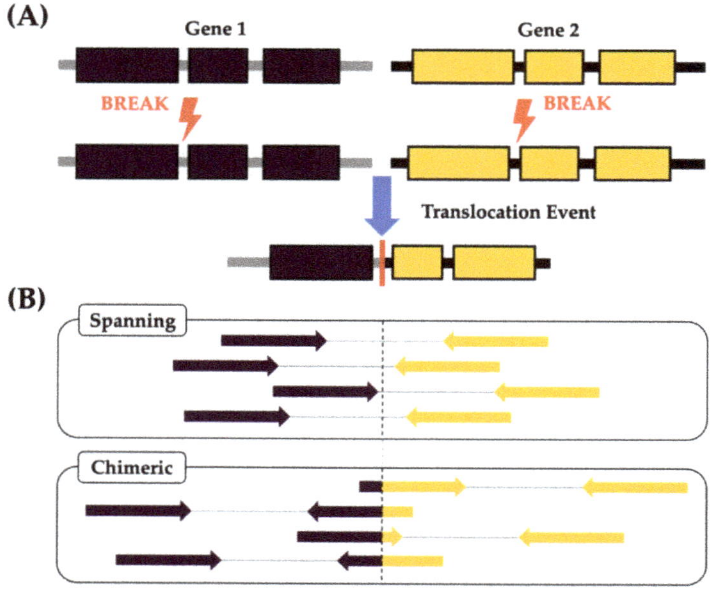

Figure 1. (**A**) Schematic of a gene fusion event, in which two separate genes located on the same or different chromosomes become juxtaposed, following a chromosomal rearrangement or translocation event. (**B**) Fusion events can be identified through the alignment of paired-end mRNA-seq reads to the reference genome, when each end of the paired read maps entirely to two different genomic regions (Spanning) or when one end of the read overlaps the fusion breakpoint (Chimeric).

While relying on spanning reads and junction reads is adequate for confirming most gene fusion events that occur at exon–exon boundaries, this is not the case for *IGH* fusions. Located in the sub-telomeric region of chromosome 14q, *IGH* is responsible for producing an individual's highly variable repertoire of antibodies and comprises multiple gene regions [16]. These gene regions undergo somatic recombination during early B-cell differentiation, resulting in an *IGH* gene rearrangement [17,18]. The aberrant recombination of *IGH* can result in a gene or gene segment from another chromosomal location being spliced upstream of an *IGH* enhancer, resulting in the upregulation of the partner gene, which acts as an oncogenic driver. A consequence of this aberrant recombination is the insertion of non-template nucleotides at fusion breakpoints [17]. These additional non-template nucleotides, along with the limitations of short-read sequencing technologies [15,16,19,20], often result in suboptimal read mapping across the *IGH* fusion breakpoints, leading to the under-reporting of these fusions by standard diagnostic and transcriptomic analysis methods.

IGH fusions also have a diverse range of partner genes [21–23]. Whilst the biological significance and clinical implications vary depending on the partner gene, many *IGH* fusions are indicative of a poor prognosis. In 2014, Russel et al. [4] successfully identified 14 different *IGH* partner genes, including *CRLF2* and *EPOR*, across 75 B-ALL patients, all of which were associated with high-risk subtypes. However, the partner gene remained unknown for a further 84 patients who tested positive for an *IGH* translocation via FISH probe. As a result of the increased detection sensitivity through the implementation of mRNA-seq analysis, the number of successfully identified *IGH* partner genes has risen in the intervening years to also include the cytogenetically cryptic *DUX4* [2,5,24].

The identification of gene fusions in patient samples in a time-efficient manner is crucial for effective risk stratification and personalised treatment planning. Current mRNA-seq analyses are time-consuming, at times exceeding 20 h to analyse one sample [25], and require significant personnel, specialised expertise, and computational resources to establish and execute them in a routine clinical context. In recent years, the Bioinformatics and Clinical Genomics community has attempted to address these issues by using state-of-the-art analysis workflow tools that can be implemented in routine sequencing and research labs [26,27]. However the careful consideration of parameter and filtering selection may still be required to achieve detection sensitivity to potential gene fusion events. In this study, we developed a reproducible mRNA-seq analysis workflow to accurately identify B-ALL gene fusions using the Nextflow workflow system [28]. We assessed the pipeline's accuracy, speed, and computational requirements when analysing the B-ALL patient samples harbouring *IGH* fusions. By assessing these difficult-to-detect fusions through mRNA-seq analyses, we aim to identify potential areas for improvement in sensitivity and accuracy.

2. Materials and Methods

The *RIGHT* (Recovering *IGH* fusion Transcripts) workflow (Figure 2) was developed using the workflow management executor Nextflow, version 21.10.6 [28]. Nextflow facilitates the parallel resolution of the implemented algorithms, namely STAR-Fusion, version 1.10.0 [24], Arriba, version 2.1.0 [25], and FusionCatcher, version 1.33 [29], thus optimising the processing time and enabling reproducibility across distributed computing infrastructures. STAR-Fusion and Arriba are often used together owing to their high accuracy and short execution times on both simulated and real data [24,25]. Adherence to the recommended best practice for mRNA-seq data analysis involves employing at least two distinct gene fusion calling algorithms, with intersected results for improved accuracy [25]. The GRCh37 human reference genome [30,31] was used with the Ensemble reference transcript annotation [32].

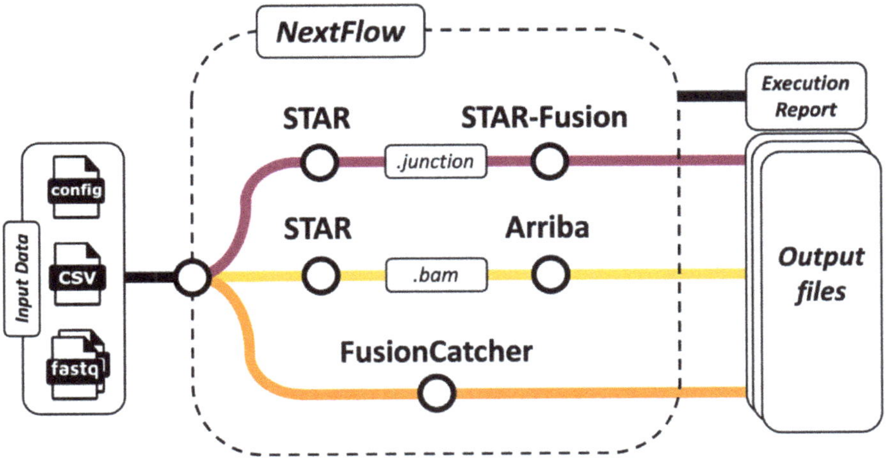

Figure 2. Schematic of the *RIGHT* workflow. STAR-Fusion, Arriba and FusionCatcher algorithms are all executed using the Nextflow system, taking an initial. csv sample manifest as input, which contains directory links and file base names for paired-end RNA-seq FASTQ files. The config file contains information regarding the resources requested, the scheduler used, e.g., Conda, Slurm, and any container options, such as Docker or Singularity. Arriba and STAR-Fusion have different formatting requirements for their alignment inputs, necessitating two separate STAR alignment runs.

To evaluate the ability of the workflow to efficiently analyse *IGH* fusions, a subset of 35 Australian B-ALL patient samples that were referred to the South Australian Health and Medical Research Institute (SAHMRI) (Adelaide, Australia) for genomic testing were selected (Supplementary Table S1), all of which were confirmed to harbour *IGH* fusions (*IGH::CRLF2* n = 17, *IGH::DUX4* n = 15, *IGH::EPOR* n = 3). These 3 gene fusions were chosen as they are the most common *IGH* fusions seen at SAHMRI. *IGH::CRLF2* fusions were confirmed via fluorescent in situ hybridization (FISH) using two separate break-apart probes, a Vysis IGH dual colour probe (Abbott) and a *CRLF2* dual colour probe (Cytocell). Gene expression profiling was used to confirm *IGH::DUX4* fusions, and the visual inspection of BAM files in the Integrative Genomics Viewer (IGV) was needed to confirm the presence of *IGH::EPOR* (Supplementary Data S1). We also analysed a second subset of 25 B-ALL patient samples that contained non-*IGH* gene fusion events, and non-translocated samples (Supplementary Table S9) as a control. These 60 samples were chosen from a previously published cohort of 180 B-ALL patient samples [33] that represented a range of common genomic lesions associated with ALL subtypes (EGA Accession: EGAS00001006460) [34]. The process of preparing libraries for mRNA sequencing was carried out using either the TruSeq Stranded mRNA LT Kit (Illumina, CA, USA) or the Universal Plus mRNA-Seq with NuQuant (Tecan, CA, USA). This was performed using 400 ng of total RNA, as per the instructions provided by the manufacturers. Subsequently, the samples underwent sequencing on either the Illumina HiSeq 2000 or NextSeq 500 platforms. The outcome of this sequencing approach yielded paired-end (PE) reads with a length of 75 bases, and an average read depth of 70 million reads.

To assess the sensitivity of the developed workflow, we processed the patient samples using the default parameters for each algorithm (Supplementary Data S2). Given the initial output files, we compared the reporting rates for *IGH* fusions for each caller and determined that STAR-Fusion had the lowest reporting rate. We then assessed the output files that STAR-Fusion produced following each stage of filtering to determine why the number of reported *IGH* fusions was lower than the other callers. STAR-Fusion produces intermediate output files during filtering comprising pre- and post-blast-filter files, listing each gene fusion detected and whether they passed filtering or not. If they did not pass filtering, the filtering step at which failure occurred was listed, and why. Given this, we were able to trace each *IGH* fusion and determine which filtering steps failed. We were then able to adjust the appropriate parameters in STAR-Fusion and process the samples again to reassess the reporting rates (Supplementary Data S3). While we used the GRCh37 reference genome, as this is currently the primary reference used at SAHMRI when analysing B-ALL patient samples, this pipeline is also compatible with the newer reference genome, GRCh38.

3. Results

3.1. Using RIGHT to Detect IGH Gene Fusion Events

Initially, we processed the 35 patient samples through the *RIGHT* workflow using the default parameters for each algorithm (Supplementary Data S2). Between the three algorithms, all *IGH* fusions were detected (Figure 3 and Supplementary Table S2), with 74% being detected by at least two of the tools. Arriba and FusionCatcher significantly outperformed STAR-Fusion, with the two tools successfully reporting all *IGH::EPOR* (n = 3) fusions, while the cytogenetically cryptic *IGH::DUX4* fusions (n = 15), which frequently go undetected, were reported in 93% (n = 14) of samples by Arriba and in 80% (n = 12) by FusionCatcher. In contrast, STAR-Fusion failed to detect any of the *IGH::EPOR* fusions and only reported 33% (n = 5) of the *IGH::DUX4* fusions. Of the 17 samples harbouring *IGH::CRLF2* fusions, FusionCatcher and Arriba reported 94% (n = 16) and 70% (n = 12), respectively, while STAR-Fusion again underperformed with only 29% (n = 5) of the fusions being detected.

A trade-off exists between high sensitivity and an increased number of overall predicted fusions, many of which are not clinically relevant or potential false positives. While STAR-Fusion demonstrated lower sensitivity, this was balanced with fewer total predictions, an average of 12 fusions per sample, in contrast to FusionCatcher which reported an average of 259 fusions per sample (Supplementary Table S3).

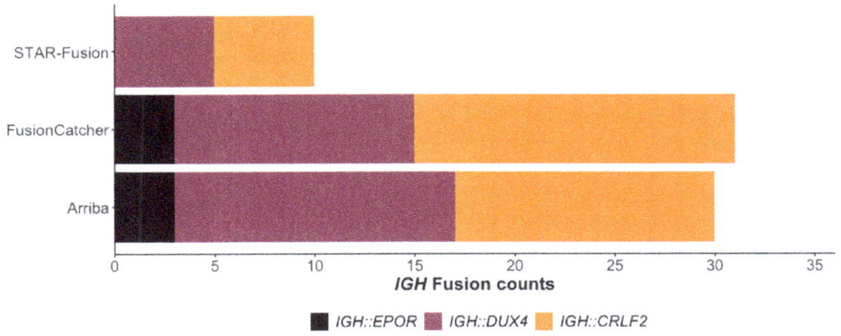

Figure 3. The number of *IGH* fusion events reported by each algorithm using default parameters (*IGH::CRLF2* n = 17, *IGH::DUX4* n = 15, *IGH::EPOR* n = 3).

3.2. Improving STAR-Fusions Performance when Detecting IGH Gene Fusions

An examination of the intermediary files generated by STAR-Fusion revealed that 33 of 35 *IGH* fusions were initially predicted, but most were subsequently excluded as they did not meet one or more of the default filtering parameters. This included insufficient junction read support and/or novel junction read support (nine samples for each criterion). For example, one sample had a read support depth of 1298 spanning fragments, but no junction reads, leading to exclusion from further filtering (Supplementary Table S4). To evaluate the effect the default values for the minimum number of supporting reads had on the overall fusion reporting rate, we decreased the values of these parameters and re-ran STAR-Fusion (Figure 4, Supplementary Data S3 and Table S5).

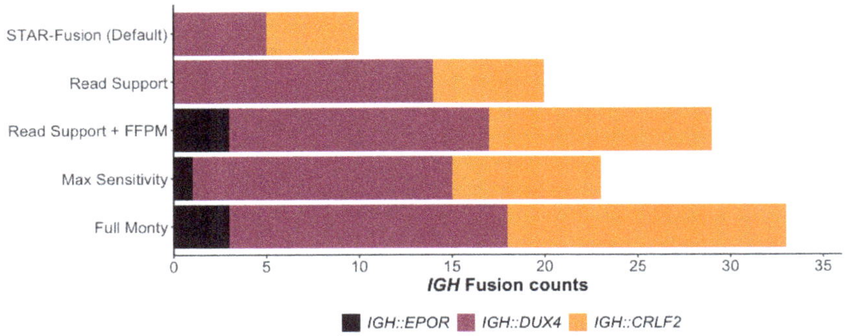

Figure 4. The number of *IGH* gene fusions reported by STAR-Fusion with the default parameter values vs. the altered parameter values. Read Support includes novel junction support reads and junction support reads, and FFPM is the fusion fragments per million reads.

The number of reported *IGH::DUX4* fusions increased following the initial parameter changes, with an almost three-fold increase (n = 14) in reported fusions when both the junction read and novel junction support read values were altered. The number of *IGH::CRLF2* fusions reported increased as well (n = 6), while *IGH::EPOR* fusions remained undetected. The overall reporting rate increased from 29% using default values to 60%, still lower than that of Arriba and FusionCatcher. Additionally, despite increasing sensitivity, the total number of fusion events detected decreased compared to the default settings, averaging 10 fusions per sample (Supplementary Table S6). It is unclear why this occurred.

We attempted to trace the select fusion events reported when using default parameters that were subsequently dropped when using altered parameters, but no pattern emerged.

STAR-Fusion implements an expression filter to normalise the number of RNA-seq reads supporting a fusion breakpoint based on the overall sequencing depth, represented as fusion fragments per million total mRNA-seq fragments (FFPM). By default, a candidate fusion breakpoint must have an FFPM value greater than 0.1, equating to one supporting read per 10 million mRNA-seq reads. We found that 10 candidate fusions were subsequently rejected because of an FFPM value lower than 0.1. By reducing the minimum FFPM in combination with the lowered minimum read support, the number of *IGH::DUX4* fusions reported stayed the same (n = 14) while the *IGH::CRLF2* fusions increased (n = 12), with STAR-Fusion also reporting all *IGH::EPOR* (n = 3), for an overall reporting rate of 82.9% (n = 29) (Figure 4). We also observed a significant increase in the total number of fusion events reported by STAR-Fusion, averaging 162.4 fusions per sample (Supplementary Table S6). Despite resulting in more predicted fusions, these results were still significantly lower than those of FusionCatcher, which reported almost 9100 total fusion events across the 35 samples, averaging nearly 260 fusions per sample, while Ariba also had more predicted fusions, with an average of 48 per sample (Supplementary Table S3).

In addition to extensive parameter customization, STAR-Fusion offers pre-set parameter bundles that are designed for maximum sensitivity. To assess the impact of these pre-set bundles on *IGH* fusion reporting, we conducted two additional tests using these undocumented parameter bundles (Figure 4, Supplementary Data S3 and Table S5). Surprisingly, using the Max Sensitivity parameter bundle resulted in fewer *IGH::CRLF2* and *IGH::EPOR* fusions being detected than when individually reducing FFPM and read support thresholds. We also observed a considerable increase in the total number of gene fusion events reported, with a total of 44,801 reported, averaging 1280 per sample. When applying the Full Monty parameter bundle, 94% of *IGH* fusions were detected, more than that achieved with any other STAR-Fusion settings tested, but at the expense of a substantial increase in the total number of fusion events reported, which amounted to 2,464,365, an average of 70,410 per sample (Supplementary Table S6).

3.3. Runtime and Resources

The *RIGHT* workflow was run on a HPC cluster, comprising seven nodes, each node running Intel(R) Xeon(R) Silver 4309Y CPU (@2.80 GHz) with 32 threads and 128 GB of memory, with Ubuntu 20.04.5 LTS as its operating system. *RIGHT* offers a runtime that is solely dependent on the slowest algorithm, by allowing all tools to be executed in parallel and independently of each other. Among the algorithms used, Arriba demonstrated the shortest runtime, averaging 15 min per sample (Tables 1 and S7) due to its one-pass filtering technique and its ability to extract candidate reads during the alignment process. FusionCatcher displayed the lengthiest average runtime of 2 h 39 min, while the default STAR-Fusion averaged 55 min. Memory consumption was comparable between each algorithm, with FusionCatcher using the least memory, with an average of 24.9 GB, while STAR-Fusion and Arriba used slightly more memory, at 38 GB and 35.8 GB, respectively. Finally, the modifications made to enhance STAR-Fusion's sensitivity only marginally increased its runtime and resource usage (Supplementary Table S8). At most, the average runtime increased by 8 min per sample for the Full Monty parameter bundle, while the average memory usage remained between 38.2–38.5 GB.

3.4. Ensemble Filtering Approaches to Identify IGH Fusions

The current recommended best practice for RNA-seq data analysis involves employing a minimum of two different gene fusion calling algorithms and reporting the intersected results [25]. We therefore compared the proportion of *IGH* fusions detected by multiple callers using both the default STAR-fusion settings and the more sensitive Full Monty setting (Figure 5).

Table 1. The maximum, minimum and mean values for the time taken for each algorithm to run, and the resident set size (RSS) required.

	Time			RSS (GB)		
	Max	**Mean**	**Min**	**Max**	**Mean**	**Min**
Arriba	27 m 44 s	15 m	6 m 43 s	38.2	35.8	34.5
FusionCatcher	4 h 25 m 21 s	2 h 39 m	1 h 23 m 50 s	27.5	24.9	22.5
STAR-Fusion (Default)	1 h 38 m 6 s	55 m	27 m 37 s	39.2	38.3	37.5
Read Support	1 h 33 m 6 s	57 m	26 m 35 s	39.2	38.3	37.4
Read Support + FFPM	1 h 29 m 18 s	56 m	27 m 4 s	39.2	38.3	37.4
Max Sensitivity	2 h 11 m 36 s	1 h 3 m	26 m 21 s	39.2	38.3	37.5
Full Monty	2 h 11 s	1 h 3 m	26 m 52 s	39.2	38.5	37.4

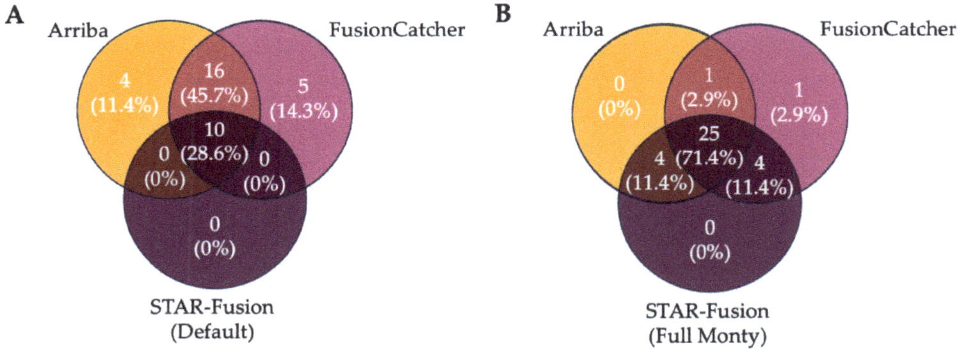

Figure 5. The intersection of gene fusion events reported by each algorithm, from (**A**) the full default pipeline, (**B**) Arriba, FusionCatcher, and the best-performing STAR-Fusion test (Full Monty).

The default *RIGHT* workflow results in 74.3% (n = 26) of *IGH* gene fusion events being reported by two or more callers, but this decreased to 28.6% (n = 10) when detected by all three callers (Figure 5A). When using STAR-Fusion with the Full Monty bundle, the number of gene fusion events detected by all algorithms increased to 71.4% (n = 25), with 97.1% (n = 34) detected by at least two callers (Figure 5B). While this is a marked improvement, the pipeline was still limited by the slowest-running algorithm, FusionCatcher. We then compared this result to only the intersection of the two fastest algorithms, in a bid to decrease the overall processing time. By using only Arriba and STAR-Fusion Full Monty, we saw 85.3% (n = 29) of gene fusion events reported by both, while also decreasing the average processing time by 1 h 36 min per sample. Given this, it can be argued that using only Arriba and the optimised STAR-Fusion, and reporting the intersection of their results, can lead to reduced processing times and improved reporting when compared to the initial default pipeline, while still adhering to the current best practice. If the processing time is not of concern, the use of all three callers is recommended; however, the combination of Arriba and FusionCatcher is also a practical option, and results in 74.3% of fusions being detected by both callers. Regardless of the combination of algorithms used, all *IGH* fusions present in the samples are detected by at least one of the callers (Supplementary Tables S2 and S5).

To ensure that the STAR-Fusion parameter optimisation that was implemented to improve the detection rate of *IGH* gene fusions did not affect the detection rate of non-*IGH* gene fusion and non-translocated cases, we processed 25 samples through the default workflow and the optimised workflow. These samples represented a range of B-ALL subtype defining alterations, including *ETV6::RUNX1*, *BCR::ABL1*, *PAX5::JAK2*, *KMT2A::AFF1* and *EP300::ZNF384* gene fusions, as well as PAX5.P80R and IKZF1.N159Y (Supplementary Table S9). For these 25 samples, all three algorithms with default parameters, as well as the optimised STAR-Fusion, found all 19 expected gene fusion events (Supplementary Table S10), and no pathogenic fusions were reported for samples that did not harbour translocation events. To ensure no additional pathogenic gene fusion events were reported when using the optimised STAR-Fusion parameters, we filtered the results against an extensive list of known pathogenic translocation events seen in B-ALL (Supplementary Table S11), and no additional pathogenic gene fusions were reported.

4. Discussion

The accurate and rapid identification of gene fusion events is crucial for assessing a patient's prognosis to facilitate efficient risk stratification and treatment. As there is no single universally accepted gold standard tool for gene fusion detection, current transcriptomic analysis approaches rely on the use of multiple algorithms and tools [8], resulting in a time-consuming process that requires significant personnel and computational resources to establish and execute in a routine clinical context. With this, we have provided a best-case computational pipeline for detecting gene fusion events in B-ALL patient samples, with a particular focus on those involving the hypervariable and highly repetitive *IGH* locus, which are notoriously difficult to detect, using a combination of specific algorithms and parameters.

The default parameters employed by standard gene fusion detection algorithms generally demonstrate adequacy in identifying gene fusion events in B-ALL, as is shown here when analysing patient samples that harbour translocation events involving distinct exon-exon breakpoints (Supplementary Table S10). However, our research here has also shown that *IGH* gene fusion events, owing to their highly variable nature, necessitate a more refined and sensitive parameter set. Our findings demonstrate that by adjusting merely three parameters, STAR-Fusion achieved a substantial enhancement in *IGH* fusion detection (94%), surpassing both Arriba and FusionCatcher (85.7% and 88.6%, respectively). This remarkable improvement can be attributed to the insufficiency of standard minimum filtering parameters, which fail to exhibit the necessary sensitivity for detecting many of these events due to the absence of distinct exon-exon breakpoints in *IGH* fusions. However, the trade-off between sensitivity and specificity must be considered, as higher sensitivity can also lead to an increase in prospective fusions, which would be unfeasible to manually curate. Moreover, despite the potential value of identifying all gene fusion events in a given patient sample, the number of clinically actionable fusions remains low [35], making it crucial to strike a balance between filtering sensitivity and accuracy, so that prognostically significant fusions are not missed and false positives are limited.

Reducing the time taken for disease classification is imperative when undertaking risk assessment and personalised patient treatment planning. Ensemble detection approaches using Nextflow allow tools to be run in parallel, reducing the overall processing time. As seen here, Arriba had an average runtime of 15 min, STAR-Fusion's runtime averaged 55 min, while FusionCatcher's average runtime was 2 h 39 min. However, by parallelising these processes, the time is only limited by the longest running algorithm. Even the changes made to STAR-Fusion increased its average runtime by only 8 min. And yet, we showed that it was possible to use only Arriba and the optimised STAR-Fusion and obtain a higher reporting rate of *IGH* gene fusion events detected by at least two algorithms compared to the default pipeline (85.3% vs. 74.3%) (Figure 5), while decreasing the processing time to 1 h per sample. While this time difference may seem negligible for an individual sample, processing multiple samples simultaneously results in a substantial improvement.

The identification of gene fusion events, particularly high-risk *IGH* fusions, is critical for B-ALL treatment and research, as they are often therapeutically targetable and frequently associated with the development and progression of various subtypes of the disease. Therefore, selecting the best-case parameters for a given algorithm, in order to achieve the most clinically significant results, is of paramount importance. However, while manually testing combinations of parameters, as seen here, can be time-consuming, machine learning and deep learning algorithms are rapidly evolving and have the potential to provide a more efficient means of identifying biomarkers in multi-omics datasets for personalised medicine [36,37]. Ultimately, future directions for precision medicine in B-ALL may involve the use of machine learning to identify the specific diagnostic markers present in an individual patient sample, and automatically select the optimal parameters for a given diagnostic algorithm.

In the present study, while our findings show promising insights into the detection of *IGH* gene fusions through bioinformatic analysis, it is imperative to address some limitations that have potential implications for the interpretation of our results. The use of short-read sequencing technology presents an acknowledged constraint. Short reads have been shown to exhibit lower accuracy in comparison to long reads [38,39], potentially impacting the sensitivity and specificity of *IGH* gene fusion detection. Additionally, the rapidly evolving landscape of bioinformatics introduces the consideration of newer gene fusion calling algorithms that might offer enhanced accuracy and sensitivity. The evaluation and incorporation of such algorithms, specifically those that have been tailored for the detection of difficult-to-identify gene fusions, warrant exploration to comprehensively assess their performance in our context [40–42].

5. Conclusions

The accurate and rapid detection of gene fusions is vital for assessing prognosis and guiding treatment in B-ALL. However, the lack of a universally accepted detection tool necessitates using multiple algorithms, leading to a time-consuming process in clinical practice. Our study showed that through curated parameter values for specific algorithms, detecting gene fusions involving the hypervariable *IGH* locus can be improved when compared to default values. However, balancing sensitivity and specificity is crucial to avoid a disproportionate number of fusions that are not clinically relevant. By using an ensemble detection approach and Nextflow, the workflow manager, we increased the detection rate of *IGH* fusions and significantly reduced the processing time. With the use of optimised algorithms determined through machine learning, the future holds promise for the efficient identification of biomarkers and parameter selection in personalised medicine for B-ALL.

Supplementary Materials: The following supporting information can be downloaded at: https://www.mdpi.com/article/10.3390/cancers15194731/s1, Data S1: Identification of *IGH::EPOR* gene fusions. *IGH::EPOR* fusions were confirmed through inspection of the sequencing reads in the BAM using IGV (Integrative Genomics Viewer); Data S2: The default commands used to run the standard pipeline; Data S3: The default and altered values for the parameters used for each test of STAR-Fusion; Table S1: Patient information, clinical information and reported genomic alterations for patients in the study cohort; Table S2: *IGH* gene fusion events reported by each caller in the default pipeline; Table S3: Total number of gene fusion events reported by each caller in the default pipeline; Table S4: Read counts for *IGH* gene fusions reported by the default pipeline and the additional STAR-Fusion parameters; Table S5: *IGH* gene fusion events reported by STAR-Fusion following each parameter change, compared to the default STAR-Fusion parameters; Table S6: Total number of gene fusion events reported by STAR-Fusion following each parameter change, compared to the default STAR-Fusion parameters; Table S7: Resources and processing time for the default pipeline; Table S8: Resources and processing time for the alternate STAR-Fusion parameters; Table S9: Patient information, clinical information and reported genomic alterations for control patients in the study cohort; Table S10: Gene fusion events reported by each caller in the default and altered pipeline; Table S11: White list of known B-ALL pathogenic gene fusion events used to filter reported events found using he optimised STAR-Fusion parameters.

Author Contributions: Conceptualization, A.J.T. and J.B.; Data curation, A.J.T. and J.A.R.; Formal analysis, A.J.T.; Funding acquisition, D.T.Y. and D.L.W.; Investigation, S.L.H., L.N.E., E.C.P., C.S., B.J.M., R.S., L.D.-P., A.S.M., M.G., R.S.K., C.Y.F. and A.S.M.Y.; Methodology, A.J.T. and J.B.; Project administration, J.B.; Resources, D.L.W.; Software, A.J.T.; Supervision, D.T.Y., J.B. and D.L.W.; Visualization, A.J.T.; Writing—original draft, A.J.T.; Writing—review & editing, J.A.R., S.L.H., L.N.E., E.C.P., C.S., B.J.M., R.S., L.D.-P., A.S.M., M.G., R.S.K., C.Y.F., A.S.M.Y., D.T.Y., J.B. and D.L.W. All authors have read and agreed to the published version of the manuscript.

Funding: This work was supported by funding from the Australian Genomics Health Alliance (AGHA) (1113531 to D.L.W.), Medical Research Future Fund (MRFF) (2007441 D.L.W.), Beat Cancer (Project grant x2 & Translational Research Package) (D.L.W., www.cancersa.org.au), and the Leukaemia Foundation (D.L.W., www.leukaemia.org.au). D.L.W. is an NHMRC R.D. Wright II Fellow (1160833) and a Beat Cancer Principal Research Fellow. D.T.Y. is an NHMRC Early Career Fellow (1146253). S.L.H. is The Kids' Cancer Project Fellow (www.thekidscancerproject.org.au). L.N.E. is the Peter Nelson Leukaemia Research Fellow (www.cancersa.org.au). The funders had no role in the study design, data collection and analysis, decision to publish, or preparation of the manuscript.

Institutional Review Board Statement: Ethical approval for sample collection and analysis was granted by the following Human Research Ethics Committees (HRECs) within South Australia; the Central Adelaide Local Health Network (CALHN) Human Research Ethics Committee and the Women's and Children's Health Network (WCHN) Human Research Ethics Committee.

Informed Consent Statement: Informed written consent was obtained from patients, or in the case of children, their legal parent/guardian.

Data Availability Statement: Genome–phenome Archive (accession numbers EGAD00001004461 and Raw FASTQ files for ALL samples in the study cohort are available from Genome-phenome Archive (EGAS00001006460). Code and additional scripts needed to reproduce the method seen here can be found in the Git repository (https://github.com/ashleethomson/The-RIGHT-Workflow).

Acknowledgments: The authors would like to acknowledge the South Australian Genomics Centre (SAGC, SA, AUS) and the ACRF Cellular Imaging and Cytometry Core Facility (SAHMRI, SA, AUS) for their sequencing and imaging services. Finally, we would like to thank the patients, their families and treating clinicians for their participation in this study.

Conflicts of Interest: The authors declare no conflict of interest.

References

1. Terwilliger, T.; Abdul-Hay, M. Acute lymphoblastic leukemia: A comprehensive review and 2017 update. *Blood Cancer J.* **2017**, *7*, e577. [CrossRef] [PubMed]
2. Roberts, K.G. Genetics and prognosis of ALL in children vs. adults. *Hematology* **2018**, *2018*, 137–145. [CrossRef] [PubMed]
3. Australian Institute of Health and Welfare (AIHW). Cancer Data in Australia. 2022. Available online: https://www.aihw.gov.au/reports/cancer/cancer-data-in-australia/data?page=3 (accessed on 25 August 2022).
4. Russell, L.J.; Enshaei, A.; Jones, L.; Erhorn, A.; Masic, D.; Bentley, H.; Laczko, K.S.; Fielding, A.K.; Goldstone, A.H.; Goulden, N.; et al. IGH@ translocations are prevalent in teenagers and young adults with acute lymphoblastic leukemia and are associated with a poor outcome. *J. Clin. Oncol.* **2014**, *32*, 1453–1462. [CrossRef] [PubMed]
5. Inaba, H.; Greaves, M.; Mullighan, C.G. Acute lymphoblastic leukaemia. *Lancet* **2013**, *381*, 1943–1955. [CrossRef]
6. Li, J.-F.; Dai, Y.-T.; Lilljebjörn, H.; Shen, S.-H.; Cui, B.-W.; Bai, L.; Liu, Y.-F.; Qian, M.-X.; Kubota, Y.; Kiyoi, H.; et al. Transcriptional landscape of B cell precursor acute lymphoblastic leukemia based on an international study of 1223 cases. *Proc. Natl. Acad. Sci. USA* **2018**, *115*, E11711–E11720. [CrossRef] [PubMed]
7. Schwab, C.; Harrison, C.J. Advances in B-cell precursor acute lymphoblastic leukemia genomics. *HemaSphere* **2018**, *2*, e53. [CrossRef]
8. Schröder, J.; Kumar, A.; Wong, S.Q. Overview of Fusion Detection Strategies Using Next-Generation Sequencing. *Methods Mol. Biol.* **2019**, *1908*, 125–138.
9. Ryan, S.L.; Peden, J.F.; Kingsbury, Z.; Schwab, C.J.; James, T.; Polonen, P.; Mijuskovic, M.; Becq, J.; Yim, R.; Cranston, R.E.; et al. Whole genome sequencing provides comprehensive genetic testing in childhood B-cell acute lymphoblastic leukaemia. *Leukemia* **2023**, *37*, 518–528. [CrossRef]
10. Tran, T.H.; Langlois, S.; Meloche, C.; Caron, M.; Saint-Onge, P.; Rouette, A.; Bataille, A.R.; Jimenez-Cortes, C.; Sontag, T.; Bittencourt, H.; et al. Whole-transcriptome analysis in acute lymphoblastic leukemia: A report from the DFCI ALL Consortium Protocol 16-001. *Blood Adv.* **2022**, *6*, 1329–1341. [CrossRef]

11. Kim, J.C.; Zuzarte, P.C.; Murphy, T.; Chan-Seng-Yue, M.; Brown, A.M.K.; Krzyzanowski, P.M.; Smith, A.C.; Notta, F.; Minden, M.D.; McPherson, J.D. Cryptic genomic lesions in adverse-risk acute myeloid leukemia identified by integrated whole genome and transcriptome sequencing. *Leukemia* **2020**, *34*, 306–311. [CrossRef]
12. Coudray, A.; Battenhouse, A.M.; Bucher, P.; Iyer, V.R. Detection and benchmarking of somatic mutations in cancer genomes using RNA-seq data. *PeerJ* **2018**, *6*, e5362. [CrossRef] [PubMed]
13. Conesa, A.; Madrigal, P.; Tarazona, S.; Gomez-Cabrero, D.; Cervera, A.; McPherson, A.; Szcześniak, M.W.; Gaffney, D.J.; Elo, L.L.; Zhang, X.; et al. A survey of best practices for RNA-seq data analysis. *Genome Biol.* **2016**, *17*, 13. [CrossRef]
14. Schroeder, H.W.; Cavacini, L. Structure and function of immunoglobulins. *J. Allergy Clin Immunol.* **2010**, *125*, S41–S52. [CrossRef] [PubMed]
15. Watson, C.T.; Breden, F. The immunoglobulin heavy chain locus: Genetic variation, missing data, and implications for human disease. *Genes Immun.* **2012**, *13*, 363–373. [CrossRef]
16. Chi, X.; Li, Y.; Qiu, X. V(D)J recombination, somatic hypermutation and class switch recombination of immunoglobulins: Mechanism and regulation. *Immunology* **2020**, *1*, 233–247. [CrossRef] [PubMed]
17. Jung, D.; Giallourakis, C.; Mostoslavsky, R.; Alt, F.W. Mechanism and control of V(D)J recombination at the immunoglobulin heavy chain locus. *Annu. Rev. Immunol.* **2006**, *24*, 541–570. [CrossRef]
18. Ozsolak, F.; Milos, P.M. RNA sequencing: Advances, challenges and opportunities. *Nat. Rev. Genet.* **2011**, *12*, 87–98. [CrossRef]
19. Gadala-Maria, D.; Gidoni, M.; Marquez, S.; Vander Heiden, J.A.; Kos, J.T.; Watson, C.T.; O'Connor, K.C.; Yaari, G.; Kleinstein, S.H. Identification of Subject-Specific Immunoglobulin Alleles From Expressed Repertoire Sequencing Data. *Front. Immunol.* **2019**, *10*, 129. [CrossRef]
20. Jackson, M.; Kavoussanakis, K.; Wallace, E.W.J. Using prototyping to choose a bioinformatics workflow management system. *PLoS Comput. Biol.* **2021**, *17*, e1008622. [CrossRef]
21. Chapiro, E.; Radford-Weiss, I.; Cung, H.-A.; Dastugue, N.; Nadal, N.; Taviaux, S.; Barin, C.; Struski, S.; Talmant, P.; Vandenberghe, P.; et al. Chromosomal translocations involving the IGH@ locus in B-cell precursor acute lymphoblastic leukemia: 29 new cases and a review of the literature. *Cancer Genet.* **2013**, *206*, 162–173. [CrossRef]
22. Russell, L.J.; Jones, L.; Erhorn, A.; Ensahei, A.; Masic, D.; Bentley, H.; Laczko, K.S.; Harrison, C.J. Immunoglobulin Heavy Chain Locus (IGH@) Translocations in Childhood B-Cell Precursor Acute Lymphoblastic Leukemia (BCP-ALL): Incidence and Risk Stratification. *Blood* **2012**, *120*, 1274. [CrossRef]
23. Dyer, M.J.S.; Akasaka, T.; Capasso, M.; Dusanjh, P.; Lee, Y.F.; Karran, E.L.; Nagel, I.; Vater, I.; Cario, G.; Siebert, R. Immunoglobulin heavy chain locus chromosomal translocations in B-cell precursor acute lymphoblastic leukemia: Rare clinical curios or potent genetic drivers? *Blood* **2010**, *115*, 1490–1499. [CrossRef]
24. Haas, B.J.; Dobin, A.; Li, B.; Stransky, N.; Pochet, N.; Regev, A. Accuracy assessment of fusion transcript detection via read-mapping and de novo fusion transcript assembly-based methods. *Genome Biol.* **2019**, *20*, 213. [CrossRef] [PubMed]
25. Uhrig, S.; Ellermann, J.; Walther, T.; Burkhardt, P.; Fröhlich, M.; Hutter, B.; Toprak, U.H.; Neumann, O.; Stenzinger, A.; Scholl, C.; et al. Accurate and efficient detection of gene fusions from RNA sequencing data. *Genome Res.* **2021**, *31*, 448–460. [CrossRef]
26. Wratten, L.; Wilm, A.; Göke, J. Reproducible, scalable, and shareable analysis pipelines with bioinformatics workflow managers. *Nat. Methods* **2021**, *18*, 1161–1168. [CrossRef] [PubMed]
27. Spišaková, V.; Hejtmánek, L.; Hynšt, J. Nextflow in bioinformatics: Executors performance comparison using genomics data. *Future Gener. Comput. Syst.* **2023**, *142*, 328–339. [CrossRef]
28. Di Tommaso, P.; Chatzou, M.; Floden, E.W.; Barja, P.P.; Palumbo, E.; Notredame, C. Nextflow enables reproducible computational workflows. *Nat. Biotechnol.* **2017**, *35*, 316–319. [CrossRef]
29. Nicorici, D.; Şatalan, M.; Edgren, H.; Kangaspeska, S.; Murumägi, A.; Kallioniemi, O.; Virtanen, S.; Kilkku, O. FusionCatcher—A tool for finding somatic fusion genes in paired-end RNA-sequencing data. *bioRxiv* **2014**, 011650. [CrossRef]
30. Genome Reference Consortium. Available online: https://www.ncbi.nlm.nih.gov/grc (accessed on 15 July 2022).
31. Church, D.M.; Schneider, V.A.; Graves, T.; Auger, K.; Cunningham, F.; Bouk, N.; Chen, H.-C.; Agarwala, R.; McLaren, W.M.; Ritchie, G.R.; et al. Modernizing reference genome assemblies. *PLoS Biol.* **2011**, *9*, e1001091. [CrossRef]
32. Cunningham, F.; Allen, J.E.; Allen, J.; Alvarez-Jarreta, J.; Amode, M.R.; Armean, I.M.; Austine-Orimoloye, O.; Azov, A.G.; Barnes, I.; Bennett, R.; et al. Ensembl 2022. *Nucleic Acids Res.* **2022**, *50*, D988–D995. [CrossRef]
33. Rehn, J.; Mayoh, C.; Heatley, S.L.; McClure, B.J.; Eadie, L.N.; Schutz, C.; Yeung, D.T.; Cowley, M.J.; Breen, J.; White, D.L. RaScALL: Rapid (Ra) screening (Sc) of RNA-seq data for prognostically significant genomic alterations in acute lymphoblastic leukaemia (ALL). *PLoS Genet.* **2022**, *18*, e1010300. [CrossRef] [PubMed]
34. RaScALL: Rapid Screening of RNA-Seq in Acute Lymphoblastic Leukaemia—EGA European Genome-Phenome Archive. Available online: https://ega-archive.org/studies/EGAS00001006460 (accessed on 27 February 2023).
35. Selvam, P.; Kelly, K.; Hesse, A.N.; Spitzer, D.; Reddi, H.V. Evaluating gene fusions in solid tumors—Clinical experience using an RNA based 53 gene next-generation sequencing panel. *Cancer Genet.* **2019**, *233–234*, 32–42. [CrossRef] [PubMed]
36. Painuli, D.; Bhardwaj, S.; Köse, U. Recent advancement in cancer diagnosis using machine learning and deep learning techniques: A comprehensive review. *Comput. Biol. Med.* **2022**, *146*, 105580. [CrossRef] [PubMed]

37. Dhillon, A.; Singh, A.; Bhalla, V.K. A Systematic Review on Biomarker Identification for Cancer Diagnosis and Prognosis in Multi-omics: From Computational Needs to Machine Learning and Deep Learning. *Arch. Comput. Methods Eng.* **2023**, *30*, 917–949. [CrossRef]
38. van Dijk, E.L.; Naquin, D.; Gorrichon, K.; Jaszczyszyn, Y.; Ouazahrou, R.; Thermes, C.; Hernandez, C. Genomics in the long-read sequencing era. *Trends Genet.* **2023**. [CrossRef]
39. Tian, L.; Shao, Y.; Nance, S.; Dang, J.; Xu, B.; Ma, X.; Li, Y.; Ju, B.; Dong, L.; Newman, S.; et al. Long-read sequencing unveils IGH-DUX4 translocation into the silenced IGH allele in B-cell acute lymphoblastic leukemia. *Nat. Commun.* **2019**, *10*, 2789. [CrossRef]
40. Tian, L.; Li, Y.; Edmonson, M.N.; Zhou, X.; Newman, S.; McLeod, C.; Thrasher, A.; Liu, Y.; Tang, B.; Rusch, M.C.; et al. CICERO: A versatile method for detecting complex and diverse driver fusions using cancer RNA sequencing data. *Genome Biol.* **2020**, *21*, 126. [CrossRef]
41. Davidson, N.M.; Chen, Y.; Sadras, T.; Ryland, G.L.; Blombery, P.; Ekert, P.G.; Göke, J.; Oshlack, A. JAFFAL: Detecting fusion genes with long-read transcriptome sequencing. *Genome Biol.* **2022**, *23*, 10. [CrossRef] [PubMed]
42. Su, X.; Malouf, G. P482: Accufusion: A Highly Scalable Software Tool for Detecting Gene Fusions By Rna-Seq in Leukemia. *HemaSphere* **2023**, *7*. [CrossRef]

cancers

MDPI

Article

Chronic Periodontitis and the Potential Likelihood of Gastric Cancer: A Nested Case-Control Study in the Korean Population Utilizing a National Health Sample Cohort

Mi Jung Kwon [1], Ho Suk Kang [2], Min-Jeong Kim [3], Nan Young Kim [4], Hyo Geun Choi [5] and Hyun Lim [2,*]

1 Department of Pathology, Hallym University Sacred Heart Hospital, Hallym University College of Medicine, Anyang 14068, Republic of Korea; mulank@hanmail.net
2 Division of Gastroenterology, Department of Internal Medicine, Hallym University Sacred Heart Hospital, Hallym University College of Medicine, Anyang 14068, Republic of Korea; hskang76@hallym.or.kr
3 Department of Radiology, Hallym University Sacred Heart Hospital, Hallym University College of Medicine, Anyang 14068, Republic of Korea; drkmj@hallym.or.kr
4 Hallym Institute of Translational Genomics and Bioinformatics, Hallym University Medical Center, Anyang 14068, Republic of Korea; honeyny78@gmail.com
5 Suseo Seoul E.N.T. Clinic and MD Analytics, Seoul 06349, Republic of Korea; mdanalytics@naver.com
* Correspondence: hlim77@hallym.or.kr

Simple Summary: This research investigates the potential link between gum disease and stomach cancer in the Korean population. In this study, we analyzed data from over 10,000 people with gastric cancer and 40,000 healthy individuals. The results indicate that individuals who had gum disease in the past one to two years were more likely to develop stomach cancer. This association was consistently observed in different groups, such as men under 65 years old. The study emphasizes the importance of regular screening for stomach cancer, particularly for those at high risk, such as individuals with a history of gum disease. These findings contribute to our understanding of the connection between oral health and stomach cancer and may guide future preventive measures.

Abstract: There is limited information regarding the potential association between chronic periodontitis (CP) and gastric cancer, especially in the Korean population. This study aimed to explore this relationship. This nested case–control study analyzed data from 10,174 patients with gastric cancer and 40,696 controls from the Korean National Health Insurance Service–National Sample Cohort using propensity score matching. Standardized differences were used to compare baseline characteristics between study groups. Logistic regression analyses adjusted for confounders were conducted to assess the association between history of CP and gastric cancer occurrence. CP histories and comprehensive subgroup analyses in the 1- and 2-year periods preceding the index date were evaluated. Individuals with a history of CP within the 1-year and 2-year periods showed an increased likelihood of developing gastric cancer. Subgroup analyses consistently supported these findings in male participants aged <65 years and individuals with various income levels or living in residential areas. However, no significant associations were observed among participants aged ≥65 years. In conclusion, CP may be a potential risk factor for gastric cancer development in the Korean population. Regular screening for gastric cancer may be necessary for high-risk individuals, specifically men aged <65 years with a history of CP.

Keywords: gastric cancer; chronic periodontitis; nested case–control study; national healthcare data

1. Introduction

Gastric cancer is the fifth most prevalent cancer and a significant cause of cancer-related mortality in Korea [1], which is among the regions with the highest risk of stomach cancer worldwide [1]. Gastric cancer develops through a complex process involving multiple factors and stages [2], the key contributors of which include Helicobacter pylori infection, geographic variations, and lifestyle choices [2]. Over the past two decades, the implementation of a mandatory national endoscopic screening program for gastric cancer, conducted every two years for adults above 40 years of age, has contributed to a reduction in gastric cancer mortality [3]. Despite ongoing efforts, gastric cancer remains the most commonly diagnosed malignancy among adult men in Korea, and its incidence continues to increase with age in both males and females in Korea [1]. These trends highlight that relying solely on screening measures may not be sufficient to fully control the incidence of stomach cancer; hence, identifying modifiable risk factors associated with gastric cancer is crucial for establishing a foundation for fundamental prevention approaches.

Chronic periodontitis (CP) is a prevalent inflammatory condition that primarily affects the gums and is commonly observed in adults aged 30 years and older, with higher rates observed in individuals aged over 50 years [4]. In this condition, there is an infiltration of immune-inflammatory cells into the deep structures of the periodontium, causing progressive devastation of the periodontal tissues and underlying alveolar bone, which is responsible for supporting the teeth [5,6]. This process contributes significantly to tooth loss in adults [4], significantly affecting their overall quality of life [5,6]. The potential connection between CP and various systemic disorders, including cancer, has attracted considerable attention [7]. Epidemiological studies worldwide have consistently reported a potential link between CP and an elevated risk of gastric cancer [8–14]. The foundation of this connection lies in the substantial roles of inflammation and dysbiosis observed under both conditions [15]. Local chronic inflammation may be a key factor underlying this association, as multiple studies have established a correlation between chronic inflammation and various gastrointestinal cancers such as gastric cancer [16]. This correlation raises concerns regarding the potential risk of developing comorbid gastric cancer, particularly among elderly individuals, given the high prevalence of gastric cancer in Korea [1]. However, there is insufficient information regarding this association, particularly among the Korean population.

In contrast with these positive findings, previous studies have reported the null relevance of CP in gastric cancer [17–19]. These studies often had imbalanced sample sizes between the study and comparison groups and included cohorts with different demographics, such as age, sex, ethnicity, education level, or income level [18,19]. Furthermore, some studies included a small number of gastric cancer cases [18,19]. While a meta-analysis that included various gastrointestinal cancers observed a significant association between CP, including tooth loss, and overall gastrointestinal cancer [20], the specific impact of CP on the incidence of gastric cancer has not been thoroughly explored, as the primary focus of the meta-analysis was not solely on gastric cancer [20]. Another meta-analysis specifically investigating gastric cancer found a notable link between CP and gastric cancer, which was limited by a considerable degree of heterogeneity among the included studies [21]. To accurately assess the potential impact of CP on the risk of developing gastric cancer, further research using validated and well-balanced large-scale cohort data that specifically focuses on gastric cancer is required.

We hypothesized that a history of CP could negatively influence the development of gastric cancer and that there might be specific risk factors associated with CP that could predict the occurrence of gastric cancer in the Korean population. This study aimed to explore these relationships by conducting a nationwide cohort study using a meticulously matched nested case–control design and comprehensive subgroup analyses to examine the potential effects of CP on the development of stomach cancer.

2. Materials and Methods

The ethics committee of Hallym University approved this study under the reference number 2022-10-008. Written informed consent was not required, as the analysis was conducted using anonymous data. The data sources used in this study were provided by the Korean National Health Insurance Service-National Sample Cohort (KNHIS-NSC) [22].

This database comprised 1,108,369 participants and 219,673,817 medical claims codes recorded between January 2002 and December 2019. The KNHIS-NSC was generated by the Korea National Health Insurance Service, which applied a systematic sampling procedure to create a prototypical sample of 1,025,340 people in 2002, accounting for approximately 2.2% of all Korean citizens. These individuals were followed up for 17 years, until 2019. Further details regarding the representativeness of the data and the cohort can be found elsewhere [22].

To investigate the relationship between the history of subjects and the presence or absence of exposure in outcome status, a nested case–control study design was deemed appropriate [23]. The National Health Insurance database employs the International Classification of Diseases, 10th revision (ICD-10) codes as a standardized reference for disease diagnosis and healthcare information organization within the database. In this study, participants who were newly diagnosed with stomach cancer were initially selected based on their diagnosis of gastric cancer (ICD-10 codes: C16.0–C16.9) and the presence of a special claim code indicating serious cancer (V193 or V194) between 2005 and 2019 (n = 10,174). A special claims code indicating a serious illness that makes cancer patients eligible for payment reduction has been implemented in the national healthcare service since 2005. Individuals not diagnosed with gastric cancer from 2005 to 2019 were included in the control group (n = 1,098,195). Individuals in the control group who were diagnosed with stomach cancer at least once (n = 2412) were excluded from the study.

To minimize disparities in baseline demographic and clinical characteristics between the gastric cancer and counterpart groups, propensity score matching was performed [24,25]. The matching process entailed pairing participants with gastric cancer with control participants who exhibited similar propensity scores, which were based on 4 covariates (sex, age, income, and region of residence) [24,25]. The index date for each patient diagnosed with stomach cancer was established as the day when both the ICD-10 codes for stomach cancer and the special claim code indicating a serious cancer illness (V193 or V194) were electronically recorded in the health care datasets [25]. For the control group, the index date was defined as the index date of the matched patients with stomach cancer [25]. As a result, each matched patient and control group shared an identical index date. During matching, 1,055,087 participants were excluded. Ultimately, 10,174 stomach cancer patients were matched in a 1:4 ratio with 40,696 controls (Figure 1). We then surveyed patients with a history of CP in both 1-year and 2-year periods before the index date in both groups.

2.1. Exposure (Chronic Periodontitis)

To ensure the accuracy of the analysis and eliminate false-positive cases, only participants who were treated for CP by dentists and diagnosed according to the ICD-10 code (K05.3) were included in the study [26]. The number of CP treatments received by each participant was documented until the day preceding both the 1-year and 2-year periods prior to the index date, and a meticulous approach was adopted to enhance the reliability of the association between CP and the outcomes under investigation.

2.2. Outcome (Gastric Cancer)

To maintain the precision of the analysis and avoid false-positive cases, stomach cancer cases were determined employing specific ICD-10 codes (C16.0–C16.9) allocated as the diagnosis [malignant neoplasm of the cardia (C16.0), fundus (C16.1), body (C16.2), pyloric antrum (C16.3), pylorus (C16.4), lesser curvature, unspecified (C16.5), greater curvature, unspecified (C16.6), overlapping sites of the stomach (C16.8), and the stomach, unspecified (C16.9)] [25]. Additionally, a special claims code indicating serious cancer illness (V193 or V194) was utilized to confirm eligibility for reduced payments from the national healthcare service.

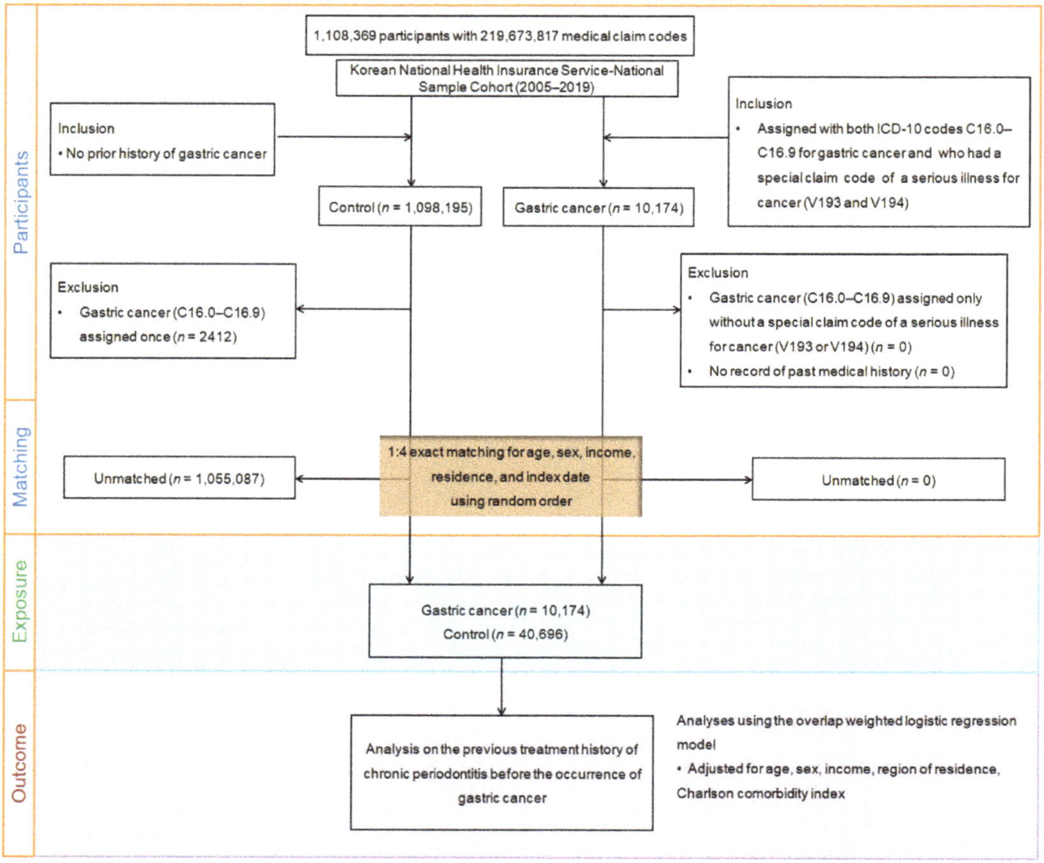

Figure 1. A schematic illustration of the participant selection process employed in this study. Out of the initial cohort of 1,108,369 participants, 10,174 individuals with gastric cancer were matched with 40,696 control participants based on age, sex, income, and region of residence.

2.3. Covariates

Participants were classified into 10 age categories, each illustrating a 5-year gap, and were distributed into five income categories, ranging from class 1 (lowest income) to 5 (highest income). Residential locations were categorized into 16 groups based on administrative districts and subsequently reorganized into urban or rural areas [26]. The Charlson Comorbidity Index (CCI) is a commonly employed tool for assessing the overall burden of comorbid conditions, calculated as a sum score ranging from 0 to 29, considering 17 potential comorbidities [27,28]. CCI score was included as a covariate in the analysis, excluding cases of gastric cancer. This was performed to consider the potential influence of comorbidities on the development of gastric cancer [28].

2.4. Statistical Analyses

Standardized differences were applied to compare baseline features between the study groups. An absolute standardized difference of less than 0.20 was considered indicative of achieving satisfactory balance [29]. The propensity score was computed using multivariate logistic regression, incorporating all relevant covariates. In the overlap weighting approach, participants with gastric cancer were weighted based on the propensity score probability, while control participants were weighted based on the probability of 1 minus the propensity score. This overlap weighting, ranging between 0 and 1, was utilized to achieve optimal balance and enhance the precision of the analyses [30–32]. The analysis of the overlap-weighted odds ratios (ORs) involved computing odds ratios with 95% confidence intervals (CIs) for gastric cancer in relation to the number of treatments for chronic periodontitis (per 10 treatments), both in the crude (unadjusted) and overlap weighted models (adjusted for age, sex, income, residence area, and CCI). Additionally, subgroup analyses were conducted based on age, sex, income, and region of residence.

Statistical analyses were conducted using SAS version 9.4 (SAS Institute Inc., Cary, NC, USA). Two-tailed analyses were performed, and statistical significance was determined at a significance level of $p < 0.05$.

3. Results

Table 1 provides the demographic characteristics of 10,174 patients diagnosed with gastric cancer, along with a comparison group of 40,696 individuals at baseline. The table includes data both before and after conducting overlap weighting adjustments for propensity score matching. Prior to adjustment, the covariates age, residence, sex, and income exhibited a standardized difference of 0.00, indicating no significant disparities between the gastric cancer and control groups. Other basic characteristics, such as the number of CP treatments for 1 year and 2 years before the index date, were not significantly different (both standardized differences = 0.01). However, the gastric cancer group had higher CCI scores than the control group (standardized difference = 0.67). After implementing overlap-weighting adjustments, these discrepancies were notably reduced, with each covariate achieving a standardized difference of <0.2. This indicates a well-balanced distribution of demographic attributes between the gastric cancer and control groups.

Table 1. General characteristics of participants after and before propensity score overlap weighting adjustment.

Characteristics	Before PS Overlap Weighting Adjustment			After PS Overlap Weighting Adjustment		
	Gastric Cancer	Control	Standardized Difference	Gastric Cancer	Control	Standardized Difference
Age (y), n (%)			0.00			0.00
5–9	1 (0.01)	4 (0.01)		1 (0.01)	1 (0.01)	
10–14	3 (0.03)	12 (0.03)		2 (0.02)	2 (0.02)	
20–24	1 (0.01)	4 (0.01)		1 (0.01)	1 (0.01)	
25–29	19 (0.19)	76 (0.19)		13 (0.17)	13 (0.17)	
30–34	95 (0.93)	380 (0.93)		63 (0.85)	63 (0.85)	
35–39	205 (2.01)	820 (2.01)		140 (1.91)	140 (1.91)	
40–44	466 (4.58)	1864 (4.58)		334 (4.56)	334 (4.56)	
45–49	711 (6.99)	2844 (6.99)		505 (6.89)	505 (6.89)	
50–54	994 (9.77)	3976 (9.77)		701 (9.56)	701 (9.56)	
55–59	1197 (11.77)	4788 (11.77)		856 (11.68)	856 (11.68)	
60–64	1449 (14.24)	5796 (14.24)		1041 (14.21)	1041 (14.21)	
65–69	1463 (14.38)	5852 (14.38)		1058 (14.43)	1058 (14.43)	
70–74	1490 (14.65)	5960 (14.65)		1085 (14.80)	1085 (14.80)	
75–79	1071 (10.53)	4284 (10.53)		784 (10.69)	784 (10.69)	
80–84	693 (6.81)	2772 (6.81)		512 (6.99)	512 (6.99)	
85+	316 (3.11)	1264 (3.11)		235 (3.20)	235 (3.20)	
Sex, n (%)			0.00			0.00
Male	6834 (67.17)	27,336 (67.17)		4927 (67.23)	4927 (67.23)	
Female	3340 (32.83)	13,360 (32.83)		2401 (32.77)	2401 (32.77)	
Income, n (%)			0.00			0.00
1 (lowest)	1959 (19.25)	7836 (19.25)		1399 (19.09)	1399 (19.09)	
2	1260 (12.38)	5040 (12.38)		896 (12.23)	896 (12.23)	
3	1621 (15.93)	6484 (15.93)		1165 (15.89)	1165 (15.89)	

Table 1. *Cont.*

Characteristics	Before PS Overlap Weighting Adjustment			After PS Overlap Weighting Adjustment		
	Gastric Cancer	Control	Standardized Difference	Gastric Cancer	Control	Standardized Difference
4	2144 (21.07)	8576 (21.07)		1535 (20.95)	1535 (20.95)	
5 (highest)	3190 (31.35)	12,760 (31.35)		2334 (31.84)	2334 (31.84)	
Region of residence, n (%)			0.00			0.00
Urban	4310 (42.36)	17,240 (42.36)		3107 (42.40)	3107 (42.40)	
Rural	5864 (57.64)	23,456 (57.64)		4221 (57.60)	4221 (57.60)	
CCI score, mean (SD)	2.40 (2.70)	0.92 (1.58)	0.67	1.71 (1.88)	1.71 (0.97)	0.00
The number of CP treatments for 1 year before index date, mean (SD)	0.52 (1.31)	0.51 (1.36)	0.01	0.54 (1.13)	0.49 (0.56)	0.05
The number of CP treatments for 2 year before index date, mean (SD)	1.00 (2.09)	0.98 (2.08)	0.01	1.03 (1.78)	0.94 (0.86)	0.06

Abbreviations: PS—propensity score; CCI—Charlson Comorbidity Index; SD—standard deviation; CP—chronic periodontitis.

To ensure the reliability of our findings, we conducted a rigorous analysis by evaluating CP histories at both 1-year and 2-year periods before the index date (Table 2). The results consistently showed a meaningful positive relationship between a history of CP and incident gastric cancer. The OR 1 year was 1.31 (95% CI = 1.15–1.49, $p < 0.001$), indicating a 31% enhanced probability of gastric cancer. Similarly, for 2 years, the OR was 1.24 (95% CI = 1.14–1.35, $p < 0.001$), suggesting a 24% elevated chance.

Table 2. Crude and overlap propensity score-weighted odds ratios for gastric cancer in relation to the treatments for chronic periodontitis within two different time periods from the index date, with subgroup analyses according to age, sex, income, and region of residence.

Characteristics	Odd Ratios for Gastric Cancer (95% Confidence Interval)			
	Crude	*p*-Value	Overlap Weighted Model †	*p*-Value
From the index date to the before the 1-year period				
Total participants (n = 50,870)	1.04 (0.88–1.21)	0.671	1.31 (1.15–1.49)	<0.001 *
Age < 65 years old (n = 25,705)	1.20 (0.97–1.50)	0.095	1.50 (1.25–1.80)	<0.001 *
Age ≥ 65 years old (n = 25,165)	0.88 (0.69–1.11)	0.27	1.10 (0.90–1.33)	0.346
Male (n = 34,170)	1.06 (0.88–1.27)	0.556	1.32 (1.13–1.54)	<0.001 *
Female (n = 16,700)	0.98 (0.72–1.34)	0.884	1.25 (0.97–1.62)	0.091
Low-income group (n = 24,200)	1.01 (0.80–1.28)	0.936	1.33 (1.09–1.62)	0.005 *
High-income group (n = 26,670)	1.06 (0.85–1.31)	0.616	1.29 (1.08–1.55)	0.005 *
Urban residents (n = 21,550)	1.09 (0.87–1.36)	0.465	1.33 (1.10–1.60)	0.003 *
Rural residents (n = 29,320)	0.98 (0.78–1.24)	0.891	1.28 (1.06–1.55)	0.009 *
From the index date to the before the 2-year period				
Total participants (n = 50,870)	1.04 (0.94–1.15)	0.456	1.24 (1.14–1.35)	<0.001 *
Age < 65 years old (n = 25,705)	1.16 (1.00–1.33)	0.049 *	1.38 (1.22–1.55)	<0.001 *
Age ≥ 65 years old (n = 25,165)	0.93 (0.80–1.08)	0.357	1.09 (0.96–1.23)	0.168
Male (n = 34,170)	1.05 (0.93–1.19)	0.396	1.25 (1.13–1.38)	<0.001 *
Female (n = 16,700)	1.00 (0.82–1.23)	0.966	1.20 (1.02–1.42)	0.028 *
Low-income group (n = 24,200)	1.04 (0.89–1.22)	0.592	1.32 (1.17–1.51)	<0.001 *
High-income group (n = 26,670)	1.04 (0.90–1.19)	0.602	1.18 (1.05–1.32)	0.006 *
Urban residents (n = 21,550)	1.07 (0.93–1.24)	0.343	1.26 (1.11–1.42)	<0.001 *
Rural residents (n = 29,320)	1.01 (0.87–1.17)	0.927	1.22 (1.08–1.37)	0.001 *

* Significance at $p < 0.05$. † Adjusted for age, sex, income, region of residence, and Charlson Comorbidity Index.

Subgroup analyses were conducted to examine associations within specific demographic categories. In the evaluation of CP history within the 1-year period prior to the index date, a significant association persisted among participants aged <65 years, males, and individuals across different income levels or residence areas. However, no significant association was observed among participants aged ≥65 years.

Similarly, in the evaluation of CP history within the 2-year period before the index date, consistent findings were observed across subgroups. CP was significantly associated with gastric cancer in participants aged <65 years, males, females, those with low or high income, and both urban and rural residents. However, similar to the 1-year period analysis, no significant association was found in the age ≥65 years subgroup.

4. Discussion

In this extensive nationwide cohort study, we conducted a rigorous evaluation by examining two distinct periods to establish a reliable association between CP and gastric cancer. These results consistently indicated that individuals who had previously experienced CP had a slightly but significantly elevated probability of developing gastric cancer. Specifically, within 1 year preceding the index date, there was a 30% increased likelihood of gastric cancer development (95% CI = 1.15–1.49), while the increased likelihood was 24% (95% CI = 1.14–1.35) within 2 years prior to the index date, which provides further support for the strong relationship between the two conditions. This association was more pronounced in males aged <65 years, regardless of income or residence. However, no such association was observed among individuals aged ≥65 years. Based on our study findings, regular screening for gastric cancer may be particularly necessary for high-risk individuals, specifically men aged <65 years with a history of CP.

Our findings appear to align with the results of previous studies conducted in various countries, including China [8], Finland [9], Iran [10], Japan [11], Sweden [13], the USA [14], and Turkey [12], which may further strengthen the evidence supporting a strong relationship between CP and gastric cancer. In a substantial prospective cohort study conducted in a rural area of China, involving 28,868 individuals aged 40–69, it was discovered that tooth loss due to CP was significantly associated with an 80% increased risk (95% CI = 1.1–3.0) of gastric cancer, particularly in non-cardiac locations [8]. In another prospective cohort study conducted in Finland that included male smokers (n = 29,124), edentulous individuals with CP were found to have a significant (1.65-fold) increased risk of gastric noncardia adenocarcinoma (95% CI = 1.09–2.49) [9]; however, the participants self-reported their dental history in questionnaires, which may introduce recall bias, and the exclusive enrollment of males may limit the study's generalizability to the overall population [9]. In another study conducted in the USA, which combined two independent studies involving both male and female health professionals, a history of periodontal disease was found to be associated with a 52% greater risk of stomach cancer [14]; however, health-professional-only cohorts may cause selection bias [14]. Similarly, a case–control study conducted in Hokkaido, Japan, including 242 gastric cancer cases and 484 matched controls, revealed that the CP accompanied by loss of more than 10 teeth showed a 1.73-times aggravated likelihood of developing stomach cancer (95% CI = 1.23–2.43) [11]. The generalizability of previous studies on the association between CP and gastric cancer may be diminished due to their reliance on community-based cohorts [8,10–13], which may not fully represent the entire population. Our study used a nationwide organized dataset covering a wide range of participants, which enabled us to minimize confounding effects and enhance the generalizability of our findings. The increased probability of gastric cancer associated with CP was consistently reproduced in our study, which involved a robust sample size with a balanced distribution of 10,174 patients with gastric cancer matched with 40,696 control participants.

Throughout our analysis, we consistently found a positive association indicating an increased likelihood of developing gastric cancer in CP individuals aged <65 years and in men, irrespective of income or residence, highlighting the importance of age and sex considerations in the association between CP and gastric cancer. These results remained consistent across the two different time periods studied. The association between CP and gastric cancer appears to vary based on different age groups. We observed a 38% higher likelihood of the occurrence of stomach cancer in patients under the age of 65 (95% CI = 1.22–1.55), while no such relevance was found in the older age group of over 65 years (OR 1.09; 95% CI = 0.96–1.23). The fact that there is an exclusively positive association between age <65 years in CP patients and incident gastric cancer is intriguing, especially considering the higher prevalence of periodontitis in subjects aged 70 to 81 years compared to those aged 50 to 59 years [33]. The incidence of CP is more prominent in older adults aged 65 years or above, with approximately two-thirds (68%) of individuals in this age group being affected [33]. Despite this, our findings seem to align with those of two previous studies that also demonstrated an elevated gastric cancer risk in younger individuals <65 years with CP [8,13]. A Swedish study indicated a 4.24-fold increased risk for individuals aged 50 (95% CI = 1.83–9.80), which gradually decreased by approximately 4% per year, resulting in a diminished magnitude of 1.54 (95% CI = 0.90–2.64) for individuals aged 75 [13]. Similarly, a Chinese study observed a decreased relative risk of gastric cancer with increasing age among participants with CP, with the strongest association observed in individuals aged <50 years [8]. The authors noted that in this region, a considerable number of individuals experience tooth loss at an early stage of life [8]. Coincidentally, this population also exhibits exceptionally high rates of esophageal and gastric cardia cancer [8], suggesting that the presence of CP in younger individuals could potentially serve as an early indicator of upper gastrointestinal cancer. Other studies from Finland and Iran also identified age as a significant factor influencing the association between the two diseases [9,10].

Our data consistently revealed a positive association in men, regardless of the two different time periods considered. This finding suggests that men and women with CP may indeed have differing degrees of risk of developing gastric cancer. Specifically, in the period from the index date to before the 2-year period, females showed a 20% higher likelihood of stomach cancer occurrence (95% CI = 1.02–1.42), whereas no statistically significant relevance was found in the period from the index date to before the 1-year period (OR 1.25; 95% CI = 0.97–1.62). Considering the male gender as an acknowledged risk factor in both CP and gastric cancer [1,4], our results may suggest that a subset of women who experience CP for a long-term period of over 2 years might be associated with a higher likelihood of developing gastric cancer.

Disparities in the prevalence and severity of periodontal disease have been linked to socioeconomic factors, including education and income [34]. Epidemiological reports consistently demonstrate an inverse relationship between periodontal disease and education and income, even after controlling for age and gender [34,35]. Additionally, socioeconomic status is known to be a risk factor for gastric cancer [36], with individuals of lower socioeconomic status facing a higher risk of gastric cancer and poorer survival rates [36,37]. As a result, it has been suggested that socioeconomic status or residential areas could potentially confound the interpretation of the association between CP and gastric cancer. In our present study, we made a notable observation of an increased likelihood of developing gastric cancer in individuals with CP who were men and aged <65 years, regardless of income or residential area. This association remained significant even after adjusting for potential confounding factors. These findings indicate that factors related to socioeconomic status or residential areas do not fully explain the association between CP and gastric cancer in our study population. There is currently a lack of studies that have conducted comprehensive subgroup analyses considering sex, income, or residential area to determine the probability of developing gastric cancer shown in our study. It may be advisable to conduct clinical risk evaluations for gastric cancer in individuals with CP, particularly in men aged <65 years, within the Korean population. Further research and comprehensive subgroup analyses are warranted to fully elucidate the potential factors influencing this association and to develop targeted preventive strategies for at-risk populations.

In contrast, several studies have reported conflicting outcomes regarding the relationship between CP and the incidence of gastric cancer. These studies, conducted in Japan [38], Taiwan [17], and the USA [18,19], did not specifically focus on gastric cancer but included it as part of a broader range of cancers [17–19,38]. Therefore, the number of stomach cancer cases in these studies may have been insufficient for a comprehensive evaluation. The inconsistencies in research outcomes could be attributed to various factors, including varying definitions of CP, data collection methods (e.g., self-reported cancer diagnosis or CP history), variations in study cohort characteristics, differences in study designs and statistical analysis methods, geographic variations between regions for the incidence rates of gastric cancer, chance discoveries, discrepancies in exposure assessment, and variations in the adjustment for confounding factors [10,14,18,19]. A meta-analytic study focusing solely on gastric cancer identified a stronger association between CP and stomach cancer among the Asian population (OR 1.35; 95% CI = 1.14–1.59) than the European (OR 1.30; 95% CI = 0.75–2.26) or American populations (OR 0.96; 95% CI = 0.56–1.64) [21]. This suggests that the effects of CP on gastric cancer may vary depending on the geographic region, potentially owing to differences in gastric cancer incidence rates.

However, the mechanisms linking CP to subsequent gastric cancer remain unknown. Several hypotheses, including chronic inflammation, oral bacterial translocation, immune response, and alterations in the oral and gut microbiomes, have been suggested to explain this connection [7,39,40]. First, the release of proinflammatory cytokines and inflammatory mediators from the inflamed gums of CP can lead to systemic inflammation throughout the body [7,39]. The prolonged presence of inflammatory molecules may promote cancer development and progression of gastric cancer [16]. Elevated levels of inflammatory markers, including interleukin-1 beta (IL-1β), C-reactive protein (CRP), and tumor necrosis factor-alpha (TNF-β), have been identified in CP and gastric cancer [41–44]. Second, bacteria present in the oral cavity, which are associated with CP, can potentially migrate or translocate from the mouth to the stomach [16,40]. The translocation of pathogens from the oral cavity to the stomach can stimulate an immune response, leading to sustained inflammation and consequent damage to stomach tissues [15] or the potential tumorigenesis of gastric cancer [16,40]. Certain oral bacteria, including *Streptococcus anginosus*, *Tannerella forsythia*, and *Peptostreptococcus stomatis*, have been detected in stomach cancers and are associated with an increased risk of developing gastric cancer [16]. Finally, CP can disturb the equilibrium of the oral microbiome, leading to an imbalance in the bacterial composition within the oral cavity [45]. Research indicates that modifications to the oral microbiome can affect the composition of the gut microbiome [45,46]. These alterations in the gut microbiome are associated with the development of gastrointestinal cancers [47]. Thus, it is plausible that an imbalance in the gut microbiota resulting from CP could play a role in the pathogenesis of gastric cancer [40].

The strength of this study is that the results could be drawn from a very large cohort that represents the entire Korean population. The NHIS-NSC database provides extensive access to participants' medical histories from healthcare facilities nationwide, thus improving the generalizability and accuracy of the study outcomes. Through overlap-weighted propensity score matching, we achieved a precise pairing of patients (n = 10,174) and control (n = 40,696). Although CP is more prevalent in men, the elderly, individuals with low socioeconomic status, rural residents, and those with a high CCI score [12,17,19], our study successfully achieved a balanced distribution of age, sex, income, residence, and CCI score among the participants, which effectively minimized selection bias and created study groups that closely resembled those observed in randomized clinical trials [23]. Demographic heterogeneity among participants may have influenced the magnitude of the associations observed between the original characteristics of the research groups [48].

Our study has some limitations. First, the retrospective observational design prevented us from establishing a definitive causal relationship between CP and stomach cancer. Second, our study specifically focused on the Korean population and relied on diagnosis codes from the Korean Health Insurance data, which may have led to the exclusion of unmeasured confounding variables not being accounted for and may have hindered the extrapolation of our results to other demographic groups. Finally, the NHIS-NSC database does not contain detailed information on the severity of CP, *Helicobacter pylori* infection status, stage of gastric cancer, histology, differentiation, family history, genetic data, or lifestyle factors. Therefore, the analysis conducted in this study did not account for the missing data.

5. Conclusions

This study provides the initial evidence of a potential association between CP and stomach cancer in the Korean population. Specifically, men aged <65 years with a history of CP may be at higher risk, and regular clinical screening for gastric cancer may be necessary. However, further research is necessary to validate and expand upon these findings and to investigate the mechanisms underlying this association.

Author Contributions: H.L., project administration, writing—original draft, review and editing, funding acquisition; M.J.K., investigation, funding acquisition, writing—original draft, review and editing; H.S.K. and M.-J.K., validation; N.Y.K., formal analysis; H.G.C., software and methodology. All persons designated as authors qualify for authorship, and all those who qualify for authorship are listed. All authors have read and agreed to the published version of the manuscript.

Funding: This research was funded by the National Research Foundation of Korea (NRF) grant of the Korea government (MSIT) (no. 2022R1G1A1012542 to Hyun Lim and no. 2022R1F1A1065335 to Mi Jung Kwon). The APC was funded by NRF-2022R1G1A1012542.

Institutional Review Board Statement: The study was conducted according to the guidelines of the Declaration of Helsinki and approved by the Institutional Review Board of Hallym University, Republic of Korea (protocol code 2022-10-008).

Informed Consent Statement: Patient consent was waived because all analyses used anonymous data.

Data Availability Statement: All data were obtained from the database of the National Health Insurance Sharing Service (NHISS) and are available at https://nhiss.nhis.or.kr/ (accessed 15 November 2022). The NHISS allows access to all data (downloaded from the website) for any researcher who agrees to follow the research ethics and pays a processing fee.

Conflicts of Interest: The authors declare no conflict of interest.

References

1. Jung, K.W.; Won, Y.J.; Hong, S.; Kong, H.J.; Im, J.S.; Seo, H.G. Prediction of Cancer Incidence and Mortality in Korea, 2021. *Cancer Res. Treat.* **2021**, *53*, 316–322. [CrossRef]
2. Ilic, M.; Ilic, I. Epidemiology of stomach cancer. *World J. Gastroenterol.* **2022**, *28*, 1187–1203. [CrossRef]
3. Jun, J.K.; Choi, K.S.; Lee, H.Y.; Suh, M.; Park, B.; Song, S.H.; Jung, K.W.; Lee, C.W.; Choi, I.J.; Park, E.C.; et al. Effectiveness of the Korean National Cancer Screening Program in Reducing Gastric Cancer Mortality. *Gastroenterology* **2017**, *152*, 1319–1328.e7. [CrossRef]
4. Pihlstrom, B.L.; Michalowicz, B.S.; Johnson, N.W. Periodontal diseases. *Lancet* **2005**, *366*, 1809–1820. [CrossRef]
5. Tahamtan, S.; Shirban, F.; Bagherniya, M.; Johnston, T.P.; Sahebkar, A. The effects of statins on dental and oral health: A review of preclinical and clinical studies. *J. Transl. Med.* **2020**, *18*, 155. [CrossRef]
6. Hajishengallis, G.; Korostoff, J.M. Revisiting the Page & Schroeder model: The good, the bad and the unknowns in the periodontal host response 40 years later. *Periodontol. 2000* **2017**, *75*, 116–151. [CrossRef]
7. Michaud, D.S.; Fu, Z.; Shi, J.; Chung, M. Periodontal Disease, Tooth Loss, and Cancer Risk. *Epidemiol. Rev.* **2017**, *39*, 49–58. [CrossRef]
8. Abnet, C.C.; Qiao, Y.L.; Mark, S.D.; Dong, Z.W.; Taylor, P.R.; Dawsey, S.M. Prospective study of tooth loss and incident esophageal and gastric cancers in China. *Cancer Causes Control* **2001**, *12*, 847–854. [CrossRef]
9. Abnet, C.C.; Kamangar, F.; Dawsey, S.M.; Stolzenberg-Solomon, R.Z.; Albanes, D.; Pietinen, P.; Virtamo, J.; Taylor, P.R. Tooth loss is associated with increased risk of gastric non-cardia adenocarcinoma in a cohort of Finnish smokers. *Scand. J. Gastroenterol.* **2005**, *40*, 681–687. [CrossRef]
10. Shakeri, R.; Malekzadeh, R.; Etemadi, A.; Nasrollahzadeh, D.; Abedi-Ardekani, B.; Khoshnia, M.; Islami, F.; Pourshams, A.; Pawlita, M.; Boffetta, P.; et al. Association of tooth loss and oral hygiene with risk of gastric adenocarcinoma. *Cancer Prev. Res.* **2013**, *6*, 477–482. [CrossRef]

11. Watabe, K.; Nishi, M.; Miyake, H.; Hirata, K. Lifestyle and gastric cancer: A case-control study. *Oncol. Rep.* **1998**, *5*, 1191–1194. [CrossRef] [PubMed]
12. Demirer, T.; Icli, F.; Uzunalimoglu, O.; Kucuk, O. Diet and stomach cancer incidence. A case-control study in Turkey. *Cancer* **1990**, *65*, 2344–2348. [CrossRef] [PubMed]
13. Ndegwa, N.; Ploner, A.; Liu, Z.; Roosaar, A.; Axell, T.; Ye, W. Association between poor oral health and gastric cancer: A prospective cohort study. *Int. J. Cancer* **2018**, *143*, 2281–2288. [CrossRef] [PubMed]
14. Lo, C.H.; Kwon, S.; Wang, L.; Polychronidis, G.; Knudsen, M.D.; Zhong, R.; Cao, Y.; Wu, K.; Ogino, S.; Giovannucci, E.L.; et al. Periodontal disease, tooth loss, and risk of oesophageal and gastric adenocarcinoma: A prospective study. *Gut* **2021**, *70*, 620–621. [CrossRef]
15. Lopes, C.; Almeida, T.C.; Pimentel-Nunes, P.; Dinis-Ribeiro, M.; Pereira, C. Linking dysbiosis to precancerous stomach through inflammation: Deeper than and beyond imaging. *Front. Immunol.* **2023**, *14*, 1134785. [CrossRef]
16. Coker, O.O.; Dai, Z.; Nie, Y.; Zhao, G.; Cao, L.; Nakatsu, G.; Wu, W.K.; Wong, S.H.; Chen, Z.; Sung, J.J.Y.; et al. Mucosal microbiome dysbiosis in gastric carcinogenesis. *Gut* **2018**, *67*, 1024–1032. [CrossRef]
17. Chou, S.H.; Tung, Y.C.; Wu, L.S.; Chang, C.J.; Kung, S.; Chu, P.H. Severity of chronic periodontitis and risk of gastrointestinal cancers: A population-based follow-up study from Taiwan. *Medicine* **2018**, *97*, e11386. [CrossRef]
18. Michaud, D.S.; Liu, Y.; Meyer, M.; Giovannucci, E.; Joshipura, K. Periodontal disease, tooth loss, and cancer risk in male health professionals: A prospective cohort study. *Lancet Oncol.* **2008**, *9*, 550–558. [CrossRef]
19. Hujoel, P.P.; Drangsholt, M.; Spiekerman, C.; Weiss, N.S. An exploration of the periodontitis-cancer association. *Ann. Epidemiol.* **2003**, *13*, 312–316. [CrossRef]
20. Zhang, Y.; Sun, C.; Song, E.J.; Liang, M.; Shi, T.; Min, M.; Sun, Y. Is periodontitis a risk indicator for gastrointestinal cancers? A meta-analysis of cohort studies. *J. Clin. Periodontol.* **2020**, *47*, 134–147. [CrossRef]
21. Yin, X.H.; Wang, Y.D.; Luo, H.; Zhao, K.; Huang, G.L.; Luo, S.Y.; Peng, J.X.; Song, J.K. Association between Tooth Loss and Gastric Cancer: A Meta-Analysis of Observational Studies. *PLoS ONE* **2016**, *11*, e0149653. [CrossRef]
22. Lee, J.; Lee, J.S.; Park, S.H.; Shin, S.A.; Kim, K. Cohort Profile: The National Health Insurance Service-National Sample Cohort (NHIS-NSC), South Korea. *Int. J. Epidemiol.* **2017**, *46*, e15. [CrossRef] [PubMed]
23. Song, J.W.; Chung, K.C. Observational studies: Cohort and case-control studies. *Plast. Reconstr. Surg.* **2010**, *126*, 2234–2242. [CrossRef] [PubMed]
24. Kwon, M.J.; Kim, J.H.; Kang, H.S.; Lim, H.; Kim, M.J.; Kim, N.Y.; Kim, S.H.; Choi, H.G.; Kim, E.S. Possible Incidental Parkinson's Disease following Asthma: A Nested Case-Control Study in Korea. *J. Pers. Med.* **2023**, *13*, 718. [CrossRef]
25. Kwon, M.J.; Kang, H.S.; Kim, J.H.; Kim, J.H.; Kim, S.H.; Kim, N.Y.; Nam, E.S.; Min, K.W.; Choi, H.G. Association between Statin Use and Gastric Cancer: A Nested Case-Control Study Using a National Health Screening Cohort in Korea. *Pharmaceuticals* **2021**, *14*, 1283. [CrossRef]
26. Kwon, M.J.; Byun, S.H.; Kim, J.H.; Kim, J.H.; Kim, S.H.; Kim, N.Y.; Park, H.R.; Choi, H.G. Longitudinal follow-up study of the association between statin use and chronic periodontitis using national health screening cohort of Korean population. *Sci. Rep.* **2022**, *12*, 5504. [CrossRef]
27. Quan, H.; Sundararajan, V.; Halfon, P.; Fong, A.; Burnand, B.; Luthi, J.-C.; Saunders, L.D.; Beck, C.A.; Feasby, T.E.; Ghali, W.A. Coding algorithms for defining comorbidities in ICD-9-CM and ICD-10 administrative data. *Med. Care* **2005**, *43*, 1130–1139. [CrossRef] [PubMed]
28. Quan, H.; Li, B.; Couris, C.; Fushimi, K.; Graham, P.; Hider, P.; Januel, J.; Sundararajan, V. Practice of epidemiology: Updating and validating the Charlson comorbidity index and score for risk adjustment in hospital discharge abstracts using data from 6 countries. *Am. J. Epidemiol.* **2011**, *173*, 676–682. [CrossRef] [PubMed]
29. Austin, P.C. Balance diagnostics for comparing the distribution of baseline covariates between treatment groups in propensity-score matched samples. *Stat. Med.* **2009**, *28*, 3083–3107. [CrossRef]
30. Li, F.; Thomas, L.E.; Li, F. Addressing Extreme Propensity Scores via the Overlap Weights. *Am. J. Epidemiol.* **2019**, *188*, 250–257. [CrossRef]
31. Thomas, L.E.; Li, F.; Pencina, M.J. Overlap Weighting: A Propensity Score Method That Mimics Attributes of a Randomized Clinical Trial. *JAMA* **2020**, *323*, 2417–2418. [CrossRef]
32. Li, F.; Morgan, K.L.; Zaslavsky, A.M. Balancing Covariates via Propensity Score Weighting. *J. Am. Stat. Assoc.* **2018**, *113*, 390–400. [CrossRef]
33. Eke, P.I.; Dye, B.A.; Wei, L.; Slade, G.D.; Thornton-Evans, G.O.; Borgnakke, W.S.; Taylor, G.W.; Page, R.C.; Beck, J.D.; Genco, R.J. Update on Prevalence of Periodontitis in Adults in the United States: NHANES 2009 to 2012. *J. Periodontol.* **2015**, *86*, 611–622. [CrossRef]
34. Borrell, L.N.; Crawford, N.D. Socioeconomic position indicators and periodontitis: Examining the evidence. *Periodontol. 2000* **2012**, *58*, 69–83. [CrossRef] [PubMed]
35. Li, A.; Vermaire, J.H.; Chen, Y.; van der Sluis, L.W.M.; Thomas, R.Z.; Tjakkes, G.E.; Schuller, A.A. Trends in socioeconomic inequality of periodontal health status among Dutch adults: A repeated cross-sectional analysis over two decades. *BMC Oral. Health* **2021**, *21*, 346. [CrossRef]
36. Sarkar, S.; Dauer, M.J.; In, H. Socioeconomic Disparities in Gastric Cancer and Identification of a Single SES Variable for Predicting Risk. *J. Gastrointest. Cancer* **2022**, *53*, 170–178. [CrossRef] [PubMed]

37. Wu, C.C.; Hsu, T.W.; Chang, C.M.; Yu, C.H.; Wang, Y.F.; Lee, C.C. The effect of individual and neighborhood socioeconomic status on gastric cancer survival. *PLoS ONE* **2014**, *9*, e89655. [CrossRef] [PubMed]
38. Hiraki, A.; Matsuo, K.; Suzuki, T.; Kawase, T.; Tajima, K. Teeth loss and risk of cancer at 14 common sites in Japanese. *Cancer Epidemiol. Biomark. Prev.* **2008**, *17*, 1222–1227. [CrossRef]
39. Vanoli, A.; Parente, P.; Fassan, M.; Mastracci, L.; Grillo, F. Gut inflammation and tumorigenesis: Every site has a different tale to tell. *Intern. Emerg. Med.* **2023**. [CrossRef] [PubMed]
40. Sun, J.; Zhou, M.; Salazar, C.R.; Hays, R.; Bedi, S.; Chen, Y.; Li, Y. Chronic Periodontal Disease, Periodontal Pathogen Colonization, and Increased Risk of Precancerous Gastric Lesions. *J. Periodontol.* **2017**, *88*, 1124–1134. [CrossRef]
41. Kim, M.R.; Kim, A.S.; Choi, H.I.; Jung, J.H.; Park, J.Y.; Ko, H.J. Inflammatory markers for predicting overall survival in gastric cancer patients: A systematic review and meta-analysis. *PLoS ONE* **2020**, *15*, e0236445. [CrossRef] [PubMed]
42. Rodrigues, W.F.; Miguel, C.B.; Lazo-Chica, J.E.; Trindade da Silva, C.A.; Vieira, C.U.; Clemente-Napimoga, J.T.; Freire Oliveira, C.J.; Napimoga, M.H. Interleukin-6, tumor necrosis factor-alpha, C-reactive protein, and hematological parameters in experimental periodontal disease after beta-adrenergic blockade. *J. Indian Soc. Periodontol.* **2019**, *23*, 511–516. [CrossRef] [PubMed]
43. Yin, S.; Lan, C.; Pei, H.; Zhu, Z. Expression of interleukin 1beta in gastric cancer tissue and its effects on gastric cancer. *OncoTargets Ther.* **2016**, *9*, 31–35. [CrossRef] [PubMed]
44. Saremi, L.; Shafizadeh, M.; Esmaeilzadeh, E.; Ghaffari, M.E.; Mahdavi, M.H.; Amid, R.; Kadkhodazadeh, M. Assessment of IL-10, IL-1ss and TNF-alpha gene polymorphisms in patients with peri-implantitis and healthy controls. *Mol. Biol. Rep.* **2021**, *48*, 2285–2290. [CrossRef]
45. Bao, J.; Li, L.; Zhang, Y.; Wang, M.; Chen, F.; Ge, S.; Chen, B.; Yan, F. Periodontitis may induce gut microbiota dysbiosis via salivary microbiota. *Int. J. Oral. Sci.* **2022**, *14*, 32. [CrossRef]
46. Kunath, B.J.; Hickl, O.; Queiros, P.; Martin-Gallausiaux, C.; Lebrun, L.A.; Halder, R.; Laczny, C.C.; Schmidt, T.S.B.; Hayward, M.R.; Becher, D.; et al. Alterations of oral microbiota and impact on the gut microbiome in type 1 diabetes mellitus revealed by integrated multi-omic analyses. *Microbiome* **2022**, *10*, 243. [CrossRef]
47. Li, J.; Zhang, A.H.; Wu, F.F.; Wang, X.J. Alterations in the Gut Microbiota and Their Metabolites in Colorectal Cancer: Recent Progress and Future Prospects. *Front. Oncol.* **2022**, *12*, 841552. [CrossRef]
48. Kendall, B.E.; Fox, G.A.; Fujiwara, M.; Nogeire, T.M. Demographic heterogeneity, cohort selection, and population growth. *Ecology* **2011**, *92*, 1985–1993. [CrossRef]

cancers

MDPI

Article

Vessel Delineation Using U-Net: A Sparse Labeled Deep Learning Approach for Semantic Segmentation of Histological Images

Lukas Glänzer [1], Husam E. Masalkhi [1], Anjali A. Roeth [2,3], Thomas Schmitz-Rode [1] and Ioana Slabu [1,*]

[1] Institute of Applied Medical Engineering, Helmholtz Institute, Medical Faculty, RWTH Aachen University, Pauwelsstraße 20, 52074 Aachen, Germany; glaenzer@ame.rwth-aachen.de (L.G.); husam.masalkhi@rwth-aachen.de (H.E.M.); smiro@ame.rwth-aachen.de (T.S.-R.)

[2] Department of Visceral and Transplantation Surgery, University Hospital RWTH Aachen, Pauwelsstrasse 30, 52074 Aachen, Germany; aroeth@ukaachen.de

[3] Department of Surgery, Maastricht University, P. Debyelaan 25, 6229 Maastricht, The Netherlands

* Correspondence: slabu@ame.rwth-aachen.de; Tel.: +49-2418-089-102

Simple Summary: In our study, we aimed to create an accurate segmentation algorithm of blood vessels within histologically stained tumor tissue using deep learning. Blood vessels are crucial for supplying nutrients to tumor cells, and accurately identifying them is essential for understanding tumor development and designing effective treatments. We conducted a comprehensive investigation by comparing various deep learning architectural methods. Additionally, we reduced the time spent for data annotation and introduced a sparse labeling technique, by which only a limited amount of data was labeled for training the model. We showed that U-Net with a combination of attention gates and residual links yielded the highest precision and accuracy compared to other tested architectures. This demonstrates that our approach, even with sparse labeling, can effectively identify blood vessels and provide accurate segmentation within tumor tissue. These findings are promising for improving our understanding of tumor vasculature and potentially contributing to improved treatment strategies.

Abstract: Semantic segmentation is an important imaging analysis method enabling the identification of tissue structures. Histological image segmentation is particularly challenging, having large structural information while providing only limited training data. Additionally, labeling these structures to generate training data is time consuming. Here, we demonstrate the feasibility of a semantic segmentation using U-Net with a novel sparse labeling technique. The basic U-Net architecture was extended by attention gates, residual and recurrent links, and dropout regularization. To overcome the high class imbalance, which is intrinsic to histological data, under- and oversampling and data augmentation were used. In an ablation study, various architectures were evaluated, and the best performing model was identified. This model contains attention gates, residual links, and a dropout regularization of 0.125. The segmented images show accurate delineations of the vascular structures (with a precision of 0.9088 and an AUC-ROC score of 0.9717), and the segmentation algorithm is robust to images containing staining variations and damaged tissue. These results demonstrate the feasibility of sparse labeling in combination with the modified U-Net architecture.

Keywords: deep learning; semantic segmentation; U-Net; histological images

1. Introduction

Deep learning is the leading artificial intelligence (AI) method for a wide range of tasks, including medical imaging problems. It is the state of the art for several computer vision tasks and has been used for medical imaging tasks, like the classification of Alzheimer's, lung cancer detection, retinal disease detection, detection of abnormalities in modalities, like MRI, CT, X-ray, or ultrasound, and semantic segmentation of medical images [1,2].

Deep learning techniques have been used in the analysis of medical images in computer-assisted imaging contexts and offer a variety of solutions and improvements in the analysis of these images supporting radiologists and other specialists at diagnosis [3–6].

Semantic segmentation of vascular structures in histological images plays a pivotal role in various biomedical research fields and holds significant importance in advancing the understanding of complex biological systems. The intricate network of blood vessels is fundamental for tissue development and maintenance, as it facilitates the perfusion of nutrients and oxygen to cells. Accurately delineating and analyzing vascular structures are of paramount importance for the design and development of 3D in vitro systems that mimic the physiological conditions of human tissues [7–10].

In the field of image processing, the analysis of stained tissues to extract the information on vascular structures presents a formidable challenge due to the vast amount of data generated by high-resolution imaging techniques [11]. Additionally, vascular structures have to be segmented within in an ambiguous and heterogeneous tissue environment. Manual segmentation of vascular structures is labor-intensive, time-consuming, and prone to inter-observer variability [12].

The need for automated and reliable segmentation algorithms is paramount to unlock the full potential of these large-scale datasets. Semantic segmentation techniques, particularly employing deep learning approaches, like U-Net [13], have demonstrated their capability in efficiently and accurately segmenting vascular structures from stained tissue images [14]. Such approaches enable handling "big data", extracting valuable information from complex tissue samples, and advancing the understanding of disease processes [9], but there are several challenges that must be addressed, like limited data availability, overfitting of the network, or a high class imbalance in the training data. To overcome these challenges, this work uses a deep learning approach based on U-Net with sparsely labeled training data (see architecture in Figure 1).

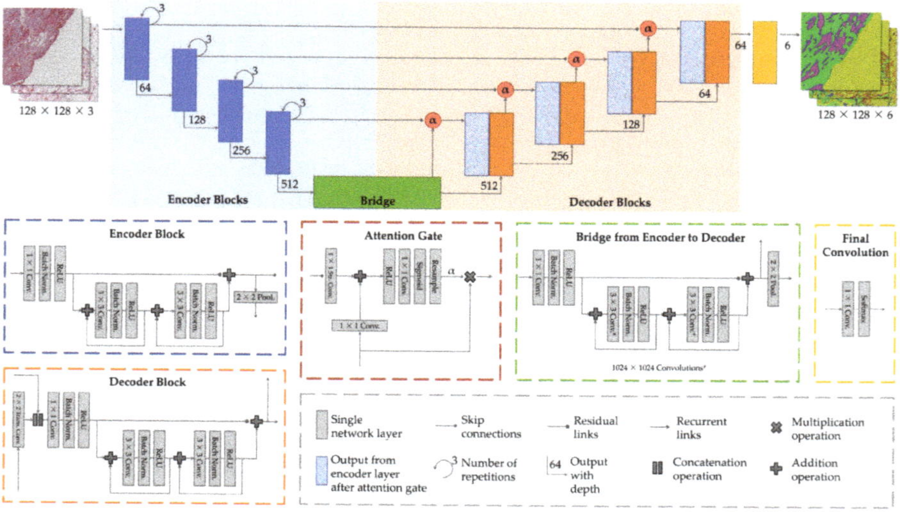

Figure 1. The network architecture. The network is based on the U-Net architecture, i.e., a four-level encoder/decoder convolutional network extended by attention gates, residual links, and recurrent blocks. The network segments six classes in histological tumor images. Arbitrary images can be handled by cutting them in patches with sizes of 128 px × 128 px × 3 (RBG color-coded), and after processing, stitching them back together to the original image. Details on the individual network architecture elements are given in the lower boxes. Their individual functionality is depicted within the main text (Section 2.3).

Numerous applications can be identified, for which sophisticated semantic segmentation of vascular structures becomes vital. Notably, the development of 3D in vitro systems heavily relies on a comprehensive understanding of vasculature. These systems aim to mimic the intricate vascular architecture necessary for sustained cellular growth and function. Semantic segmentation of histological images enables the precise mapping of vascular networks within engineered tissues [15], aiding in the design and implementation of artificial perfusion to provide nutrients and oxygen to cells [16], thereby promoting their growth and viability. By replicating the intricate architecture of blood vessels, these systems can facilitate the perfusion of nutrients and efficient delivery of oxygen, closely resembling the conditions found in natural tissues. Another application is drug testing and development. Correctly delineating vascular structures in histology images aids in the development of 3D in vitro systems for drug testing [17,18]. By incorporating vascular networks into these systems, interactions of the therapeutic agents with blood vessels, drug efficacy, and potential side effects can be assessed [19]. This information is valuable for predicting drug behavior in the human body [20] and improving the accuracy of preclinical testing, ultimately leading to the development of safer and more effective treatments.

Image segmentation in general is an important task in computer vision, with applications in a variety of fields, including medical imaging and its analysis and processing, e.g., in computer-guided therapy and diagnostics, including:

1. Organ Segmentation: Segmentation of various organs in medical images, such as liver, kidney, pancreas, gall bladder, and lung [21–23]. This provides important support for diagnosing, surgical planning, and disease monitoring. However, these methods are based on CT or MRI data and are focused on localization of a target structure not on a precise segmentation [23].
2. Cell Segmentation: Segmentation of various cell types in microscopy images [24], such as detection of metastases in histopathology images [25], segmentation of cells' nuclei [26,27], and segmentation of blood cells in microscopic images [28,29]. These methods are focused on localization rather than on an accurate segmentation and are applied to very homogeneous images.
3. Tumor Segmentation: Tumor segmentation in different types of medical images, such as ultrasound [30], computed tomography (CT) [31–35], and magnetic resonance imaging (MRI) scans [36,37]. Accurate segmentation of tumors is crucial for diagnosing, treatment planning, and monitoring of cancer patients. Conventionally, the image types for tumor segmentation are gained from ultrasound, CT, and MRI, showing characteristics that cannot directly be transferred to histological images.
4. Vessel Segmentation: Segmentation of blood vessels in various medical images, such as magnetic resonance angiography (MRA) scans [38], retinal images [39–41], and brain scans [42], which is important for the diagnosis and treatment of various diseases, such as diabetic retinopathy and stroke. Vessel segmentation is applied to various image modalities, yet the vessels are mostly homogeneous in structure. Typically, segmented images express two classes. Thus, for histological images, a scalable multiclass model that can be extended to classes specific to the desired application must be built.

Convolutional neural networks (CNNs) have shown remarkable success in image segmentation tasks, with the U-Net architecture being one of the most popular and effective CNN models for this task [14]. The U-Net architecture by Ronneberger et al. [13] is a U-shaped network that consists of an encoder and a decoder network connected by skip connections. The encoder network is a traditional CNN that consists of multiple convolutional and pooling layers. The decoder network is also a CNN, using transposed convolutions (also known as deconvolutions) to upsample the feature maps produced by the encoder network. One of the key features of the U-Net architecture is the use of skip connections between the encoder and decoder networks. These connections allow the decoder to access information from earlier layers of the encoder, which helps to preserve spatial information and leads to better segmentation results.

The focus of this work lies on the semantic segmentation with U-Net-based neural networks of blood vessels from histological human pancreatic tumor images. Pancreatic ductal adenocarcinoma is a type of cancer with limited treatment options due to its chemotherapy resistance [43]. Thus, new therapeutic options are required. Based on a dataset labeled with a novel sparse labelling technique, a set of 169 histological tumor images is fully segmented into six classes, two of which identify the vessels of the underlying tumor. Such data will provide valuable insights into tumor vascularization and angiogenesis and, furthermore, allow for in vitro and in silico analysis of tumor development and maintenance. U-Net has shown great promise for analyzing biomedical data [14]. Thus, to handle the described challenges, in addition to the original U-Net, this work incorporates attention mechanisms, dropout during the training to be more robust to the heterogenic data, a multiclass harmonic mean loss function, as well as data augmentation and under-/oversampling to resolve class imbalance. The semantic segmentation method is applied to histological tumor images. The modified U-Net architecture is discussed, and the results of the segmentation are evaluated using various metrics demonstrating precision of the segmentation results and thus its suitability for various applications.

All in all, this work introduces a deep neural network architecture that can segment histological images very precisely and thus enables various applications in the field of 3D in vitro systems in the generation of which detailed tissue structures are required. Additionally, a novel labeling technique that enables data annotation for segmentations of medical images within strongly reduced time and effort is introduced.

2. Materials and Methods

2.1. Sample Acquisition

With informed consent of the patient and permission of the local IRB (EK206/09), a specimen, a human pancreatic ductal adenocarcinoma, was resected and fixed in a 3.5% formaldehyde solution (Otto-Fischar GmbH, Saarbrücken, Germany), then embedded in paraffin wax, and sliced into 169 sections using a microtome (HM 340 E, Thermo Fisher Scientific Inc., Waltham, MA, USA) at a thickness of 2.5 μm per slice. These slices were then placed manually onto slides (Starforst, Engelbrecht Medizin- und Labortechnik, Edermünde, Germany) and dried overnight at 56 °C. Subsequently, the sections were stained with the "von Willebrandt factor" antibody (DakoCytomation, Glostrup, Denmark) using the ZytoChem Plus AP Polymer System (Mouse/Rabbit) (Zytomed Systems, Berlin, Germany) and Hematoxylin (Zytomed Systems, Berlin, Germany) and then covered with Vitro-Clud (R. Langenbrinck GmbH, Emmendingen, Germany). The slide images were digitalized using a microscope (Axio Imager.Z2, Carl Zeiss Microscopy Deutschland GmbH, Oberkochen, Germany) and cropped to a size of 13,020 × 10,422 px^2, resulting in images with a pixel size of 0.5 μm.

2.2. Data Preparation

To reduce the network's complexity, i.e., the number of trained parameters, the network's input layer was limited to images with a size of 128 px × 128 px. To handle arbitrary image resolutions, images were cut into patches, which were processed independently and were re-aligned after processing and stitched back together. For the training, 7500 patches were randomly selected from the images and manually labeled.

All further preprocessing, the training steps were performed on these patches. For training, the patches were split into fractions of 60-20-20 for the training set, test set, and validation set, respectively. Data splitting is a fundamental step in machine learning model development, involving the division of data into training, validation, and test sets [44]. The training set is used to train the model by optimizing its parameters through iterative learning. The validation set serves as an independent subset for tuning hyperparameters and assessing the model performance during training. It aids in making informed decisions on model architecture and hyperparameter settings. Finally, the test set, which remains unseen during development, provides an unbiased evaluation of the model's performance on real-world data. By using separate datasets, this data splitting strategy enables the prevention of overfitting, the assessment of generalization capabilities, and fair comparisons with other models or benchmarks.

To obtain reliable training data, there were many challenges that are especially prominent for deep learning applications in medical imaging. One major challenge was limited data availability, as only 169 slices from a single tumor were available, which makes it difficult to train deep learning models effectively. Another challenge was noisy and heterogeneous image data. In combination with limited data, this makes it challenging to train more universal models applicable to similar image data, as potentially many variations in image characteristics are not present in the training data. Class imbalance, i.e., the underrepresentation of important classes, is also a common issue in biomedical datasets [45] and was very prominent in the histological images introducing difficulties in-training models that can accurately classify all classes, e.g., pixels with very different characteristics belonging to the same class or vice versa. Lastly, a big challenge in deep learning was the need for large amounts of labeled data, which is time-consuming and expensive to obtain.

To cope with the abovementioned challenge of limited data, class imbalance, and labeling times, extensions to U-Net were incorporated, and a novel labeling technique was used. As vessels can take complex forms and are not homogeneous in their appearance, a distinction between vessel lumen and vessel wall was made. The remaining parts of the images were further subdivided into background, tissue, destroyed or corrupted tissue, and debris. Examples for each of those classes are shown in Figure 2b–g. Looking at the whole image slide in Figure 2a, the classes' background and tissue are highly overrepresented, whereas the other classes, including the most relevant vessel lumen and vessel wall, are underrepresented leading to a high class imbalance. To counteract this imbalance, the overrepresented classes (background and tissue) were undersampled in labeling, and the classes' vessel lumen and vessel wall were oversampled. Oversampling minority classes and undersampling majority classes are the best approaches to tackle class imbalance [46]. Both oversampling and undersampling were performed manually during labeling. Throughout testing, misclassified structures were identified, i.e., positive and negative hard mining [47,48], and added to the labeling to increase performance. This typically results in a patch as shown in Figure 3a. The labels in the exemplary patch show the sparse labeling used for the segmentation training. The classes' vessel wall (dark purple) and vessel lumen (light purple) were extensively labeled, i.e., almost all pixels belonging to these classes were labeled for training. In contrary, the classes tissue (light green) and background (yellow) were highly undersampled. For this patch, this leads to a nearly equal label distribution for each class. During the manual labeling, there were intrinsic properties of the data that needed to be clearly identifiable by the network:

1. Vessel walls are fine but continuous structures: Walls are always labeled completely, indicating that there are no gaps, even with low image intensity.
2. Vessel lumens are separated from the tissue by a vessel wall: Vessel lumens are also labeled by drawing a line on the inside of the enclosing wall. Also, a line on the outside of the wall as tissue is labeled to indicate the separation from tissue and lumen by a wall. The remaining lumen is labeled by lines crossing the whole area of the lumen.
3. Remaining blood cells within the vessel lumen should be labeled as lumen: The labeled lines within the lumen go across the remaining cells to identify them as part of the lumen.
4. The tissue is a large continuous structure making up most part of the image: Tissue is labeled by long lines across the heterogeneous areas of tissue. These lines indicate its continuousness and penalize frequent changes in the segmentation.
5. The background is also large and continuous and located at the images' edges: The background is also labeled with long lines across its area. A separating line at the tissue border indicates the transition from tissue to background.

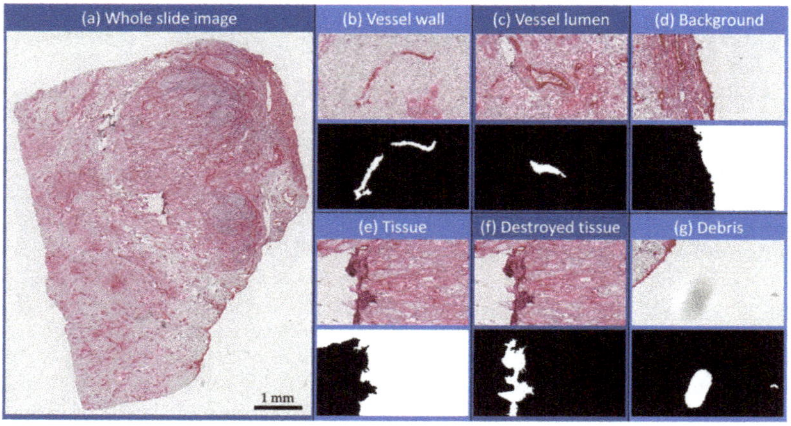

Figure 2. Input image and examples for each chosen class classification with an original excerpt on the top and the segmentation in black and white below. White shows the segmented regions of the respective classes, whereas black includes all other classes: (**a**) an exemplary whole-slide histological image with stained vessels; (**b**) two-vessel walls from elongated vessels; (**c**) vessel lumen with cells; (**d**) background; (**e**) intact tumor tissue; (**f**) corrupted/destroyed tissue; (**g**) debris on the slide (can also be occluded tissue). These examples show clearly that the segmented classes are very heterogeneous and not always distinguishable from one another without spatial localization.

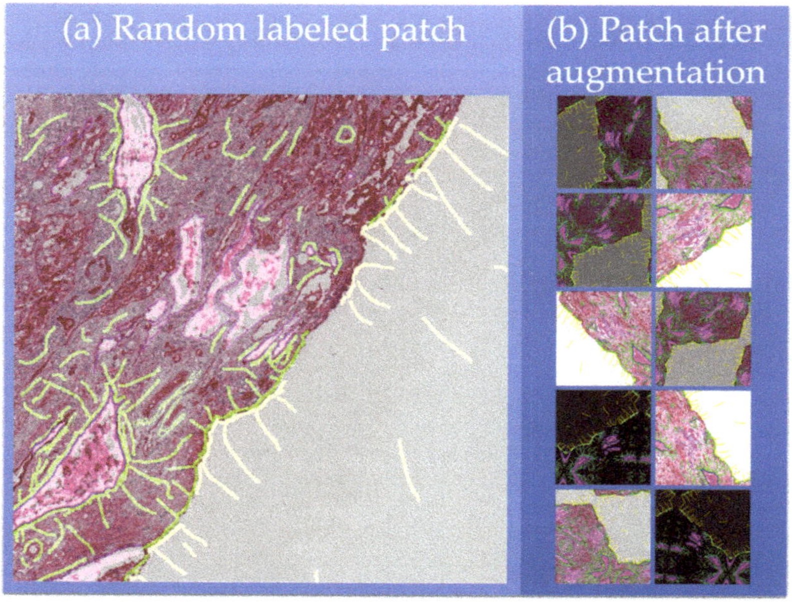

Figure 3. (**a**) Typical patch with sparse labeling and (**b**) patch after applying 10 different random augmentations with random contrast, brightness, zoom, rotation, and flip. When zooming or rotating, empty image parts are filled by mirroring, and the result is cropped to the original size of 128 px × 128 px. Each class is color-coded. Vessel walls: dark purple; vessel lumen: light purple; tissue: light green; background: yellow.

These properties highlight the difficulties of segmenting vascular structures in a heterogeneous tissue environment and give indications on what aspects should be included during labeling.

As a final measure to handle class imbalance and lack of data, extensive data augmentation was applied to the training patches, which helped to increase the size of image datasets and improve model performance. U-Net's architecture is particularly well-suited for data augmentation [13] because the skip connections allow for the incorporation of small image patches into the model without losing spatial resolution. This can help to address the challenge of limited data availability, as more training examples can be generated by applying transformations, such as rotations, flips, and zooms, to the original images [25,49]. This can improve the model's applicability to similar data and its sensitivity to detect subtle features that may be missed by other architectures. Each patch was randomly augmented 10 times within the following parameter ranges:

1. Contrast: random increase or decrease in contrast by up to 90%;
2. Brightness: random increase or decrease in the brightness by up to 30%;
3. Zoom: random scaling between 50% and 200% of the original size, where x and y directions are scaled independently;
4. Rotation: random angle between -90° and 90°;
5. Flipping: no flipping, horizontal or vertical flipping.

Contrast and brightness are typical variations due to inhomogeneous staining of the tissue during preparation. Varying these aids the network in learning features that are invariant to contrast and brightness, such as vessel shapes or tissue borders. Zoom, rotation, and flipping additionally create more variation in the dataset counteracting the sparse data by introducing more feature variations. Figure 3b shows augmentations of an exemplary patch. Due to this manifold augmentation, the network becomes more robust when segmenting new images as more variations are seen during training than are in the labeled data. The 10 augmentations per patch lead to a total of 45000 training patches.

2.3. *Network Architecture*

The segmentation network is based on the original U-Net architecture introduced by Ronneberger et al. [13]. The U-Net architecture consists of an encoder network (Figure 1, blue), a bridge (Figure 1, green), and a decoder network (Figure 1, orange). The encoder network consists of a series of convolutional layers that progressively downsample the input image and extract high-level features. The output of the encoder network is a set of feature maps that represent the high-level features of the input image. The bridge connects the encoder network to the decoder network and typically consists of a single or double convolutional layer. The decoder network consists of a series of deconvolutional layers that upsample the feature maps to produce the final segmentation map. The decoder network is also characterized by its skip connections, which concatenate the feature maps from the encoder network with the upsampled feature maps from the decoder network. These skip connections allow the decoder network to recover spatial information from the encoder network and improve the segmentation performance. To improve the semantic segmentation of histological images, several extensions were considered that have proven effective when dealing with medical images.

2.3.1. Attention Gates

Incorporating attention gates in the network provides the ability to selectively focus on regions of interest in the image [50,51]. The advantage of attention gates lies in their ability to assign different weights to different regions of the image based on their importance in the segmentation task [52] and thus aid in counteracting class imbalance. Attention gates also improve the model's ability to handle complex images with high levels of noise, blur, or low contrast [14]. The application of attention gates in medical image segmentation has been shown to improve the segmentation accuracy by focusing the network's attention on the most informative regions of the image [23,35,51,52]. Here, attention gates allow overweighting more complex classes, i.e., the fine-structured vessel wall and vessel lumen or the heterogeneous tissue, compared to a simple one, like the homogeneous background in the image (see Figure 1, dashed red box).

2.3.2. Recurrent Links

Recurrent links allow the model to propagate information across the frames and capture the temporal dependencies between them [53]. The use of recurrent links in the network enables the incorporation of temporal information into the segmentation task. This is particularly useful in the case of histological images, where the segmentation over time of the vascular structures is an essential aspect of the segmentation task. Especially for the segmentation of histological images, recurrent links have proven useful and are widely incorporated in modern architectures [26,37,54–56]. As shown in Figure 4, each convolutional unit (3×3 convolution, batch normalization, activation) is extended to form a recurrent unit and can be repeated three times following the recurrent link.

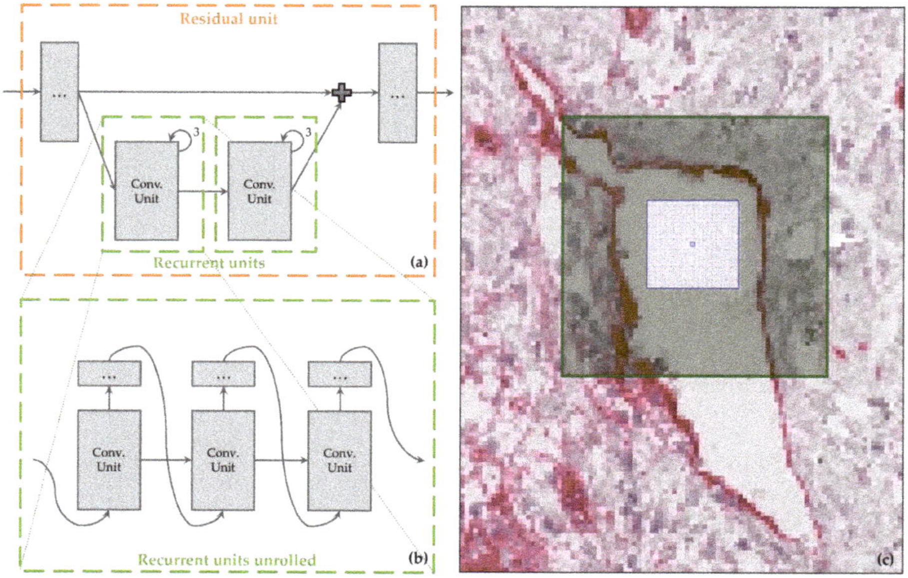

Figure 4. (**a**) The residual units bypass the two recurrent units in their encoder/decoder level (cf. Figure 1 for definition of symbols). (**b**) Unrolling the three-fold recurrent units visualizes the stacking of convolutions (conv.) and their effect on the receptive field. (c) Considering the blue pixel in the center, without recurrence, the networks receptive field corresponds to the blue grid of size 21 px $\times$ 21 px. Using recurrence increases the receptive field to the green area of size 61 px $\times$ 61 px, giving more spatial context to the convolutions.

The main purpose of recurrent links is capturing temporal dependencies; however, as a side effect of stacking 3×3 convolutions, the receptive field is also increased enabling the detection of larger structures. This becomes important when the network needs to distinguish a large vessel lumen from background. Using the formulas introduced by Araujo et al. [57], the receptive field for a pixel in the output layer can be computed as

$$r_0 = \sum_{l=0}^{L} \left((k_l - 1) \prod_{i=1}^{l-1} s_i \right) + 1 \quad (1)$$

where r_0 stands for the receptive field in level 0 of the network, L for the total number of layers, k_l for the kernel size used in layer l, and s_i for the stride used in level i. Using

(1) without recurrence, the receptive field of the blue pixel (Figure 4c) in the center is highlighted by the blue grid of size 21 px × 21 px. It can be observed that for the given pixel, the network has no spatial information to distinguish between background and vessel lumen. Introducing recurrence, the receptive field becomes larger, i.e., 61 px × 61 px, highlighted by the green square. The network now has far more spatial information and can more easily distinguish between the background and a lumen.

2.3.3. Residual Links

The addition of residual links in the network preserves low-level (i.e., small-scale) features by allowing the network to bypass certain layers and propagate information directly from the input to the output [58]. So, similar to the skip connections where information from one encoder layer is passed directly to the corresponding layer in the decoder to preserve spatial information, the data are passed down/up to lower/higher layers (cf. Figure 1). This can be useful in medical image segmentation tasks, where small details, i.e., vascular structures, can be crucial in the future application. Additionally, residual links can prevent vanishing gradients, a common problem in deep learning networks with many layers, which may lead to a stop in a network's learning after a certain number of layers [58]. Residual links have been shown to improve the segmentation performance in various medical image segmentation tasks [37,59–61], usually in combination with the other mechanisms (attention gates, recurrent links) incorporated here. In the implementation, each encoder/decoder block has one residual unit bypassing both its recurrent units (see Figure 4).

2.3.4. Loss Function

A loss function is a crucial component in training a neural network as it quantifies the error between predicted and true values. In the case of segmenting histological images, a loss function that emphasizes accurate boundary prediction is necessary due to the complex and irregular shapes of the vascular structures. U-Net can be extended by a weighted loss function [62,63] to address class imbalance by using class weighting or by oversampling under-represented classes during training [46,64,65]. This can help to ensure that the model is able to accurately classify all classes, even those that are less frequent in the training data. Two of the most commonly used error metrics are precision and recall [66]. Precision (PREC, Equation (2)) describes the fraction of correctly identified pixels among all pixels predicted for that class, whereas recall (RECL, Equation (3)) is the fraction of correctly identified pixels among all pixels labeled for that class:

$$PREC = \frac{TP + \sigma}{TP + FP + \sigma} \tag{2}$$

$$RECL = \frac{TP + \sigma}{TP + FN + \sigma} \tag{3}$$

Here, TP stands for true positive, i.e., all correctly predicted pixels, FP (false positive) for all pixels from another class predicted to be in the considered class, and FN (false negative) for all pixels of the considered class predicted to be in another class. σ is a smoothing operator for numerical stability. Combining both metrics with a harmonic mean yields the typically used F1 score or Dice score [54]:

$$DICE = \frac{2 + \sigma}{\frac{1}{PREC} + \frac{1}{RECL} + \sigma} = \frac{2TP + \sigma}{2TP + FP + FN + \sigma}. \tag{4}$$

As this work proposes a multiclass segmentation network, the loss function evaluates the Dice score for each of the six classes separately, combines them by a harmonic mean and turns the score into a loss. A harmonic mean is very sensitive to variations in each of its values, so as a loss function, it penalizes unprecise segmentations and misclassifications and forces the network to minimize the classification error on all classes, which is needed here due to a high class imbalance. So, for each class $c \in C$ where C is the set of the defined six classes, the total loss of the network can then be calculated using

$$L = 1 - \frac{|C|}{\sum_{c \in C} \left(\frac{1}{PREC_c} + \frac{1}{RECL_c} + \frac{1}{DICE_c} \right)} \quad (5)$$

thus, combining all individual class scores and normalizing the loss to the range [0, 1].

In addition to the metrics precision, recall, and Dice, a fourth metric called specificity [66] (also called inverse recall) is measured. The specificity gives the true negative (TN) rate, i.e., the fraction of correctly identified pixels among all pixels labeled as not belonging to that class and is defined as

$$SPEC = \frac{TN + \sigma}{TN + FP + \sigma} \quad (6)$$

The specificity is not part of the loss function but is used as an evaluation metric.

2.3.5. Hyperparameters

Hyperparameters determine the behavior of the training algorithm and directly affect the performance of the model. Performing a grid search on hyperparameters is essential, regarding the defined loss function, to identify the optimal configuration of hyperparameters for a deep learning network.

In the proposed deep learning network, a grid search on five hyperparameters was performed: batch size, dropout, learning rate and the activation of attention gates, residual links, and recurrent links. For the batch size, 1, 2, 4, 8, 16, and 32 were tested. For the dropout, four values, i.e., 0, 0.125, 0.25, and 0.375, were tested. For the learning rate, 1×10^{-2}, 1×10^{-3}, and 1×10^{-4} were tested. Additionally, the activation of attention gates, residual links, and recurrent links were tested as binary options. All combinations of these hyperparameters were assessed using a training and validation set, and the optimal configuration of hyperparameters was selected based on the performance metrics on the validation set. The optimal hyperparameters according to multiple runs of this grid search were identified as:

- Batch size: 16 (for all architectures);
- Dropout: 0.25 (for Recurrent U-Net) and 0.125 (for all other architectures);
- Learning rate: 1×10^{-4} (for all architectures).

The implementation uses a dynamic learning rate approach for the deep learning model. Specifically, the initial learning rate is set to 1×10^{-4}, according to the grid search, but instead of using a fixed learning rate throughout the training process, it is reduced by a factor of 0.1 whenever the loss of the network plateaued for 10 epochs. This approach allowed fine-tuning the learning rate as the model learned more about the data and prevented the model from getting stuck in sub-optimal local minima. Additionally, early stopping was employed to further prevent overfitting of the model. After four consecutive plateaus in the loss, the training process was stopped, with a maximum of 300 epochs.

The use of dropout regularization in the network also prevents overfitting by randomly dropping out a fraction of the layer outputs during training, thus, forcing the network to learn more robust features. Dropout regularization prevents the network from memorizing the training data and improves the generalization performance of the model [67,68]. After each encoder and decoder block, the respective dropout is applied.

2.4. *Used Software and Hardware*

For the development of the network, the open-source TensorFlow library and Keras library together with TensorBoard for evaluation and visualization of the network's performance were used [69,70]. The evaluation graphs were created with matplotlib [71].

Data labeling was performed manually with the Medical Image Labeler from MATLAB's Medical Imaging Toolbox™ (The MathWorks, Inc., Natick, MA, USA).

For training, all computations were performed with computing resources granted by RWTH Aachen University. The RWTH Aachen University High Performance Cluster (RWTH Aachen University, Aachen, NRW, Germany) provides access to computational nodes with access to 2 GPU-cards of type V100-SXM2.

3. Results

In this section, results of a quantitative analysis of an ablation study are presented, giving an overview of the network's performance. The common coefficients Dice, precision, recall/sensitivity, and specificity are used for evaluation. In the ablation study, each of the added architectural mechanisms, namely attention gates, residual links, and recurrent links, are tested individually and in combination. Additionally, the number of training parameters are listed for further comparison among the different models. Furthermore, to assess the segmentation separately for each class, AUC ROC evaluations, elevated for a multiclass approach, are presented. In a qualitative analysis, the segmentations are compared visually, indicating strengths and deficits of each model.

3.1. *Quantitative Ablation Study*

From the perspective of a quantitative analysis, an ablation study for six different architectural variants was performed and evaluated. From the results shown in Table 1, it becomes evident that the sparse labeling in combination with different U-Net architectures yields very accurate segmentation results on histological data. The performance results of each architectural variant are summarized in Table 1. Additionally, in Supplement Figure S1, a confusion matrix for each architecture is given. The baseline model, a basic U-Net, already achieved high scores with a precision of 0.9032, a recall of 0.8601, a specificity of 0.9877, and a Dice coefficient of 0.8432. Introducing attention gates to the U-Net architecture led to slight improvements in precision (0.9053) and recall (0.8621), while maintaining a high specificity of 0.9864. The Dice coefficient increased to 0.8524, indicating an enhanced segmentation performance. Incorporating residual links into the U-Net architecture impacts the precision slightly, decreasing it to 0.8961, but the recall remained reasonable at 0.8435. The specificity remained high at 0.9879. However, the Dice coefficient showed a moderate decrease to 0.8197, suggesting a slight reduction in segmentation accuracy compared to the baseline. The addition of recurrent links in the U-Net architecture resulted in a lower precision of 0.8058 and recall of 0.8080. Despite this, the specificity remained high at 0.9782. However, the Dice coefficient noticeably decreased to 0.7436, indicating a notable decrease in segmentation accuracy compared to the basic U-Net.

Table 1. Performance comparison for each variant investigated in the ablation study. Each variant was trained three times, and the values are reported as average and standard deviation. Bold numbers indicate the best performance for the respective metric. Precision, recall, specificity, and Dice range from 0 to 1, with 1 being a perfect segmentation with no errors. See Supplementary Materials for the confusion matrices leading to these evaluations.

Method/Metric	Precision (Equation (2))	Recall/ Sensitivity (Equation (3))	Specificity (Equation (6))	Dice (Equation (4))	Trained Parameters	Trained Epochs	Dropout Regularization
Basic U-Net	0.9032 (± 0.0144)	0.8601 (± 0.068)	0.9877 (± 0.007)	0.8432 (± 0.0657)	31,055,622	212	0.125
U-Net + Attention gates	0.9053 (± 0.0069)	**0.8621 (± 0.0041)**	0.9864 (± 0.0008)	**0.8524 (± 0.0022)**	31,778,762	245	0.125
U-Net + Residual links	0.8961 (± 0.0048)	0.8435 (± 0.0129)	**0.9879 (± 0.001)**	0.8197 (± 0.0148)	32,463,174	191	0.125
U-Net + Recurrent links	0.8058 (± 0.0481)	0.8080 (± 0.0113)	0.9782 (± 0.0038)	0.7436 (± 0.0415)	35,631,750	108	0.25
U-Net + Attention gates + Residual links	**0.9088 (± 0.0061)**	0.8383 (± 0.019)	0.9869 (± 0.0005)	0.8247 (± 0.0235)	33,186,314	217	0.125
U-Net + Attention gates, Residual links, Recurrent links	0.7974 (± 0.0074)	0.8117 (± 0.024)	0.9787 (± 0.0005)	0.7432 (± 0.0187)	37,762,442	86	0.125

Incorporating each of the presented architectural methods independently already suggests that the segmentation benefits from added attention gates and residual links. Adding recurrence, however, decreases the segmentation performance. The reason for this is overfitting. The more complex network can more easily learn the small dataset, as it has far more parameters than the other architectures: 35.6 million >> 31.1 million for the baseline model. Next to the number of parameters, the number of training epochs also indicates overfitting. Although the recurrence model is more complex, it takes over 100 epochs less for training, indicating an overfit to the training set. Lastly, the recurrent U-Net was the only architecture where the best dropout was identified as 0.25 (instead of 0.125), which also implies overfitting.

Combining attention gates with residual links yielded a higher precision of 0.9088, albeit with a slightly lower recall of 0.8383. The specificity remained consistently high at 0.9869. However, the Dice coefficient decreased to 0.8247, suggesting a moderate reduction in segmentation accuracy compared to the basic U-Net. Finally, incorporating attention gates, residual links, and recurrent links in the U-Net architecture led to the lowest precision (0.7974), recall (0.8117), and the Dice coefficient (0.7432). However, the specificity remained high at 0.9787. As before, the network performs well, yet with the same argumentation as before, overfitting to the small dataset has to be assumed.

Based on the quantitative analysis, the U-Net model with attention gates demonstrated improved precision, recall, and the Dice coefficient compared to the basic U-Net (cf. Table 1). The addition of residual links had varying impacts on the performance, and the inclusion of recurrent links generally resulted in lower segmentation accuracy, which is attributed to overfitting. Notably, the combination of attention gates and residual links provided a trade-off between precision and the Dice coefficient. However, the model with attention gates, residual links, and recurrent links did not perform as well, showing lower precision and Dice coefficient.

In addition to these global metrics that assess the segmentation as one, Figure 5 shows the AUC ROC curves [72] for each class. Here, the computation for ROC curves for binary classification estimation was elevated to fit the multiclass approach by the one-vs-rest method. The curves in Figure 5 clearly show that the segmentation algorithm performs well on all defined classes as the total AUC ROC values are all above 0.912. Apart from the class for destroyed tissue, all classes are segmented reliably as indicated by their AUC ROC, which was very close to 1. This was consistent for all models, indicating that there were too little training data for the class of destroyed tissue.

This class is very heterogeneous (cf. Figure 2f) and thus needs more training data to cover all class characteristics. Still, the overall performance of all models is very good. The basic U-Net sets a high baseline with a total AUC score of 0.9506. With added attention gates, the model improved its performance (AUC score of 0.9671), especially on the class of destroyed tissue. Residual links also increased the performance to an AUC score of 0.9654. As seen before, the added recurrent links decreased the performance of the model, reaching the lowest AUC score of 0.912. Although the model achieves good performance on the class of destroyed tissue, the performance on the classes of vessel walls, vessel insides, and debris significantly decreased compared to the baseline model. Being the only model that performs poorly on the class of debris again implies overfitting as seen before. The class of debris is the smallest labeled class and thus can be more easily memorized by the more complex model. The combination of attention gates and residual links led to the highest AUC score of all models of 0.9717. The model achieved the best performance on almost all individual classes. Only the classes of vessel wall and tissue are surpassed by the baseline model with 0.0016 and the attention model with 0.0004, respectively. The model with attention gate and residual and recurrent links also showed an increased performance (AUC score of 0.9602) compared to the baseline model. It showed a slightly reduced performance on the class of vessel walls yet achieves the second-to-best score on the class of destroyed tissue. Also, the decrease in the class of debris that was expressed in the model with only recurrent links is compensated through the attention gates and residual links, thus showing great promise for a better performance on a larger dataset with increased yet sparse labeling.

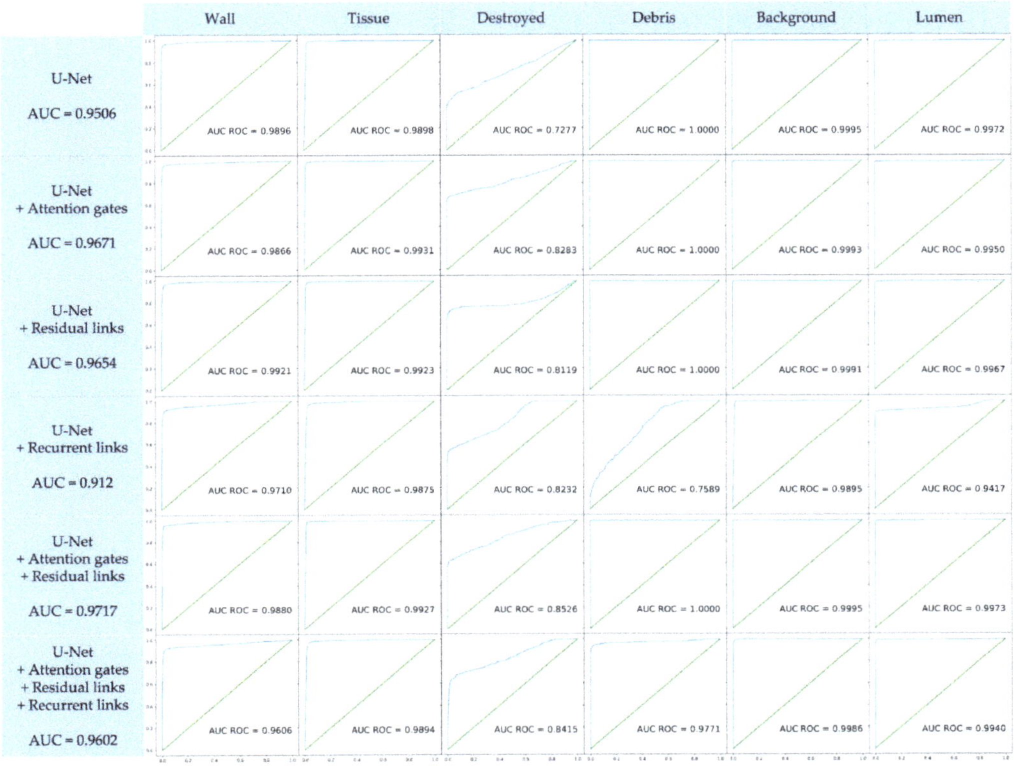

Figure 5. Comparison of the ROC curves with their AUC scores for each architecture and each individual class. The ROC curves for each class were computed using the one-vs-rest method, which indicates how good the respective network can distinguish the individual class from the other classes. Each diagram shows the AUC-ROC score for the specific combination of architecture and selected class. The AUC scores beneath the architecture configurations in the first column are the total AUC-ROC scores for the multiclass evaluation.

3.2. *Qualitative Segmentation Analysis*

The qualitative results are shown in Figure 6. Three patches are exemplarily shown to highlight the strengths and deficits of each model. Patch A shows three large and prominent vessels (marked with green circles), color variations from very bright on the left side to very dark on the right side, as well as some destroyed tissue in the bottom left area (marked with an orange circle). Patch B has also strong color variation from dark on the left to bright on the right. There are a lot of complex shaped vessels in the patch's center (marked with blue circle) that are very close to one another and contain a lot of structures (e.g., blood cells) showing a very heterogeneous lumen (marked with red circle). Patch C is very dark with little contrast. There are many elongated small vessels present with no lumen (marked with yellow circle).

For patch A, the U-Net baseline model clearly segments most vessels with their lumen in purple and their wall in dark blue. Also, the destroyed tissue in the bottom left area and in the center was correctly identified (marked red), and the tissue (marked green) covers all remaining parts of the tumor slice and has a sharp border to the background (marked yellow). However, the elongated vessel on the right is only partially segmented and was falsely identified as background. For patch B, the complex shapes and the heterogeneous lumens were correctly identified. Also, patch C shows great results, as the elongated structures are finely separated from one another.

With added attention gates, the visual results look very similar to the reference model. Vessel walls and lumens were well segmented in all three patches. The model identified more of the destroyed tissue in patch A, which is consistent with the models increased AUC-ROC score in Figure 5 for this class, as seen before. In the center of patch A, the vessel contains some blood cells that were misclassified as tissue.

The same holds for the added residual links. In patch A, the model falsely identified some vessel lumens in the destroyed tissue region but correctly segmented the vessel lumens of the center vessel.

As the metrics in Table 1 reflect, the segmentation of the U-Net with added recurrence performs less accurately than the reference model. The large vessels in patch A were missed almost completely. Also, patch B and C are missing vessels and have only partially segmented lumens. The model also falsely identified a lot more destroyed tissue, especially in the dark regions in patch C.

The combination of attention gates and residual links shows very accurate segmentations. In all patches, the complex-shaped or small vessels are identified correctly. In patch A's center vessel, the heterogeneous blood cells, apart from very few pixel errors, are completely segmented as part of the lumen. There is also more identified, destroyed tissue than in the reference model. These good results are again consistent with the metrics in Table 1 and the AUC-ROC scores in Figure 5.

Lastly, the model with added attention gates and residual and recurrent links shows good segmentations of vessels in patches A and B. In the center vessel of patch A, the heterogeneous region was partially misclassified as tissue; however, this model is the only one that almost completely identified the homogeneous elongated vessel on the right of patch A. Yet, there is an overexpression of destroyed tissue. This model tends to classify dark regions as destroyed tissue, which is very prominent in patch C. As before, this is a clear sign of overfitting, as most destroyed regions in the dataset are dark and heterogeneous. Bigger training data for such regions will be necessary to avoid the overfitting for this complex model.

3.3. Selection of the Best Architecture

The quantitative analysis showed that each of the presented architectures had their individual benefits and drawbacks. The attention gates achieved the highest scores for recall and Dice, whereas residual links achieved the highest sensitivity. The combination of both mechanisms provided a great trade-off between these scores and achieved the best precision. Although the recurrence increased the receptive field and thus yielded a good performance on large homogeneous structures as seen in Figure 6, its performance metrics were the lowest among all tested architectures, which is attributed to overfitting the small dataset. Yet, the analysis of the AUC-ROC scores showed promising qualities for including recurrence in future models, as its ability to distinguish between the different classes among the other models. With extended computational resources and further labeling, further investigations using recurrent links in semantic segmentation models will enable an even better segmentation of heterogeneous structures. The metrics in Table 1, the AUC-ROC scores in Figure 5 and the visual inspection in Figure 6 demonstrate that the model combining attention gates and residual links yields the most promising results for a semantic segmentation of histological images. Figure 7 shows three full slices from the dataset with their respective segmentation. Clearly defined structures with sharp edges and very few misclassifications allow the best applicability of these segmentation results for subsequent quantitative analysis, clinical decision-making, and advanced image-guided interventions.

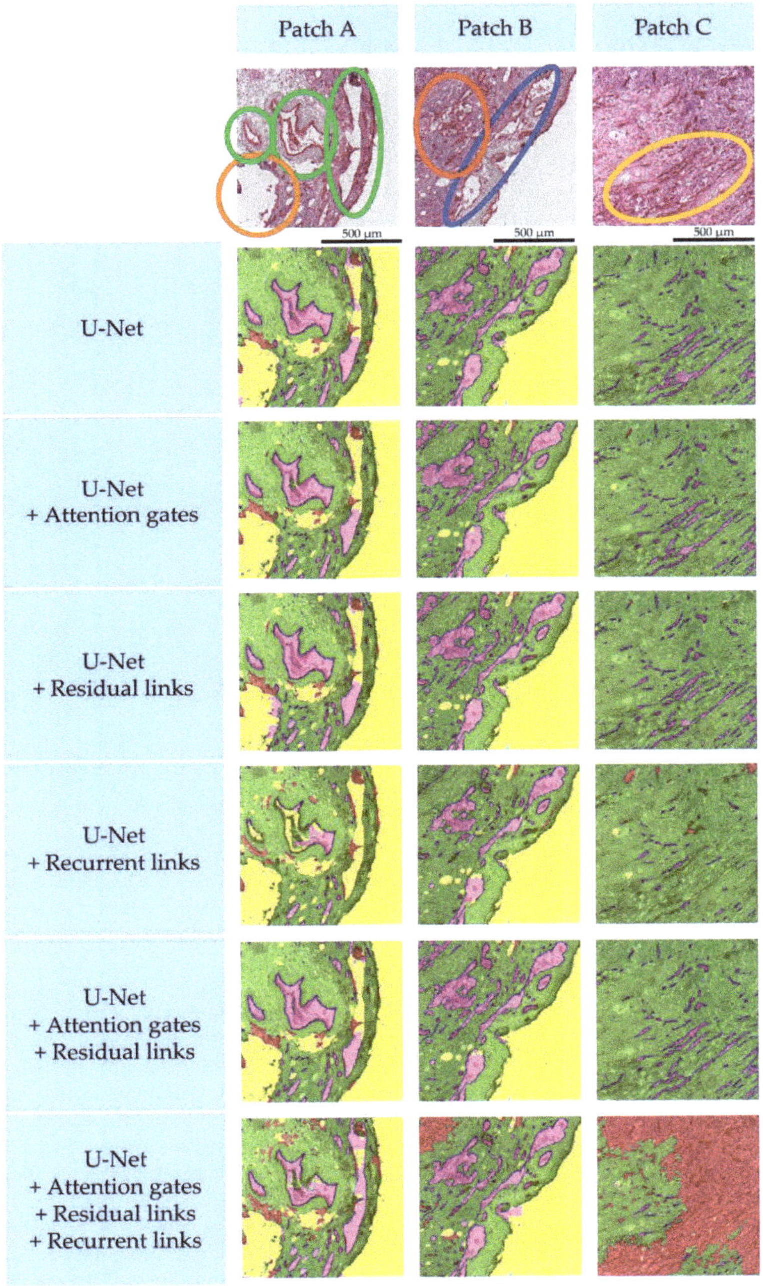

Figure 6. Qualitative segmentation results of all models shown exemplarily on three different patches. The patches on top are taken from original images. The results below show overlays of the respective patch with its segmentation result. Vessel lumens are colored purple, vessel walls are dark blue, tissue is green, destroyed tissue is red, and the background is yellow. Beneath each architecture, the AUC-ROC scores from Figure 5 are included for comparison.

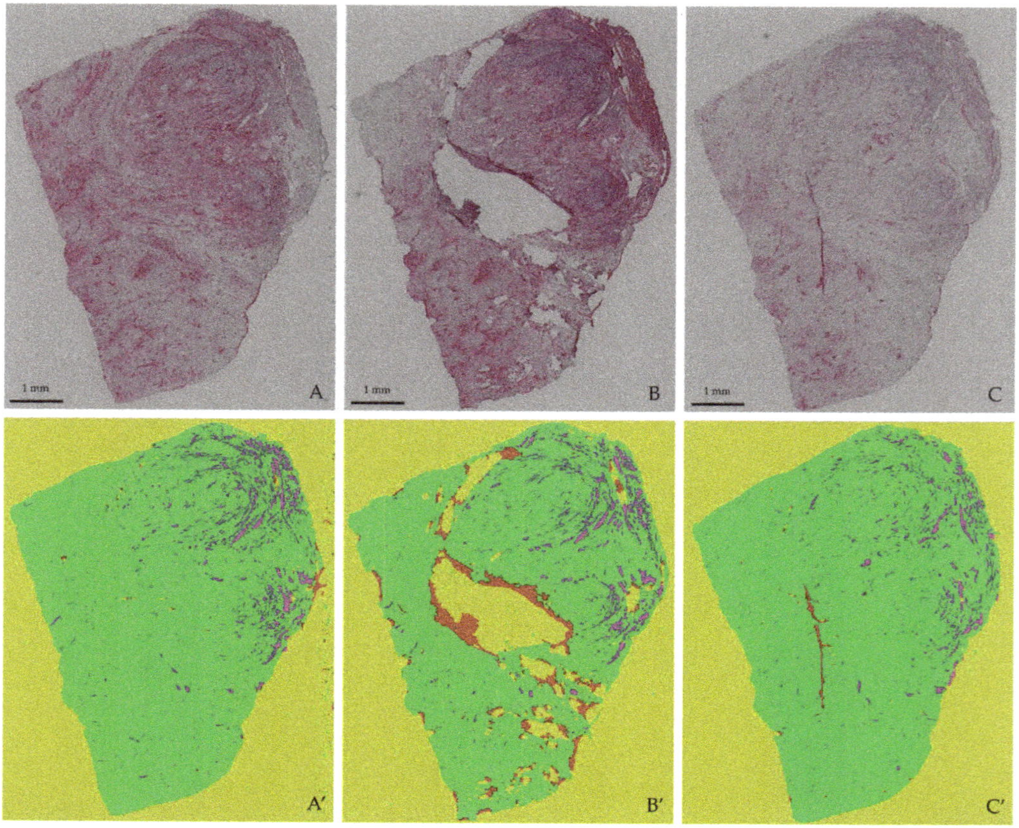

Figure 7. Three full slices segmented using U-Net with attention gates and residual links. The slices give examples of slices with high contrast (**A**), slices with intensity variations and a lot of destroyed tissue (**B**), and very bright slices with very little contrast (**C**). The model performs well on all of these difficulties. The segmentations are shown below and are denoted (**A′**), (**B′**), and (**C′**).

4. Discussion and Future Work

With this study, we presented a model that handles histological images with high contrast (Figure 7A), intensity variations, and destroyed tissue (Figure 7B), as well as very bright slices with little contrast (Figure 7C). The model was designed for segmenting histological images, yet the presented methods are versatile and can be applied to all sorts of applications in medical image segmentation. Depending on the desired application, more classes (e.g., for glands, cell nuclei, etc.) can be designed and given as new training input. To the best of our knowledge, there are no semantic segmentation algorithms that can achieve this level of accuracy and precision when delineating vascular structures in histological images. Having a precise segmentation across consecutive slices makes it possible to trace the vessels' paths through the tissue and potentially reconstruct them in a 3D model. To track the vessels' paths through the tissue, it is important that the whole slide images are registered. Several registration techniques designed to re-align medical images are available [73–83], many of which are based on SIFT [84] or SURF [85] feature point extraction, which can also be applied to histological images with stained vessels [86]. To overcome the challenge of feature extraction in highly repetitive patterns, normalized cross-correlation was used [87,88], and to improve the similarity measure, the Gaussian Laplacian second-order differential operator was additionally applied [89].

To implement the described deep learning approach, data scarcity was a major challenge in this work. The used dataset consisted of 169 histological slices that had no annotations. Fully annotating them manually is very time-consuming and would require medical experts. Therefore, a novel sparse labeling technique (cf. Section 2.2) was employed in this work. This new labeling technique enabled us to annotate a reasonably large dataset within a feasible timeframe to be able to train a deep neural network. Approaches, like unsupervised domain adaptation (UDA) [90], address the challenge of data annotation. UDA leverages knowledge from a labeled source domain, performing a so-called domain shift, to improve model performance on an unlabeled or sparsely labeled target domain. [91] In the context of medical imaging, UDA has gained increasing attention to overcome the limitations of collecting large, labeled datasets across different medical imaging modalities [90,91]. However, it is important to note that UDA may not be directly applicable to histological datasets in certain cases. Histological images present unique challenges due to their high complexity, fine-grained structures, and significant staining variations. The domain shift between different histological datasets can be highly complex and difficult to capture solely through unsupervised adaptation techniques. There are approaches to handle these challenges of complex domains via orthogonal decomposition of domain specific features [92] or disentanglement of domain invariant and domain specific modalities [93]. There are UDA approaches dealing with histological images, i.e., for general whole-slide images [94] or specific to the classification of breast cancer images [95]. Further advancements bridging domains of different imaging modalities are made [96] by, e.g., style adaptation [97] or selective entropy constraints [98] where pixels are first categorized in reliable and unreliable before the domain shift. However, all these approaches rely on a well-labeled source domain. This work targets applications that include, e.g., 3D reconstruction of in vitro models, for which a very precise pixel-wise segmentation is needed. To the best of our knowledge, there are no publicly available datasets with such detailed annotations available. In such cases, alternative approaches are more appropriate for addressing the domain shift and improving the performance of models on histological datasets. Therefore, we introduced a new labeling technique that was specifically tailored to address the identified challenges of data scarcity, class imbalance, and the data's heterogeneous structure.

With the labeled dataset, the network presented in this work was able to segment the images into six classes with high precision (cf. Table 1). The two most interesting classes regard the vascular structures of the used specimen. There are many applications, in which delineating vessels with various imaging modalities plays an important role, e.g., for early detection of severe diseases, like diabetes, hypertensive retinopathy, or retinal vessel segmentation [39–41]. Retinal images, however, consist of long and fine-grained homogeneous structures with significant lower complexity than histological tissue images. Other applications are cerebrovascular diseases, for which the detection of deformations and abnormalities in brain blood vessels with digital subtraction angiography (DSA) images is of paramount importance [42]. Similar to retinal images, DSA images are homogeneous and contain long vessel structures. More complex or heterogeneous images are encountered in X-ray angiography (XRA) segmentation. The segmentation of main coronary arteries is important for assessing coronary diseases, such as stenosis [99]. So far, a progressive perception learning framework was proposed that segments coronary arteries using boundary perception [100]. All these applications are based on image modalities containing significantly less complex vessel information. DSA, XRA, MRI, or CT have too low resolutions to capture small arteries of down to 10 nm [101,102]. This makes the model presented in this work unique in the reconstruction of 3D in vitro networks with a resolution and structural information.

However, the model accuracy may benefit from improvements. Especially concerning the areas of destroyed tissue or low contrast regions, the distinction between vessels and tissue remains challenging. By expanding the training dataset and incorporating more patches with these challenging areas, we are confident to further increase the model performance. Having more data will also allow to further incorporate recurrent links into the architecture, which was not feasible due to the identified overfitting.

Concerning the implementation of the model and its clinical use, code verification and security is required. Here, the application of formal methods and smart contracts offers a novel approach to enhance the verification and correctness of deep learning code. In the context of this work, the following ideas could be applied. By leveraging the transparency and immutability of blockchain technology, smart contracts could provide several advantages in ensuring code integrity [103–105]. Different formal methods, such as model checking or runtime verification, could be applied. With model checking [106–108], storing the deep learning code and model parameters on the blockchain could enable the verification of code execution by comparing the recorded hash or identifiers with the executed results. This would allow for easy detection of discrepancies or deviations, ensuring the correctness of the code execution. This could also facilitate the validation of model training. Recording essential training details on the blockchain, such as datasets, hyperparameters, and model architecture, could increase transparency and external verification. This would guard against manipulation or data leakage, enhancing the reliability and correctness of the model training process. By runtime verification [106,109], the continuous monitoring of model performance is made possible. By periodically receiving model predictions or metrics stored on the blockchain, comparisons with predefined benchmarks or ground truth data can be made. This could enable the early detection of issues, like model degradation or adversarial attacks, ensuring the ongoing correctness of the deep learning model's performance. Implementing such formal methods to ensure code verification, training validation, performance monitoring, and model governance will be an important part of our ongoing development for a future clinical setting. These proposed methods are ideas on how smart contracts could be used to verify a deep learning model within a sensitive medical context, as this is an emerging research field and there is no standard procedure for deep learning verification yet.

5. Conclusions

In conclusion, the deep learning network for semantic segmentation of vascular structures in histological images incorporates several techniques to improve the segmentation performance. The addition of attention gates, residual links, and recurrent links allows the network to selectively focus on regions of interest, preserve low-level features, and model the segmentation over time of the vascular structures. The use of data augmentation, under-/oversampling, and dropout regularization addresses class imbalance in the data and prevents overfitting in the network, respectively. The combination of these techniques demonstrates the feasibility of sparse labeling and thus introduces a novel labeling technique applicable for biomedical data, where a precise labeling in itself is an elaborate task and results in a deep learning network that exceeds state-of-the-art segmentation algorithms on the task of semantic segmentation of histological images.

Supplementary Materials: The following supporting information can be downloaded at: https://www.mdpi.com/article/10.3390/cancers15153773/s1, Figure S1: The confusion matrices for each of the evaluated network architectures.

Author Contributions: Conceptualization, L.G. and I.S.; methodology, L.G.; software, H.E.M.; validation, L.G. and H.E.M.; formal analysis, L.G.; investigation, L.G.; resources, A.A.R., I.S. and T.S.-R.; data curation, L.G. and I.S.; writing—original draft preparation, L.G.; writing—review and editing, L.G. and I.S.; visualization, L.G.; supervision, I.S.; project administration, I.S.; funding acquisition, I.S. All authors have read and agreed to the published version of the manuscript.

Funding: Funded by the Federal Ministry of Education and Research (BMBF) and the Ministry of Culture and Science of the German State of North Rhine-Westphalia (MKW) under the Excellence Strategy of the Federal Government and the Länder (OPSF555) and by BMBF (VIP+, Grant no.03VP10971/2).

Institutional Review Board Statement: The study was conducted according to the guidelines of the Declaration of Helsinki and approved by the Institutional Review Board of the RWTH Aachen University Hospital (EK206/09, 5 January 2010).

Informed Consent Statement: Not applicable.

Data Availability Statement: Data are available in a pseudonymized manner upon request due to ethical restrictions (patient confidentially). Therefore, the data are not available publicly.

Acknowledgments: Training of the neural networks was performed with computing resources granted by RWTH Aachen University under project rwth1291.

Conflicts of Interest: The authors declare no conflict of interest. The funders had no role in the design of the study; in the collection, analyses, or interpretation of data; in the writing of the manuscript, or in the decision to publish the results.

References

1. Singh, A.; Sengupta, S.; Lakshminarayanan, V. Explainable Deep Learning Models in Medical Image Analysis. *J. Imaging* **2020**, *6*, 52. [CrossRef] [PubMed]
2. Zhou, S.K.; Greenspan, H.; Davatzikos, C.; Duncan, J.S.; van Ginneken, B.; Madabhushi, A.; Prince, J.L.; Rueckert, D.; Summers, R.M. A Review of Deep Learning in Medical Imaging: Imaging Traits, Technology Trends, Case Studies with Progress Highlights, and Future Promises. *Proc. IEEE* **2021**, *109*, 820–838. [CrossRef]
3. Yousef, R.; Gupta, G.; Yousef, N.; Khari, M. A holistic overview of deep learning approach in medical imaging. *Multimed. Syst.* **2022**, *28*, 881–914. [CrossRef] [PubMed]
4. Suganyadevi, S.; Seethalakshmi, V.; Balasamy, K. A review on deep learning in medical image analysis. *Int. J. Multimed. Inf. Retr.* **2022**, *11*, 19–38. [CrossRef] [PubMed]
5. Ahmad, M.; Ding, Y.; Qadri, S.F.; Yang, J. Convolutional-neural-network-based feature extraction for liver segmentation from CT images. In Proceedings of the Eleventh International Conference on Digital Image Processing (ICDIP 2019), Guangzhou, China, 10–13 May 2019; Jiang, X., Hwang, J.-N., Eds.; SPIE: Bellingham, WA, USA, 2019; p. 159, ISBN 9781510630758.
6. Qadri, S.F.; Lin, H.; Shen, L.; Ahmad, M.; Qadri, S.; Khan, S.; Khan, M.; Zareen, S.S.; Akbar, M.A.; Bin Heyat, M.B.; et al. CT-Based Automatic Spine Segmentation Using Patch-Based Deep Learning. *Int. J. Intell. Syst.* **2023**, *2023*, 2345835. [CrossRef]
7. Asghar, W.; El Assal, R.; Shafiee, H.; Pitteri, S.; Paulmurugan, R.; Demirci, U. Engineering cancer microenvironments for in vitro 3-D tumor models. *Mater. Today* **2015**, *18*, 539–553. [CrossRef]
8. Sung, K.E.; Beebe, D.J. Microfluidic 3D models of cancer. *Adv. Drug Deliv. Rev.* **2014**, *79*, 68–78. [CrossRef]
9. Rodrigues, J.; Heinrich, M.A.; Teixeira, L.M.; Prakash, J. 3D In Vitro Model ®evolution: Unveiling Tumor-Stroma Interactions. *Trends Cancer* **2021**, *7*, 249–264. [CrossRef]
10. Gerardo-Nava, J.L.; Jansen, J.; Günther, D.; Klasen, L.; Thiebes, A.L.; Niessing, B.; Bergerbit, C.; Meyer, A.A.; Linkhorst, J.; Barth, M.; et al. Transformative Materials to Create 3D Functional Human Tissue Models In Vitro in a Reproducible Manner. *Adv Healthc. Mater.* **2023**, 2301030. [CrossRef]
11. Ben Hamida, A.; Devanne, M.; Weber, J.; Truntzer, C.; Derangère, V.; Ghiringhelli, F.; Forestier, G.; Wemmert, C. Deep learning for colon cancer histopathological images analysis. *Comput. Biol. Med.* **2021**, *136*, 104730. [CrossRef]
12. Mo, Y.; Wu, Y.; Yang, X.; Liu, F.; Liao, Y. Review the state-of-the-art technologies of semantic segmentation based on deep learning. *Neurocomputing* **2022**, *493*, 626–646. [CrossRef]
13. Ronneberger, O.; Fischer, P.; Brox, T. U-Net: Convolutional Networks for Biomedical Image Segmentation. *Lect. Notes Comput. Sci.* **2015**, *9351*, 234–241. [CrossRef]
14. Siddique, N.; Paheding, S.; Elkin, C.P.; Devabhaktuni, V. U-Net and Its Variants for Medical Image Segmentation: A Review of Theory and Applications. *IEEE Access* **2021**, *9*, 82031–82057. [CrossRef]
15. Bae, H.; Puranik, A.S.; Gauvin, R.; Edalat, F.; Carrillo-Conde, B.; Peppas, N.A.; Khademhosseini, A. Building vascular networks. *Sci. Transl. Med.* **2012**, *4*, 160ps23. [CrossRef] [PubMed]
16. O'Connor, C.; Brady, E.; Zheng, Y.; Moore, E.; Stevens, K.R. Engineering the multiscale complexity of vascular networks. *Nat. Rev. Mater.* **2022**, *7*, 702–716. [CrossRef]
17. Chen, E.P.; Toksoy, Z.; Davis, B.A.; Geibel, J.P. 3D Bioprinting of Vascularized Tissues for in vitro and in vivo Applications. *Front. Bioeng. Biotechnol.* **2021**, *9*, 664188. [CrossRef]
18. Lindemann, M.C.; Luttke, T.; Nottrodt, N.; Schmitz-Rode, T.; Slabu, I. FEM based simulation of magnetic drug targeting in a multibranched vessel model. *Comput. Methods Programs Biomed.* **2021**, *210*, 106354. [CrossRef]
19. Helms, F.; Haverich, A.; Wilhelmi, M.; Böer, U. Establishment of a Modular Hemodynamic Simulator for Accurate In Vitro Simulation of Physiological and Pathological Pressure Waveforms in Native and Bioartificial Blood Vessels. *Cardiovasc. Eng. Technol.* **2022**, *13*, 291–306. [CrossRef]
20. Langhans, S.A. Three-Dimensional In Vitro Cell Culture Models in Drug Discovery and Drug Repositioning. *Front. Pharmacol.* **2018**, *9*, 6. [CrossRef]

21. Kakeya, H.; Okada, T.; Oshiro, Y. 3D U-JAPA-Net: Mixture of Convolutional Networks for Abdominal Multi-organ CT Segmentation. In *Medical Image Computing and Computer Assisted Intervention—MICCAI 2018*; Frangi, A.F., Schnabel, J.A., Davatzikos, C., Alberola-López, C., Fichtinger, G., Eds.; Springer International Publishing: Cham, Switzerland, 2018; pp. 426–433. ISBN 978-3-030-00936-6.
22. Seo, H.; Huang, C.; Bassenne, M.; Xiao, R.; Xing, L. Modified U-Net (mU-Net) With Incorporation of Object-Dependent High Level Features for Improved Liver and Liver-Tumor Segmentation in CT Images. *IEEE Trans. Med. Imaging* **2020**, *39*, 1316–1325. [CrossRef]
23. Li, C.; Tan, Y.; Chen, W.; Luo, X.; He, Y.; Gao, Y.; Li, F. ANU-Net: Attention-based nested U-Net to exploit full resolution features for medical image segmentation. *Comput. Graph.* **2020**, *90*, 11–20. [CrossRef]
24. Ibtehaz, N.; Rahman, M.S. MultiResUNet: Rethinking the U-Net architecture for multimodal biomedical image segmentation. *Neural Netw.* **2020**, *121*, 74–87. [CrossRef] [PubMed]
25. Jin, Y.W.; Jia, S.; Ashraf, A.B.; Hu, P. Integrative Data Augmentation with U-Net Segmentation Masks Improves Detection of Lymph Node Metastases in Breast Cancer Patients. *Cancers* **2020**, *12*, 2934. [CrossRef]
26. Alom, M.Z.; Yakopcic, C.; Taha, T.M.; Asari, V.K. Nuclei Segmentation with Recurrent Residual Convolutional Neural Networks based U-Net (R2U-Net). In Proceedings of the NAECON 2018—IEEE National Aerospace and Electronics Conference, Dayton, OH, USA, 23–26 July 2018; IEEE: Piscataway, NJ, USA, 2018; pp. 228–233, ISBN 978-1-5386-6557-2.
27. Long, F. Microscopy cell nuclei segmentation with enhanced U-Net. *BMC Bioinform.* **2020**, *21*, 8. [CrossRef] [PubMed]
28. Benazzouz, M.; Benomar, M.L.; Moualek, Y. Modified U-Net for cytological medical image segmentation. *Int. J. Imaging Syst. Tech.* **2022**, *32*, 1761–1773. [CrossRef]
29. Zhang, M.; Li, X.; Xu, M.; Li, Q. Automated Semantic Segmentation of Red Blood Cells for Sickle Cell Disease. *IEEE J. Biomed. Health Inform.* **2020**, *24*, 3095–3102. [CrossRef]
30. Li, X.; Guo, Y.; Jiang, F.; Xu, L.; Shen, F.; Jin, Z.; Wang, Y. Multi-Task Refined Boundary-Supervision U-Net (MRBSU-Net) for Gastrointestinal Stromal Tumor Segmentation in Endoscopic Ultrasound (EUS) Images. *IEEE Access* **2020**, *8*, 5805–5816. [CrossRef]
31. Li, S.; Tso, G.K.; He, K. Bottleneck feature supervised U-Net for pixel-wise liver and tumor segmentation. *Expert Syst. Appl.* **2020**, *145*, 113131. [CrossRef]
32. Zhang, Y.; Lei, B.; Fu, C.; Du, J.; Zhu, X.; Han, X.; Du, L.; Gao, W.; Wang, T.; Ma, G. HBNet: Hybrid Blocks Network for Segmentation of Gastric Tumor from Ordinary CT Images. In Proceedings of the 2020 IEEE 17th International Symposium on Biomedical Imaging (ISBI), Iowa City, IA, USA, 3–7 April 2020; IEEE: Piscataway, NJ, USA, 2020; pp. 1–4, ISBN 978-1-5386-9330-8.
33. Wang, L.; Wang, B.; Xu, Z. Tumor Segmentation Based on Deeply Supervised Multi-Scale U-Net. In Proceedings of the 2019 IEEE International Conference on Bioinformatics and Biomedicine (BIBM), San Diego, CA, USA, 18–21 November 2019; IEEE: Piscataway, NJ, USA, 2019; pp. 746–749, ISBN 978-1-7281-1867-3.
34. Liu, Y.-C.; Shahid, M.; Sarapugdi, W.; Lin, Y.-X.; Chen, J.-C.; Hua, K.-L. Cascaded atrous dual attention U-Net for tumor segmentation. *Multimed. Tools Appl.* **2021**, *80*, 30007–30031. [CrossRef]
35. Pang, S.; Du, A.; Orgun, M.A.; Wang, Y.; Yu, Z. Tumor attention networks: Better feature selection, better tumor segmentation. *Neural Netw.* **2021**, *140*, 203–222. [CrossRef]
36. Hasan, S.M.K.; Linte, C.A. A Modified U-Net Convolutional Network Featuring a Nearest-neighbor Re-sampling-based Elastic-Transformation for Brain Tissue Characterization and Segmentation. In Proceedings of the 2018 IEEE Western New York Image and Signal Processing Workshop (WNYISPW), Rochester, NY, USA, 5 October 2018; IEEE: Piscataway, NJ, USA, 2018; pp. 1–5. [CrossRef]
37. Shi, W.; Pang, E.; Wu, Q.; Lin, F. Brain Tumor Segmentation Using Dense Channels 2D U-net and Multiple Feature Extraction Network. In *Brainlesion: Glioma, Multiple Sclerosis, Stroke and Traumatic Brain Injuries*; Crimi, A., Bakas, S., Eds.; Springer International Publishing: Cham, Switzerland, 2020; pp. 273–283. ISBN 978-3-030-46639-8.
38. Angermann, C.; Haltmeier, M. Random 2.5D U-net for Fully 3D Segmentation. In *Machine Learning and Medical Engineering for Cardiovascular Health and Intravascular Imaging and Computer Assisted Stenting*; Liao, H., Balocco, S., Wang, G., Zhang, F., Liu, Y., Ding, Z., Duong, L., Phellan, R., Zahnd, G., Breininger, K., et al., Eds.; Springer International Publishing: Cham, Switzerland, 2019; pp. 158–166. ISBN 978-3-030-33326-3.
39. Jin, Q.; Meng, Z.; Pham, T.D.; Chen, Q.; Wei, L.; Su, R. DUNet: A deformable network for retinal vessel segmentation. *Knowl. Based Syst.* **2019**, *178*, 149–162. [CrossRef]
40. Wu, Y.; Xia, Y.; Song, Y.; Zhang, D.; Liu, D.; Zhang, C.; Cai, W. Vessel-Net: Retinal Vessel Segmentation Under Multi-path Supervision. In *Medical Image Computing and Computer Assisted Intervention—MICCAI 2019*; Shen, D., Liu, T., Peters, T.M., Staib, L.H., Essert, C., Zhou, S., Yap, P.-T., Khan, A., Eds.; Springer International Publishing: Cham, Switzerland, 2019; pp. 264–272. ISBN 978-3-030-32238-0.
41. Adarsh, R.; Amarnageswarao, G.; Pandeeswari, R.; Deivalakshmi, S. Dense Residual Convolutional Auto Encoder for Retinal Blood Vessels Segmentation. In Proceedings of the 2020 6th International Conference on Advanced Computing and Communication Systems (ICACCS), Coimbatore, India, 6–7 March 2020; IEEE: Piscataway, NJ, USA, 2020; pp. 280–284, ISBN 978-1-7281-5196-0.
42. Zhang, M.; Zhang, C.; Wu, X.; Cao, X.; Young, G.S.; Chen, H.; Xu, X. A neural network approach to segment brain blood vessels in digital subtraction angiography. *Comput. Methods Programs Biomed.* **2020**, *185*, 105159. [CrossRef]

43. Palzer, J.; Mues, B.; Goerg, R.; Aberle, M.; Rensen, S.S.; Olde Damink, S.W.M.; Vaes, R.D.W.; Cramer, T.; Schmitz-Rode, T.; Neumann, U.P.; et al. Magnetic Fluid Hyperthermia as Treatment Option for Pancreatic Cancer Cells and Pancreatic Cancer Organoids. *Int. J. Nanomed.* **2021**, *16*, 2965–2981. [CrossRef]
44. James, G.; Witten, D.; Hastie, T.; Tibshirani, R. *An Introduction to Statistical Learning*; Springer: New York, NY, USA, 2013; ISBN 978-1-4614-7137-0.
45. Shakeel, F.; Sabhitha, A.S.; Sharma, S. Exploratory review on class imbalance problem: An overview. In Proceedings of the 2017 8th International Conference on Computing, Communication and Networking Technologies (ICCCNT), Delhi, India, 3–5 July 2017; IEEE: Piscataway, NJ, USA, 2017; pp. 1–8. [CrossRef]
46. Bria, A.; Marrocco, C.; Tortorella, F. Addressing class imbalance in deep learning for small lesion detection on medical images. *Comput. Biol. Med.* **2020**, *120*, 103735. [CrossRef] [PubMed]
47. Shrivastava, A.; Gupta, A.; Girshick, R. Training Region-Based Object Detectors with Online Hard Example Mining. In Proceedings of the 2016 IEEE Conference on Computer Vision and Pattern Recognition (CVPR), Las Vegas, NV, USA, 27–30 June 2016; IEEE: Piscataway, NJ, USA, 2016; pp. 761–769, ISBN 978-1-4673-8851-1.
48. Dong, Q.; Gong, S.; Zhu, X. Class Rectification Hard Mining for Imbalanced Deep Learning. In Proceedings of the 2017 IEEE International Conference on Computer Vision (ICCV), Venice, Italy, 22–29 October 2017; IEEE: Piscataway, NJ, USA, 2017; pp. 1869–1878, ISBN 978-1-5386-1032-9.
49. Dai, J.; Qi, H.; Xiong, Y.; Li, Y.; Zhang, G.; Hu, H.; Wei, Y. Deformable Convolutional Networks. In Proceedings of the 2017 IEEE International Conference on Computer Vision (ICCV), Venice, Italy, 22–29 October 2017; IEEE: Piscataway, NJ, USA, 2017; pp. 764–773, ISBN 978-1-5386-1032-9.
50. Oktay, O.; Schlemper, J.; Le Folgoc, L.; Lee, M.; Heinrich, M.; Misawa, K.; Mori, K.; McDonagh, S.; Hammerla, N.Y.; Kainz, B.; et al. Attention u-net: Learning where to look for the pancreas. *arXiv* **2018**, arXiv:1804.03999. [CrossRef]
51. Schlemper, J.; Oktay, O.; Schaap, M.; Heinrich, M.; Kainz, B.; Glocker, B.; Rueckert, D. Attention gated networks: Learning to leverage salient regions in medical images. *Med. Image Anal.* **2019**, *53*, 197–207. [CrossRef] [PubMed]
52. Vaswani, A.; Shazeer, N.; Parmar, N.; Uszkoreit, J.; Jones, L.; Gomez, A.N.; Kaiser, L.; Polosukhin, I. Attention Is All You Need. In *Advances in Neural Information Processing Systems 30 (NIPS 2017)*; Guyon, I., Luxburg, U.V., Bengio, S., Wallach, H., Fergus, R., Vishwanathan, S., Garnett, R., Eds.; Curran Associates, Inc.: New York, NY, USA, 2017; pp. 6000–6010.
53. Hochreiter, S.; Schmidhuber, J. Long short-term memory. *Neural Comput.* **1997**, *9*, 1735–1780. [CrossRef]
54. Alom, M.Z.; Yakopcic, C.; Hasan, M.; Taha, T.M.; Asari, V.K. Recurrent residual U-Net for medical image segmentation. *J. Med. Imaging* **2019**, *6*, 14006. [CrossRef]
55. Tomar, N.K.; Jha, D.; Riegler, M.A.; Johansen, H.D.; Johansen, D.; Rittscher, J.; Halvorsen, P.; Ali, S. FANet: A Feedback Attention Network for Improved Biomedical Image Segmentation. *IEEE Trans. Neural Netw. Learn. Syst.* **2022**, 1–14. [CrossRef]
56. Jiang, Y.; Wang, F.; Gao, J.; Cao, S. Multi-Path Recurrent U-Net Segmentation of Retinal Fundus Image. *Appl. Sci.* **2020**, *10*, 3777. [CrossRef]
57. Araujo, A.; Norris, W.; Sim, J. Computing Receptive Fields of Convolutional Neural Networks. *Distill* **2019**, *4*, e21. [CrossRef]
58. He, K.; Zhang, X.; Ren, S.; Sun, J. Deep Residual Learning for Image Recognition. In Proceedings of the 2016 IEEE Conference on Computer Vision and Pattern Recognition (CVPR), Las Vegas, NV, USA, 27–30 June 2016; IEEE: Piscataway, NJ, USA, 2016; pp. 770–778, ISBN 978-1-4673-8851-1.
59. Li, D.; Dharmawan, D.A.; Ng, B.P.; Rahardja, S. Residual U-Net for Retinal Vessel Segmentation. In Proceedings of the 2019 IEEE International Conference on Image Processing (ICIP), Taipei, Taiwan, 22–25 September 2019; IEEE: Piscataway, NJ, USA, 2019; pp. 1425–1429, ISBN 978-1-5386-6249-6.
60. Yu, W.; Fang, B.; Liu, Y.; Gao, M.; Zheng, S.; Wang, Y. Liver Vessels Segmentation Based on 3d Residual U-NET. In Proceedings of the 2019 IEEE International Conference on Image Processing (ICIP), Taipei, Taiwan, 22–25 September 2019; IEEE: Piscataway, NJ, USA, 2019; pp. 250–254, ISBN 978-1-5386-6249-6.
61. Zhang, J.; Lv, X.; Zhang, H.; Liu, B. AResU-Net: Attention Residual U-Net for Brain Tumor Segmentation. *Symmetry* **2020**, *12*, 721. [CrossRef]
62. Pan, L.-S.; Li, C.-W.; Su, S.-F.; Tay, S.-Y.; Tran, Q.-V.; Chan, W.P. Coronary artery segmentation under class imbalance using a U-Net based architecture on computed tomography angiography images. *Sci. Rep.* **2021**, *11*, 14493. [CrossRef]
63. Johnson, J.M.; Khoshgoftaar, T.M. Survey on deep learning with class imbalance. *J. Big Data* **2019**, *6*, 1–54. [CrossRef]
64. Wasikowski, M.; Chen, X.w. Combating the Small Sample Class Imbalance Problem Using Feature Selection. *IEEE Trans. Knowl. Data Eng.* **2010**, *22*, 1388–1400. [CrossRef]
65. Qu, W.; Balki, I.; Mendez, M.; Valen, J.; Levman, J.; Tyrrell, P.N. Assessing and mitigating the effects of class imbalance in machine learning with application to X-ray imaging. *Int. J. Comput. Assist. Radiol. Surg.* **2020**, *15*, 2041–2048. [CrossRef] [PubMed]
66. Powers, D.M.W. Evaluation: From precision, recall and F-measure to ROC, informedness, markedness and correlation. *arXiv* **2020**, arXiv:2010.16061. [CrossRef]
67. Hinton, G.E.; Srivastava, N.; Krizhevsky, A.; Sutskever, I.; Salakhutdinov, R.R. Improving neural networks by preventing co-adaptation of feature detectors. *arXiv* **2012**, arXiv:1207.0580. [CrossRef]
68. Wager, S.; Wang, S.; Liang, P.S. Dropout Training as Adaptive Regularization. In *Advances in Neural Information Processing Systems*; Burges, C.J., Bottou, L., Welling, M., Ghahramani, Z., Weinberger, K.Q., Eds.; Curran Associates, Inc.: New York, NY, USA, 2013.
69. TensorFlow Developers. *TensorFlow*; Zenodo: Geneve, Switzerland, 2023.

70. Chollet, F.; Zhu, Q.S.; Rahman, F.; Lee, T.; Qian, C.; de Marmiesse, G.; Jin, H.; Zabluda, O.; Marks, S.; Watson, M.; et al. Keras. GitHub. 2015. Available online: https://github.com/fchollet/keras (accessed on 28 June 2023).
71. Hunter, J.D. Matplotlib: A 2D Graphics Environment. *Comput. Sci. Eng.* **2007**, *9*, 90–95. [CrossRef]
72. Fawcett, T. An introduction to ROC analysis. *Pattern Recognit. Lett.* **2006**, *27*, 861–874. [CrossRef]
73. Kupfer, B.; Netanyahu, N.S.; Shimshoni, I. An Efficient SIFT-Based Mode-Seeking Algorithm for Sub-Pixel Registration of Remotely Sensed Images. *IEEE Geosci. Remote Sens. Lett.* **2015**, *12*, 379–383. [CrossRef]
74. Liu, Q.; Zhao, G.; Deng, J.; Xue, Q.; Hou, W.; He, Y. Image Registration Algorithm for Sequence Pathology Slices of Pulmonary Nodule. In Proceedings of the 2019 8th International Symposium on Next Generation Electronics (ISNE), Zhengzhou, China, 9–10 October 2019; IEEE: Piscataway, NY, USA, 2019; pp. 1–3, ISBN 978-1-7281-2062-1.
75. Lobachev, O.; Ulrich, C.; Steiniger, B.S.; Wilhelmi, V.; Stachniss, V.; Guthe, M. Feature-based multi-resolution registration of immunostained serial sections. *Med. Image Anal.* **2017**, *35*, 288–302. [CrossRef] [PubMed]
76. Saalfeld, S.; Fetter, R.; Cardona, A.; Tomancak, P. Elastic volume reconstruction from series of ultra-thin microscopy sections. *Nat. Methods* **2012**, *9*, 717–720. [CrossRef] [PubMed]
77. Hermann, J.; Brehmer, K.; Jankowski, V.; Lellig, M.; Hohl, M.; Mahfoud, F.; Speer, T.; Schunk, S.J.; Tschernig, T.; Thiele, H.; et al. Registration of Image Modalities for Analyses of Tissue Samples Using 3D Image Modelling. *Proteom. Clin. Appl.* **2020**, *15*, e1900143. [CrossRef] [PubMed]
78. Paknezhad, M.; Loh, S.Y.M.; Choudhury, Y.; Koh, V.K.C.; Yong, T.T.K.; Tan, H.S.; Kanesvaran, R.; Tan, P.H.; Peng, J.Y.S.; Yu, W.; et al. Regional registration of whole slide image stacks containing major histological artifacts. *BMC Bioinform.* **2020**, *21*, 558. [CrossRef]
79. Zhang, J.; Li, Z.; Yu, Q. Point-Based Registration for Multi-stained Histology Images. In Proceedings of the 2020 IEEE 5th International Conference on Image, Vision and Computing (ICIVC), Beijing, China, 10–12 July 2020; IEEE: Piscataway, NY, USA, 2020; pp. 92–96, ISBN 978-1-7281-6661-2.
80. Deng, R.; Yang, H.; Jha, A.; Lu, Y.; Chu, P.; Fogo, A.B.; Huo, Y. Map3D: Registration-Based Multi-Object Tracking on 3D Serial Whole Slide Images. *IEEE Trans. Med. Imaging* **2021**, *40*, 1924–1933. [CrossRef]
81. Wang, C.-W.; Chen, H.-C. Improved image alignment method in application to X-ray images and biological images. *Bioinformatics* **2013**, *29*, 1879–1887. [CrossRef]
82. Wang, C.-W.; Ka, S.-M.; Chen, A. Robust image registration of biological microscopic images. *Sci. Rep.* **2014**, *4*, 6050. [CrossRef]
83. Liu, Y.; Tian, J.; Hu, R.; Yang, B.; Liu, S.; Yin, L.; Zheng, W. Improved Feature Point Pair Purification Algorithm Based on SIFT During Endoscope Image Stitching. *Front. Neurorobot.* **2022**, *16*, 840594. [CrossRef]
84. Lowe, D.G. Distinctive Image Features from Scale-Invariant Keypoints. *Int. J. Comput. Vis.* **2004**, *60*, 91–110. [CrossRef]
85. Bay, H.; Ess, A.; Tuytelaars, T.; van Gool, L. Speeded-Up Robust Features (SURF). *Comput. Vis. Image Underst.* **2008**, *110*, 346–359. [CrossRef]
86. Schwier, M.; Böhler, T.; Hahn, H.K.; Dahmen, U.; Dirsch, O. Registration of histological whole slide images guided by vessel structures. *J. Pathol. Inform.* **2013**, *4*, S10. [CrossRef]
87. Kugler, M.; Goto, Y.; Kawamura, N.; Kobayashi, H.; Yokota, T.; Iwamoto, C.; Ohuchida, K.; Hashizume, M.; Hontani, H. Accurate 3D Reconstruction of a Whole Pancreatic Cancer Tumor from Pathology Images with Different Stains. In Proceedings of the Computational Pathology and Ophthalmic Medical Image Analysis: First International Workshop, COMPAY 2018, and 5th International Workshop, OMIA 2018, Granada, Spain, 16–20 September 2018; Stoyanov, D., Taylor, Z., Ciompi, F., Xu, Y., Martel, A., Maier-Hein, L., Rajpoot, N., van der Laak, J., Veta, M., McKenna, S., et al., Eds.; Springer: Cham, Switzerland, 2018; pp. 35–43, ISBN 9783030009496.
88. Kugler, M.; Goto, Y.; Tamura, Y.; Kawamura, N.; Kobayashi, H.; Yokota, T.; Iwamoto, C.; Ohuchida, K.; Hashizume, M.; Shimizu, A.; et al. Robust 3D image reconstruction of pancreatic cancer tumors from histopathological images with different stains and its quantitative performance evaluation. *Int. J. Comput. Assist. Radiol. Surg.* **2019**, *14*, 2047–2055. [CrossRef] [PubMed]
89. Liu, S.; Yang, B.; Wang, Y.; Tian, J.; Yin, L.; Zheng, W. 2D/3D Multimode Medical Image Registration Based on Normalized Cross-Correlation. *Appl. Sci.* **2022**, *12*, 2828. [CrossRef]
90. Kouw, W.M.; Loog, M. A Review of Domain Adaptation without Target Labels. *IEEE Trans. Pattern Anal. Mach. Intell.* **2021**, *43*, 766–785. [CrossRef]
91. Guan, H.; Liu, M. Domain Adaptation for Medical Image Analysis: A Survey. *IEEE Trans. Biomed. Eng.* **2022**, *69*, 1173–1185. [CrossRef]
92. Sun, Y.; Dai, D.; Xu, S. Rethinking adversarial domain adaptation: Orthogonal decomposition for unsupervised domain adaptation in medical image segmentation. *Med. Image Anal.* **2022**, *82*, 102623. [CrossRef]
93. Xie, Q.; Li, Y.; He, N.; Ning, M.; Ma, K.; Wang, G.; Lian, Y.; Zheng, Y. Unsupervised Domain Adaptation for Medical Image Segmentation by Disentanglement Learning and Self-Training. *IEEE Trans. Med. Imaging* **2022**, 1. [CrossRef]
94. Ren, J.; Hacihaliloglu, I.; Singer, E.A.; Foran, D.J.; Qi, X. Unsupervised Domain Adaptation for Classification of Histopathology Whole-Slide Images. *Front. Bioeng. Biotechnol.* **2019**, *7*, 102. [CrossRef]
95. Alirezazadeh, P.; Hejrati, B.; Monsef-Esfahani, A.; Fathi, A. Representation learning-based unsupervised domain adaptation for classification of breast cancer histopathology images. *Biocybern. Biomed. Eng.* **2018**, *38*, 671–683. [CrossRef]
96. Liu, X.; Yoo, C.; Xing, F.; Oh, H.; El Fakhri, G.; Kang, J.-W.; Woo, J. Deep Unsupervised Domain Adaptation: A Review of Recent Advances and Perspectives. *SIP* **2022**, *11*. [CrossRef]

97. Ge, Y.; Chen, Z.-M.; Zhang, G.; Heidari, A.A.; Chen, H.; Teng, S. Unsupervised domain adaptation via style adaptation and boundary enhancement for medical semantic segmentation. *Neurocomputing* **2023**, *550*, 126469. [CrossRef]
98. Feng, W.; Ju, L.; Wang, L.; Song, K.; Zhao, X.; Ge, Z. Unsupervised Domain Adaptation for Medical Image Segmentation by Selective Entropy Constraints and Adaptive Semantic Alignment. *AAAI* **2023**, *37*, 623–631. [CrossRef]
99. Garrone, P.; Biondi-Zoccai, G.; Salvetti, I.; Sina, N.; Sheiban, I.; Stella, P.R.; Agostoni, P. Quantitative coronary angiography in the current era: Principles and applications. *J. Interv. Cardiol.* **2009**, *22*, 527–536. [CrossRef]
100. Zhang, H.; Gao, Z.; Zhang, D.; Hau, W.K.; Zhang, H. Progressive Perception Learning for Main Coronary Segmentation in X-Ray Angiography. *IEEE Trans. Med. Imaging* **2023**, *42*, 864–879. [CrossRef]
101. Feezor, R.J.; Caridi, J.; Hawkins, I.; Seeger, J.M. *Angiography. Endovascular Surgery*; Elsevier: Amsterdam, The Netherlands, 2011; pp. 209–225. ISBN 9781416062080.
102. Ghekiere, O.; Salgado, R.; Buls, N.; Leiner, T.; Mancini, I.; Vanhoenacker, P.; Dendale, P.; Nchimi, A. Image quality in coronary CT angiography: Challenges and technical solutions. *Br. J. Radiol.* **2017**, *90*, 20160567. [CrossRef]
103. Abdellatif, T.; Brousmiche, K.-L. Formal Verification of Smart Contracts Based on Users and Blockchain Behaviors Models. In Proceedings of the 2018 9th IFIP International Conference on New Technologies, Mobility and Security (NTMS), Paris, France, 26–28 February 2018; IEEE: Piscataway, NJ, USA, 2018; pp. 1–5, ISBN 978-1-5386-3662-6.
104. Krichen, M.; Lahami, M.; Al-Haija, Q.A. Formal Methods for the Verification of Smart Contracts: A Review. In Proceedings of the 2022 15th International Conference on Security of Information and Networks (SIN), Sousse, Tunisia, 11–13 November 2022; IEEE: Piscataway, NJ, USA, 2022; pp. 1–8, ISBN 978-1-6654-5465-0.
105. Khan, S.N.; Loukil, F.; Ghedira-Guegan, C.; Benkhelifa, E.; Bani-Hani, A. Blockchain smart contracts: Applications, challenges, and future trends. *Peer Peer Netw. Appl.* **2021**, *14*, 2901–2925. [CrossRef]
106. Almakhour, M.; Sliman, L.; Samhat, A.E.; Mellouk, A. Verification of smart contracts: A survey. *Pervasive Mob. Comput.* **2020**, *67*, 101227. [CrossRef]
107. Bao, Y.; Zhu, X.-Y.; Zhang, W.; Shen, W.; Sun, P.; Zhao, Y. On Verification of Smart Contracts via Model Checking. In *Theoretical Aspects of Software Engineering*; Aït-Ameur, Y., Crăciun, F., Eds.; Springer International Publishing: Cham, Switzerland, 2022; pp. 92–112. ISBN 978-3-031-10362-9.
108. Bošnački, D.; Wijs, A. Model checking: Recent improvements and applications. *Int. J. Softw. Tools Technol. Transf.* **2018**, *20*, 493–497. [CrossRef]
109. Ellul, J. Towards Configurable and Efficient Runtime Verification of Blockchain Based Smart Contracts at the Virtual Machine Level. In *Leveraging Applications of Formal Methods, Verification and Validation: Applications*; Margaria, T., Steffen, B., Eds.; Springer International Publishing: Cham, Switzerland, 2020; pp. 131–145. ISBN 978-3-030-61466-9.

cancers

MDPI

Article

Pareto-Optimized Non-Negative Matrix Factorization Approach to the Cleaning of Alaryngeal Speech Signals

Rytis Maskeliūnas [1,*], Robertas Damaševičius [1], Audrius Kulikajevas [1], Kipras Pribuišis [2], Nora Ulozaitė-Stanienė [2] and Virgilijus Uloza [2]

[1] Faculty of Informatics, Kaunas University of Technology, 44249 Kaunas, Lithuania; robertas.damasevicius@ktu.lt (R.D.); audrius.kulikajevas@ktu.lt (A.K.)

[2] Department of Otorhinolaryngology, Academy of Medicine, Lithuanian University of Health Sciences, 44240 Kaunas, Lithuania; kipras.pribuisis@lsmuni.lt (K.P.); nora.ulozaite@lsmuni.lt (N.U.-S.); virgilijus.ulozas@lsmuni.lt (V.U.)

* Correspondence: rytis.maskeliunas@ktu.lt

Simple Summary: This paper introduces a new method for cleaning impaired speech by combining Pareto-optimized deep learning with Non-negative Matrix Factorization (NMF). The approach effectively reduces noise in impaired speech while preserving the desired speech quality. The method involves calculating the spectrogram of a noisy voice clip, determining a noise threshold, computing a noise-to-signal mask, and smoothing it to avoid abrupt transitions. Using a Pareto-optimized NMF, the modified spectrogram is decomposed into basis functions and weights, allowing for reconstruction of the clean speech spectrogram. The final result is a noise-reduced waveform achieved by inverting the clean speech spectrogram. Experimental results validate the method's effectiveness in cleaning alaryngeal speech signals, indicating its potential for real-world applications.

Abstract: The problem of cleaning impaired speech is crucial for various applications such as speech recognition, telecommunication, and assistive technologies. In this paper, we propose a novel approach that combines Pareto-optimized deep learning with non-negative matrix factorization (NMF) to effectively reduce noise in impaired speech signals while preserving the quality of the desired speech. Our method begins by calculating the spectrogram of a noisy voice clip and extracting frequency statistics. A threshold is then determined based on the desired noise sensitivity, and a noise-to-signal mask is computed. This mask is smoothed to avoid abrupt transitions in noise levels, and the modified spectrogram is obtained by applying the smoothed mask to the signal spectrogram. We then employ a Pareto-optimized NMF to decompose the modified spectrogram into basis functions and corresponding weights, which are used to reconstruct the clean speech spectrogram. The final noise-reduced waveform is obtained by inverting the clean speech spectrogram. Our proposed method achieves a balance between various objectives, such as noise suppression, speech quality preservation, and computational efficiency, by leveraging Pareto optimization in the deep learning model. The experimental results demonstrate the effectiveness of our approach in cleaning alaryngeal speech signals, making it a promising solution for various real-world applications.

Keywords: alaryngeal; voice quality; voice cleaning; voice disorders; Pareto optimization

1. Introduction

Laryngeal cancer remains the most common malignant tumor in the upper respiratory tract [1]. Despite the decreasing incidence, approximately 60% of patients present with stage III or IV disease at the initial workup [2,3]. Surgery or surgery combined with chemoradiotherapy remains the preferred treatment method for laryngeal cancer, offering an optimal 5-year survival rate [4,5]. The surgical treatment options are laryngeal-preserving or radical surgery. Laryngeal-preserving surgery options can range from endolaryngeal cordectomy with a laser to partial removal of the larynx—partial laryngectomy. The complete removal of the larynx, also known as a total laryngectomy, is the radical option. The more advanced the disease, the more radical the treatment required to achieve remission. Advanced laryngeal cancer stages limit the treatment options that can be offered to patients. In most cases, the complete removal of the larynx—total laryngectomy—is advised. Such surgery leaves the patient without the larynx, the main part of the vocal apparatus, and their vocal function is significantly impaired. Long-term voice and speech function rehabilitation is required, often with unsatisfactory results. Total laryngectomy results in the complete and permanent separation of the upper and lower airways and requires the creation of a terminal tracheostoma to breathe. The complete removal of the larynx and lack of air movement through the mouth results in patients' total loss of phonatory function [6]. After the removal of the larynx, the patient has to rely on alaryngeal speech to communicate. Alaryngeal speech can be achieved in three ways: esophageal speech, an electrolarynx, or a tracheoesophageal prosthesis (TEP). Esophageal speech and an electrolarynx benefit from low maintenance and do not require additional surgery. The TEP outperforms both methods by providing better perceptual (voice quality and intelligibility) and acoustic (maximum phonation time, fundamental frequency, and intensity) speech outcomes [7]. A TEP can be implanted through a tracheoesophageal fistula formed during laryngectomy or later [8]. It functions as a one-way valve that allows the air to move from the trachea to the esophagus but keeps the food and liquids from entering the lungs (see Figure 1).

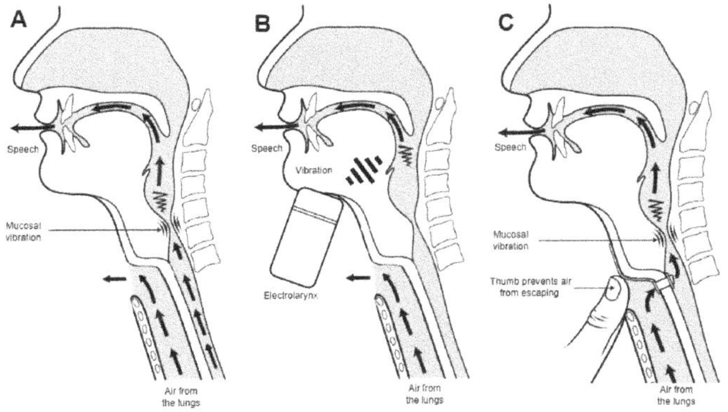

Figure 1. Types of speech production after total laryngectomy. (**A**) Esophageal speech: air is pulled in and released from the esophagus; (**B**) vibrations created by an electrolarynx; (**C**) the patient is occluding a tracheostoma to allow air to pass through the mouth. Adapted from Hurren 2015 [9].

The air moving through the TEP creates vibrations in the mucosa and generates speech [10]. The use of a pulmonary air supply to speak increases fluency and utterance lengths [11]. Despite its higher maintenance costs, the TEP is the preferred method for speech rehabilitation after total laryngectomy [12]. Alaryngeal (esophageal or TEP) speech is a patient's only verbal communication option after a total laryngectomy. Although the patient retains the ability to speak, the body begins to adapt and substitutes vocal folds with structures (aryepiglottic/ventricular folds, pharyngeal mucosa) that were not naturally intended for voice production. The downside of this adaptation is that the speech generated in this manner features frequent unintended phonatory breaks, frequency shifts, unvoiced segments, and high irregularity, and might be aperiodic (see Figure 2) [13]. It becomes even more problematic when the patient has to use the phone or speak in a loud environment, which may lead to social isolation [14,15]. The inability to communicate is most prominent in the early postoperative period before any speech rehabilitation occurs when patients have to rely on written text to communicate with their physician and family.

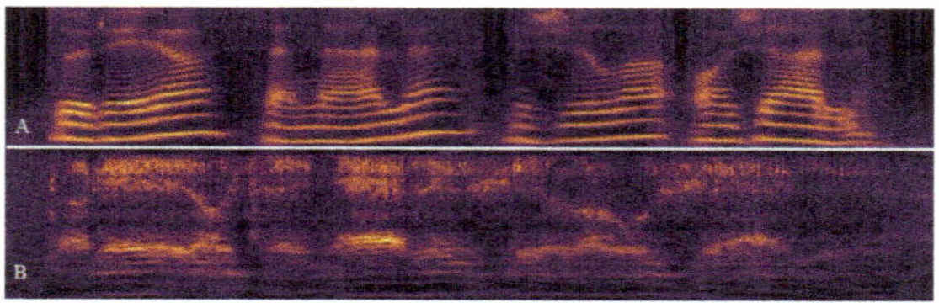

Figure 2. (**A**) Normal speech; (**B**) Speech after total laryngectomy with a tracheoesophageal prosthesis. Cochleagram deterioration and blurring between different words caused by aperiodicity, phonatory breaks, and additive noise.

It becomes even more problematic when the patient has to use the phone or speak in a loud environment, which may lead to social isolation [13,14]. The inability to communicate is most prominent in the early postoperative period before any speech rehabilitation occurs when patients have to rely on written text to communicate with their physician and family. Therefore, enhancing the signal quality of alaryngeal speech and improving a patient's speaking ability represent fundamental scientific/technical and clinical issues.

This may involve techniques such as breath control [16], pitch and tone modifications [17,18], and articulation exercises [19], including spectral subtraction [20], Wiener filtering [21], and statistical prediction model-based [22] or machine learning-based approaches [23]. However, these traditional methods often suffer from drawbacks such as introducing artifacts, suppressing the desired speech components, or being computationally expensive. With the advent of deep learning, several new approaches have been proposed that leverage the power of neural networks to address the limitations of traditional methods. Among these, non-negative matrix factorization (NMF) [24] has gained significant attention for its ability to represent non-negative data such as audio spectrograms as a linear combination of basis functions [25].

In this paper, we propose a novel approach for cleaning impaired speech signals by combining Pareto-optimized deep learning with NMF. Our method aims to balance various objectives, such as noise suppression, speech quality preservation, and computational efficiency, by leveraging Pareto optimization in a deep learning model. By incorporating Pareto optimization, we ensure that the trade-offs between different objectives are optimally balanced, ultimately improving the performance of the noise-reduction process.

The proposed method consists of several steps. First, we calculate the spectrogram of a noisy voice clip and extract its frequency statistics. Based on the desired noise sensitivity, a threshold is calculated to distinguish between the signal and noise components in the spectrogram. Next, we compute the noise-to-signal mask and smooth it to avoid abrupt transitions in noise levels. The modified spectrogram is then obtained by applying the smoothed mask to the signal spectrogram. To further enhance the speech signal, we employ a Pareto-optimized NMF to decompose the modified spectrogram into basis functions and corresponding weights. These basis functions and weights are learned to best represent the clean speech signal while achieving a balance between various objectives. Finally, the clean speech spectrogram is reconstructed using the learned basis functions and weights, and a noise-reduced waveform is obtained by inverting the clean speech spectrogram.

The main contributions of this paper are as follows:

- We propose a novel method for cleaning impaired speech signals by combining Pareto-optimized deep learning with NMF, addressing the limitations of traditional speech enhancement techniques.
- We introduce a smoothing technique for the noise-to-signal mask to avoid abrupt transitions in noise levels, resulting in a more natural-sounding output signal.
- We demonstrate the effectiveness of our approach through a series of experiments, showing significant improvements in speech quality and intelligibility compared to traditional methods.

The remainder of this paper is organized as follows. Section 2 provides a review of the related works in the field of speech enhancement. In Section 3, we describe our proposed method. Section 4 presents the experimental setup and results, followed by a discussion of the findings. Finally, Section 5 concludes the paper and suggests future research directions.

2. Review of State-of-the-Art Works

This overview of related works aims to help the reader explore the various approaches to improving speech intelligibility and quality for individuals with speech disorders. Various techniques, such as clear speech variants, adaptive filter structures, deep learning models, and speech enhancement algorithms, have been investigated to address the challenges in speech enhancement. These studies demonstrate the potential of different methods, including instruction-based interventions, signal processing, and machine learning techniques, to enhance speech intelligibility and quality across various disorders and conditions. The findings may help the reader better understand the complex relationship between speech impairments and the effectiveness of different approaches in overcoming these challenges, ultimately improving communication for affected individuals.

2.1. Assessing Speech-Signal Impairments

Evaluating the quality and intelligibility of alaryngeal speech can be difficult for several reasons [26]. First, evaluating speech quality is inherently subjective, as different people may have different opinions on what constitutes good or clear speech. Evaluators may also have biases or preconceived notions about alaryngeal speech, which can affect their judgment [27]. Second, alaryngeal speech can be complex and variable, depending on the individual's chosen method of alaryngeal speech and their level of proficiency [28], among other factors. Evaluators may need to consider multiple aspects of speech, such as pitch, tone, articulation, and prosody, which can make the evaluation more challenging [29]. Third, there is a limited amount of training data available for evaluating alaryngeal speech, as it is a relatively rare condition [30]. This can make it difficult to develop standardized evaluation methods and norms for different types of alaryngeal speech [31]. Finally, alaryngeal speech can vary widely between individuals, depending on factors such as age, gender, health status, and other individual characteristics [32]. This variability can make it difficult to develop standardized evaluation methods that are applicable to all individuals who have undergone a laryngectomy [33].

Numerous researchers have stressed the significance of selecting relevant characteristics for differentiating damaged speech [34–36]. Some researchers have investigated how speech difficulties caused by cerebral palsy and hearing impairment affect prosody, pronunciation, and voice quality. According to their findings, these factors are statistically significant for increasing the detection ability of impaired talks, with voice quality being the strongest discriminative feature for identifying speech intelligibility in damaged speech. Malini and Chandrakala [37] suggested a regularized self-representation-based compact supervector technique for assessing the intelligibility of damaged speech. On the UA-SPEECH database, their approach outperformed other methods such as hybrid GMM/SVM, supervector, x-vector, i-vector, and bag-of-models-based approaches. Albaqshi and Sagheer [38] emphasized the difficulties in dysarthric speech recognition owing to incomprehensible speech, irregular phoneme articulation, and data scarcity. Bessell et al. [39] found that a changed accent has a slower speech pace, greater consonant and vowel length, syllable-timed rhythm, and other characteristics. Moon et al. [40] sought to define the speech patterns of those suffering from hepatic encephalopathy as a possible diagnostic and monitoring tool. The subjects' maintained and damaged speech patterns, on the other hand, did not follow patterns normally linked with organic brain problems, suggesting that left-handed preference may contribute to distinctions between singing and reading vs. recitation, repetition, and spontaneous speaking. This is also often the case after an ischemic stroke. De Cock et al. [41] investigated speech features, dysarthria type, and severity, showing that unilateral upper motor neuron dysarthria is the most common type, with the majority of subjects having mild dysarthria. Similarly, Rowe et al. [42] found that variable expressions of dysarthria may impact speech performance, whereas Stipancic and Tjaden [43] found the least detectable change in sentence intelligibility in speakers with multiple sclerosis and Parkinson's disease. Rosdi et al. [44] presented fuzzy Petri nets to increase the classification accuracy of speech-intelligibility detection systems. Maskeliunas et al. suggested applying a convolutional network to help classify and asses impaired speech signals [45]. Kim et al. [46] used one- and two-dimensional convolutional neural networks to classify alaryngeal speech. Feng et al. [47] found that acoustic investigations can reveal that impaired speech has a substantially shorter voice start time for aspirated consonants, as well as a smaller vowel spacing. Vieira et al. [48] presented a non-intrusive voice-quality classifier based on the tree convolutional neural network for measuring user satisfaction with speech communication platforms. Poncelet et al. [49] suggested using an end-to-end spoken language understanding system that can be trained by the user through demonstrations and can translate impaired speech directly into semantics.

Numerous speech recognition-oriented techniques can also be used to help detect and asses speech impairment [50,51]. Gupta et al. [52] suggested a residual network-based approach for detecting dysarthria severity level based on short speech segments, whereas Latha et al. [53] employed deep learning and several acoustic cues to recognize dysarthric speech and generate discernible speech. Vishnika Veni and Chandrakala [54] researched the application of the deep neural network-hidden Markov model and lattice maximum mutual information technique for the successful identification of damaged speech. In [55], the authors suggested a histogram of states-based strategy for learning compact and discriminative embeddings for dysarthric voice detection using the deep neural network-hidden Markov model. Srinivasan et al. [56] proposed a multi-view representation-based disordered speech recognition system based on auditory image-based features and cepstral characteristics, showing improved performance in recognizing very low intelligibility words compared to conventional methods. Chandrakala et al. [57] presented a bag-of-models (BoM)-based approach that uses adjusted Gaussian mixture model (AGMM)-based embeddings for impaired speech-intelligibility evaluation. They tested the method on two datasets and discovered that it outperformed the supervector, hybrid GMM/SVM, i-vector, and x-vector-based techniques in terms of prediction error and reliability for intelligibility-level evaluation and score predictions. Fu et al. [58] created a Sch-net neural network built on a convolutional neural network for end-to-end schizophrenia speech identification using deep learning techniques, implying that it has the potential to help in the diagnosis of a particular language disability. Marini et al. [59] verified the efficacy of a speech analysis approach for dysarthria speakers by modifying the size and shift parameters of the spectral analysis window to increase ASR system performance.

2.2. Algorithms for Alaryngeal Speech Enhancement

The majority of voice restoration treatments result in hushed and monotonous speech. Aside from reduced intelligibility, this type of speech lacks expressiveness and naturalness due to (a) a lack of pitch, which results in whispered speech, and (b) artificial pitch production, which results in monotone speech. Algorithms for alaryngeal speech enhancement can be classified into two categories: classic digital signal processing (DSP) methods and methods based on artificial intelligence (AI) and machine learning (ML) [60].

The first category is the most popular as it includes filtering-based methods originally developed for noise reduction, as background noise can interfere with the clarity of alaryngeal speech [61]. DSP techniques, such as spectral subtraction, Wiener filtering, and adaptive filtering, can be used to reduce background noise and improve speech quality [62]. For example, Jaiswal et al. [63] suggested a concealed Wiener filter-based technique for voice augmentation to improve the common spectral subtraction algorithm. Pauline and Dhanalakshmi [64] presented an efficient adaptive filter structure for noise reduction in voice signals that utilized the least mean square (LMS) and normalized LMS algorithms. They evaluated the proposed filter model on both normal speech signals and speech signals from Parkinson's disease patients. In terms of the SNR, MSE, and PSNR values, their filter model outperformed existing cascaded LMS filter models. Doi et al studied how the LPC spectrum of alaryngeal speech could be used to determine the impulse response of the vocal tract. Modified harmonic amplitudes calculated using the transformation function were interpolated at the desired harmonics of the target pitch, and the transformation function was then computed using the line spectral frequencies rather than the harmonic amplitudes [65]. Pauline et al. [66] presented cascaded adaptive filter construction for speech-signal de-noising, where the best variable-stage cascaded adaptive filter model outperformed existing cascaded filter architectures, with an output SNR that was 10–15 dB higher. Panda et al. [67] suggested using spectral subtraction to improve alaryngeal speech, which was modified by Hamed et al. to include the power of noise [68]. Wei suggested using the Mel Frequency Scale as an alternative [69]. Another approach is pitch and formant manipulation, as alaryngeal speech can have a monotonous or robotic quality due to a lack of natural pitch and formant variation. DSP techniques such as pitch shifting and formant manipulation can also be used to add more natural-sounding variation to speech [70]. Giri and Rayavarapu [71] presented a combined approach for modifying the key frequency, intensity, and speech rate of dysarthric speech by utilizing time-domain pitch-synchronous overlap. They discovered that the improvement in intelligibility was significant in speakers with low initial intelligibility and modest in speakers with high intelligibility. Additionally, there are methods for articulation enhancement, as alaryngeal speech can also suffer from poor articulation, making it difficult to distinguish between different sounds. This can be combated by utilizing dynamic range compression, and equalization can be used to enhance the clarity and intelligibility of specific consonant sounds [72]. Finally, prosody modification is common, as it can help process the patterns of stress, intonation, and rhythm in speech. Alaryngeal speech can sometimes lack the natural prosody found in normal speech and prosody modification can be used to add more natural-sounding patterns of stress, intonation, and rhythm to speech [73].

The second category includes AI and ML methods that can be used for alaryngeal speech enhancement. Currently, the most popular methods are deep learning models [74], such as convolutional neural networks (CNNs), recurrent neural networks (RNNs), and generative adversarial networks (GANs), which can be trained on large datasets of alaryngeal speech to learn patterns and relationships between speech features and speech quality. These models can be used to perform classic DSP tasks such as noise reduction, pitch and formant manipulation, and prosody modification [75]. Saleem et al. [76] suggested a computationally efficient deep learning model for improving noisy voice. For magnitude estimation, their model used a U-shaped fuzzy long short-term memory, which outperformed other deep learning models and significantly enhanced speech intelligibility and quality. In contrast to traditional GAN-based approaches [77], Santjago et al. [78] suggested using a speaker-dependent GAN to enhance generated speech. Others have proposed that an adversarial acoustic regression loss should be added to encourage better extraction of features at the discriminator and employ a two-step adversarial training schedule that serves as a warm-up and fine-tune sequence. Both the objective and subjective assessments indicated that these two enhancements improved speech reconstruction by better matching the original speaker's identity and naturalness [79]. Amarjuf combined the predicted phase with deep learning approaches to increase the overall quality [80]. Reinforcement learning can be applied to train speech enhancement systems that adapt to changing environments or input signals, as well as optimize speech enhancement systems based on a reward signal that reflects the quality of the enhanced speech [81]. Gaussian mixture models are also common, as they can work as a type of generative model that can be used to model the statistical distribution of speech features such as the spectral envelope or the fundamental frequency [82]. GMMs can also be used to separate speech from noise or modify the pitch and formant of speech. Ming et al. [83] suggested a hybrid technique that includes non-negative matrix factorization with GMM. According to Xui, the Gaussian mixture model approach is also beneficial for detecting vocal nodules and laryngitis [84]. Support vector machines can be used to classify impaired speech signals into different categories such as normal speech or alaryngeal speech produced using different methods [85]. SVMs can also be used for noise reduction and speech enhancement [86]. Hidden Markov models can also be used as a generative model that models the statistical distribution of speech features over time, often to classify speech signals into different categories or generate new speech signals based on the statistical distribution of the input speech [87].

3. Materials and Methods

3.1. Dataset

Thirty native Lithuanian-speaking male patients surgically treated for histologically confirmed laryngeal cancer at the Lithuanian University of Health Sciences Department of Otorhinolaryngology provided speech samples for this study. The patients in this group had undergone a total laryngectomy with secondary TEP implantation [88,89]. These individuals were chosen because they had no larynx or vocal folds and relied solely on alaryngeal speech to communicate. The complete removal of the larynx and speech production using a TEP often result in distinct speech abnormalities with a fairly uniform functional speech handicap compared to neurodegenerative disorders, where speech patterns are more diverse and less distinct. The average age of the patients was 63.1 years (standard deviation = 28.8). The patients were free of common colds, upper respiratory infections, or other conditions that may have affected speech quality at the time of recording. Only male participants' speech samples were collected since advanced laryngeal cancer is less common in women, and recruiting an adequate number of female participants was not feasible. Endoscopic evaluation of the neopharynx, TEP canal, and trachea was performed prior to recording. Faulty or leaking prostheses were replaced prior to recording. This examination was carried out as part of standard clinical practice and contributed to the speech sample database exclusively containing speech samples from patients in remission. For at least six months following surgery, speech recordings were acquired. This ensured enough time for healing, speech adaptation, and rehabilitation [90].

Alaryngeal speech samples were recorded in a T-series quiet room (T-room, CA Tegner AB, Bromma, Sweden) using a D60S Dynamic Vocal microphone (AKG Acoustics, Vienna, Austria) placed 10.0 cm from the lips at a comfortable (about 90°) microphone-to-mouth angle. Two different speaking assignments were completed. The patient began by reading a phonetically balanced Lithuanian line: "Turėjo senelė žilą oželį" (Old grandma had a billy goat). The relative frequencies of the phonemes in the phrase were made as close as possible to the distribution of speech sounds in Lithuanian. The patient then counted from one to ten at a rate appropriate for their respiratory function. All speech activities were performed at a comfortable volume level and at the patient's own tempo. Speech was recorded at 44,100 samples per second and saved as uncompressed 16-bit waveform audio format files. Using Praat version 6.0.53, the recordings were manually prepared and contained no more than 300 ms of an unvoiced fragment at the beginning and conclusion of the recordings. To ensure the security of participants' personal data, serial numbers were assigned to the speech recordings.

3.2. Alaryngeal Speech Assessment

Several approaches were used to measure objective alaryngeal speech:

1. The artificial intelligence-based automated classifier for substitution voicing ResNet 118 was used to assign speech samples to the following classes: normal speech—Probability 0; speech with a single vocal fold—Probability 1; and alaryngeal speech with TEP—Probability 2 [91].
2. The acoustic parameter of alaryngeal speech (average voicing evidence (AVE), available in the AMPEX software [92]) was utilized to compare the alaryngeal speech samples before and after optimization using Pareto-optimized NMF software. The AVE parameter describes the average voicing evidence and the degree of regular-

ity/periodicity in the voiced frames. Since the actual background frames are usually unvoiced, the analysis is performed on all frames, not just speech frames. This approach is more robust against possible errors of the speech/background classification, which is purely energy-based. In contrast, the voicing evidence is derived from analyzing all the sub-band signals created by the auditory model.

3. The AI-based acoustic substitution voicing index (ASVI) parameter [93] was employed to quantitatively evaluate the alaryngeal speech samples before and after optimization using Pareto-optimized NMF software. This parameter includes the constant combined with statistically significant parameters from ResNet 118 (Probability 0, Probability 1, and Probability 2) combined with the AVE and mean fundamental frequency. The possible ASVI values ranged from 0 to 30, with better speech quality indicated by higher scores.

3.3. Methodology

Our approach used Pareto-optimized deep learning to evaluate the possibility of cleaning the impaired speech. The approach started by calculating the spectrogram over the entire noisy voice clip, based on which the frequency statistics were calculated. Once the statistics were calculated, a threshold based on the desired noise sensitivity was then calculated. Afterward, a signal spectrogram was calculated based on the same input noisy voice clip, which, in combination with the calculated threshold, was then used to determine the noise-to-signal mask. The mask was then smoothed by applying a filter in both frequency and time to avoid sudden jumps in noise levels. Finally, the smoothed mask was then applied to the spectrogram of the signal and inverted creating a noise-reduced waveform.

3.3.1. Non-Negative Matrix Factorization (NMF)

Given a non-negative matrix $V \in \mathbb{R}_{\geq 0}^{m \times n}$, non-negative matrix factorization (NMF) aims to find two non-negative matrices $W \in \mathbb{R}_{\geq 0}^{m \times k}$ and $H \in \mathbb{R}_{\geq 0}^{k \times n}$ such that their product approximates the original matrix V:

$$V \approx WH \tag{1}$$

The objective is to minimize the distance between V and WH, typically measured by the Frobenius norm or another divergence measure:

$$\min_{W \geq 0, H \geq 0} \|V - - - WH\| \tag{2}$$

where $\|\cdot\|$ denotes the Frobenius norm or another divergence measure, and k is the desired dimensionality of the factorization (typically, $k \ll \min(m, n)$).

3.3.2. Pareto-Optimized Non-Negative Matrix Factorization (PONMF)

We define Pareto-optimized NMF as the problem of approximating a non-negative matrix V with the product of two non-negative matrices W and H, considering multiple objectives $f_1, f_2, \ldots, f_p$. The Pareto-optimized NMF formulation seeks a solution that balances the trade-offs among these objectives, achieving a Pareto optimal solution where no objective can be improved without worsening at least one other objective.

Given a non-negative matrix $V \in \mathbb{R}_{\geq 0}^{m \times n}$, Pareto-optimized non-negative matrix factorization (NMF) aims to find two non-negative matrices $W \in \mathbb{R}_{\geq 0}^{m \times k}$ and $H \in \mathbb{R}_{\geq 0}^{k \times n}$ such that their product approximates the original matrix V:

$$V \approx WH \tag{3}$$

The objective is to find a Pareto optimal solution, considering multiple objectives $f_1, f_2, \ldots, f_p$. A Pareto optimal solution is one where it is not possible to improve any objective without worsening at least one other objective. The Pareto-optimized NMF can be formulated as:

$$\min_{W \geq 0, H \geq 0} \left(f_1(V, W, H), f_2(V, W, H), \ldots, f_p(V, W, H) \right) \tag{4}$$

subject to Pareto optimality. Here, $f_i(V, W, H)$ represents the i-th objective such as minimizing the reconstruction error, promoting sparsity, or reducing computational complexity. The goal is to find a solution that balances the trade-offs among these objectives.

The first step is to calculate the spectrogram over the entire noisy voice clip to obtain a representation of the frequency spectrum of a signal over time. The noisy voice clip is windowed and its Fourier transform is calculated to obtain a spectrogram.

Once the spectrogram is calculated, frequency statistics are calculated to obtain a better understanding of the frequency distribution of the signal. This is achieved by calculating the mean and standard deviation of the magnitude of each frequency bin over time.

Based on the desired noise sensitivity, a threshold is calculated to distinguish between the signal and noise in the spectrogram. A signal spectrogram (see an example in Figure 3) is then calculated based on the same input noisy voice clip. This is achieved by windowing the noisy voice clip and taking its Fourier transform over time. The threshold calculated earlier is used to determine the noise-to-signal mask. The mask is a binary value for each frequency bin and time frame of the spectrogram, where 1 indicates the signal and 0 indicates noise. To avoid sudden jumps in noise levels, the mask is smoothed by applying a filter in both the frequency and time domains, making the noise-to-signal mask more continuous and less abrupt. Next, the smoothed mask is applied to the spectrogram of the signal, and the signal is inverted to create a noise-reduced waveform. This is achieved by multiplying the spectrogram of the signal with the smoothed mask and then taking the inverse Fourier transform over time to obtain the noise-reduced waveform. Then, a Pareto-optimized non-negative matrix factorization (NMF)-based method is applied to decompose the spectrogram into a set of basis functions and their corresponding weights. NMF-based methods for speech enhancement involve learning the basis functions and Pareto-optimized weights that best represent the clean speech signal and then using these to reconstruct the clean speech from a noisy input signal (Algorithm 1).

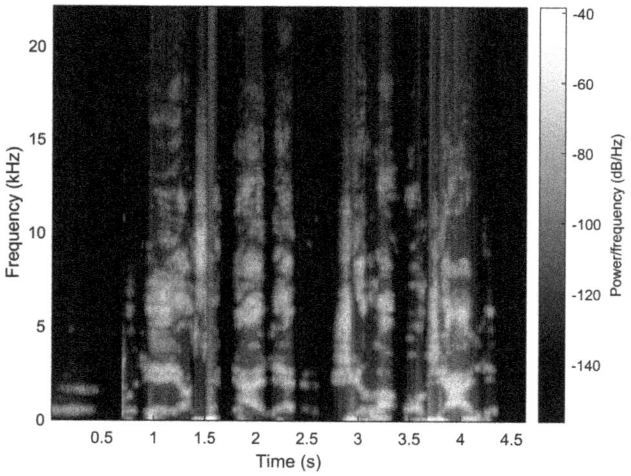

Figure 3. An example of a voice spectrogram.

Algorithm 1 Pareto-Optimized Deep Learning for Impaired Speech Cleaning

Require: Noisy voice clip V
Ensure: Noise-reduced waveform W
1: Calculate spectrogram S of noisy voice clip V
2: Compute frequency statistics F from spectrogram S
3: Calculate threshold T based on the desired noise sensitivity using frequency statistics F
4: Determine signal spectrogram S_{signal} using noisy voice clip V
5: Compute noise-to-signal mask M using threshold T and signal spectrogram S_{signal}
6: Smooth mask M by applying a filter in both the frequency and time domains to obtain smoothed mask M_{smooth}
7: Apply smoothed mask M_{smooth} to the spectrogram of signal S_{signal} to obtain modified spectrogram S_{mod}
8: Invert modified spectrogram S_{mod} to create noise-reduced waveform W
9: **return** W

3.3.3. Speech-Signal Cleaning

The updated approach to cleaning impaired speech using Pareto-optimized deep learning and non-negative matrix factorization (NMF) involves the following steps:

1. Calculate the spectrogram of the entire noisy voice clip. This is achieved by windowing the noisy voice clip and taking its Fourier transform over time to obtain a spectrogram, which is a representation of the frequency spectrum of a signal over time.
2. Compute the frequency statistics from the spectrogram. This is achieved by calculating the mean and standard deviation of the magnitude of each frequency bin over time. These statistics help in understanding the distribution and characteristics of the noise present in the voice clip.
3. Calculate a threshold based on the desired noise sensitivity. This threshold helps differentiate between the noise and signal components in the spectrogram.
4. Determine the signal spectrogram using the same input noisy voice clip. This is achieved by windowing the noisy voice clip and taking its Fourier transform over time.
5. Compute the noise-to-signal mask using the calculated threshold. The mask is a binary value for each frequency bin and time frame of the spectrogram, where 1 indicates the signal and 0 indicates noise.
6. Smooth the noise-to-signal mask by applying a filter in both the frequency and time domains. This helps avoid sudden jumps in noise levels and produces a more continuous and less abrupt mask.
7. Apply the smoothed mask to the spectrogram of the signal. This step effectively suppresses the noise components in the spectrogram while retaining the desired signal.
8. Decompose the modified spectrogram using Pareto-optimized non-negative matrix factorization (NMF). NMF-based methods for speech enhancement involve learning the basis functions and Pareto-optimized weights that best represent the clean speech signal.
9. Reconstruct the clean speech from the noisy input signal using the learned basis functions and Pareto-optimized weights.
10. Invert the reconstructed spectrogram to create a noise-reduced waveform. This final output is a cleaned version of the original impaired speech, with the noise components significantly reduced or removed.

3.3.4. Pareto-Optimized Deep Learning with NMF for Impaired Speech Cleaning

Using Pareto optimization in the deep learning model and incorporating NMF-based methods can ensure that the trade-offs between different objectives (e.g., noise suppression, speech quality, and computational efficiency) are balanced in the best possible way, ultimately improving the performance of the noise-reduction process (Algorithm 2).

Algorithm 2 Pareto-Optimized Deep Learning with NMF for Impaired Speech Cleaning

Require: Noisy voice clip V
Ensure: Noise-reduced waveform W
1: Calculate spectrogram S of noisy voice clip V
2: Compute frequency statistics F from spectrogram S
3: Calculate threshold T based on the desired noise sensitivity using frequency statistics F
4: Determine signal spectrogram S_{signal} using noisy voice clip V
5: Compute noise-to-signal mask M using threshold T and signal spectrogram S_{signal}
6: Smooth mask M by applying a filter in both the frequency and time domains to obtain smoothed mask M_{smooth}
7: Apply smoothed mask M_{smooth} to the spectrogram of signal S_{signal} to obtain modified spectrogram S_{mod}
8: Decompose modified spectrogram S_{mod} using Pareto-optimized non-negative matrix factorization (NMF) to obtain basis functions B and optimized weights W_{opt}
9: Reconstruct clean speech spectrogram S_{clean} using basis functions B and optimized weights W_{opt}
10: Invert clean speech spectrogram S_{clean} to create noise-reduced waveform W

4. Results

A statistically significant improvement in alaryngeal speech quality was observed because after applying Pareto-optimized NMF, the alaryngeal speech samples were reclassified into the lower speech disability category (see Table 1 and Figure 4).

Table 1. Evaluation results of original and optimized speech samples. Prob0—probability of healthy speech; Prob1—probability of speech with a single vocal fold; Prob2—probability of tracheoesophageal speech; AVE—average voicing evidence; ASVI—acoustic substitution voicing index; NMF—non-negative matrix factorization.

	Group	N	Mean	Std. Deviation	p
Probability 0	Original	75	4.09	19.51	0.001
	Pareto-optimized NMF	75	13.51	33.3	0.001
Probability 1	Original	75	56.18	48.66	0.454
	Pareto-optimized NMF	75	57.28	47.83	0.454
Probability 2	Original	75	39.73	47.9	0.08
	Pareto-optimized NMF	75	29.21	43.89	0.08
AVE	Original	75	0.81	0.11	0.34
	Pareto-optimized NMF	75	0.8	0.1	0.34
ASVI	Original	75	8.8	4.94	0.166
	Pareto-optimized NMF	75	10.17	6.09	0.166

To further test for improvements in the optimized speech samples, the Chi-squared test [94] was utilized to test if the proportion of speech recordings considered improved was large enough to be statistically significant. Only 4 out of 75 original speech recordings were classified as healthy, whereas 10 out of 75 were classified as healthy speech after optimization. This resulted in a statistically significant difference between the proportions (p = 0.043). These findings can be observed in Table 2.

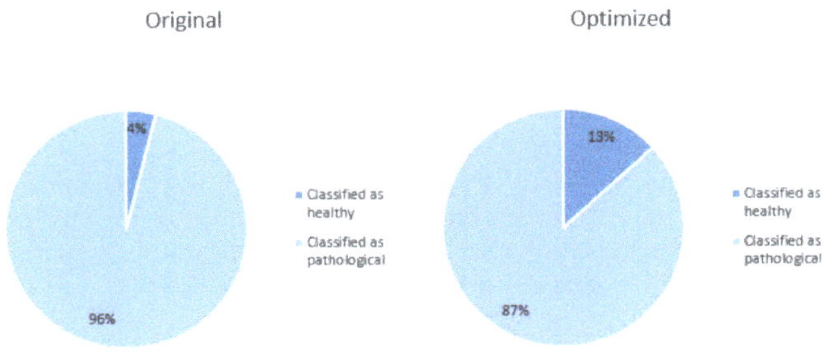

Figure 4. A pie chart illustrating the proportion of speech recordings classified as normal/pathological before and after speech-signal optimization.

Table 2. Comparison of original and optimized speech recordings. NMF—non-negative matrix factorization.

Group	Method	N	p	χ^2
Healthy speech	Original	4	4.0	0.043
	Pareto-optimized NMF	10	13.33	
Speech after laryngeal oncosurgery	Original	72	96.0	4.097
	Pareto-optimized NMF	65	86.67	

An example of the result of the alaryngeal speech-signal optimization is presented in Figure 5.

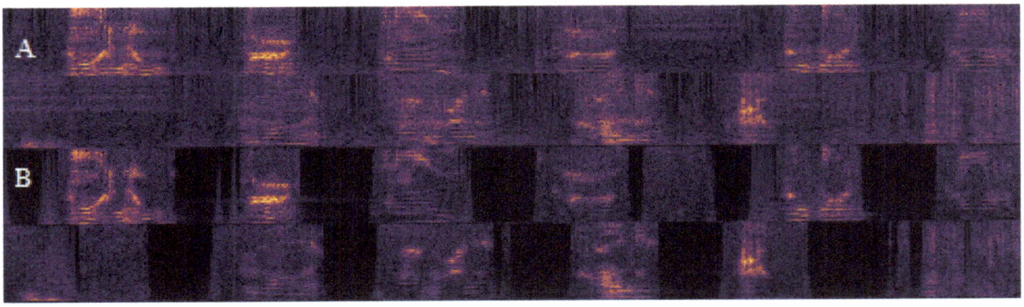

Figure 5. Cochleograms depicting a patient counting to ten with a tracheoesophageal prosthesis before (**A**) and after (**B**) speech-signal optimization. Less additive noise between separate numbers can be observed in the optimized cochleagram.

Table 3 presents the results of statistical tests (Levene's test and t-test) performed on several groups of data (Probability 0, Probability 1, Probability 2, AVE, and ASVI).

Levene's test for equality of variances checks whether the variances are equal across the groups. The null hypothesis is that the variances are equal. If the significance (sig.) is less than the threshold level (commonly 0.05), the null hypothesis is rejected, indicating that the variances are not equal. The choice between "equal variances assumed" and "equal variances not assumed" is determined by the results of Levene's test. If the variances are found to be equal (sig. > 0.05 in Levene's test), then we should refer to the t-test row for "equal variances assumed". If the variances are not equal (sig. < 0.05 in Levene's test), we should refer to the row "equal variances not assumed". The significance for each group of data was as follows:

- Probability 0: sig. = 0.000, indicating that the variances were not equal across groups.
- Probability 1: sig. = 0.454, indicating that the variances were equal.
- Probability 2: sig. = 0.008, indicating that the variances were not equal.
- AVE: sig. = 0.340, indicating equal variances across groups.
- ASVI: sig. = 0.166, indicating equal variances across groups.

The *t*-test for equality of means checks whether the means of two groups are statistically significantly different. The null hypothesis is that the means are equal. If the significance (two-tailed) is less than the threshold level (commonly 0.05), the null hypothesis is rejected. The significance value for each group of data was as follows:

- Probability 0: sig. = 0.036 (for equal variances assumed) and 0.037 (for equal variances not assumed), indicating that the means of the two groups were significantly different.
- Probability 1: sig. = 0.890 (both cases), indicating that the means were not significantly different.
- Probability 2: sig. = 0.163 (both cases), indicating that the means are not significantly different.
- AVE: sig. = 0.750 (both cases), indicating that the means are not significantly different.
- ASVI: sig. = 0.133 (for equal variances assumed) and 0.134 (for equal variances not assumed), indicating that the means are not significantly different.

The mean difference, standard error difference, and 95% confidence interval of the difference provide further details on how the means of the two groups differed and the uncertainty surrounding that difference.

Table 3. Results of statistical tests.

		Levene's Test		*t*-Test for Equality of Means						
		F	Sig.	t	df	Sig. (2-Tailed)	Mean Difference	Std. Error Difference	95% Conf. Int.	
									Lower	Upper
Probability 0	Equal variances assumed	18.313	0.000	−2.113	148	0.036	−9.41893	4.45670	−18.22592	−0.61195
	Equal variances not assumed			−2.113	119.448	0.037	−9.41893	4.45670	−18.24330	−0.59457
Probability 1	Equal variances assumed	0.563	0.454	−0.139	148	0.890	−1.09627	7.87862	−16.66538	14.47284
	Equal variances not assumed			−0.139	147.956	0.890	−1.09627	7.87862	−16.66542	14.47288
Probability 2	Equal variances assumed	7.317	0.008	1.402	148	0.163	10.51547	7.50161	−4.30864	25.33957
	Equal variances not assumed			1.402	146.885	0.163	10.51547	7.50161	−4.30957	25.34050
AVE	Equal variances assumed	0.918	0.340	0.319	148	0.750	0.005560	0.017451	−0.028926	0.040046
	Equal variances not assumed			0.319	147.237	0.750	0.005560	0.017451	−0.028927	0.040047
ASVI	Equal variances assumed	1.941	0.166	−1.509	148	0.133	−1.36607	0.90525	−3.15495	0.42281
	Equal variances not assumed			−1.509	141.961	0.134	−1.36607	0.90525	−3.15558	0.42343

To summarize, as shown in Table 1, the mean AVE of the alaryngeal speech samples decreased from 81 to 80% after optimization. The AVE proportion remained statistically significant and unchanged in the samples before and after Pareto–NMF optimization. This is understandable and expected because the Pareto-optimized NMF approach removed background noise without artificially improving the quality of the alaryngeal speech recordings by filling in the unvoiced speech segments (pauses, intended phonatory breaks, etc.).

Lastly, the speech samples were evaluated using the ASVI, which represents the scale of the objective improvement of the alaryngeal speech signals when comparing the original and Pareto-optimized NMF alaryngeal speech recordings. Although the ASVI was higher in the group after optimization, the difference was not statistically significant. A description of the aforementioned evaluation can be found in Table 1.

5. Discussion

Speech is the complex result of several systems in the body working together. First, the respiratory tract must move air through the larynx and mouth. The vocal folds need to function correctly to produce voice. Speech is produced only when the articulation occurs in the pharynx and mouth and is then processed by the speaker's neural feedback loop, which helps correct the pitch and loudness. Finally, speech is used to communicate, so it has to be pleasant or, at the very least, intelligible to the listener [95]. Disturbances in any of these steps cause various levels of speech impairment.

Total laryngectomy patients often undergo speech rehabilitation programs to learn alternative methods of speech production such as esophageal speech, an electrolarynx, or tracheoesophageal speech with a voice prosthesis. These techniques can generate additional noise during speech production, thereby affecting speech quality and intelligibility. Implementing noise-reduction strategies can help mitigate this issue by improving the overall clarity and naturalness of the patient's speech [7]. However, a speech handicap becomes more problematic when the patient has to use the phone or speak in a loud environment, which may lead to social isolation [14,15].

The suggested Pareto–NMF optimization approach helps mitigate the additive and background noise problem that is common in alaryngeal speakers. The Pareto–NMF optimization removes additive and background noise without impacting the AVE. Although minuscule for a regular speaker, this improvement benefits the TEP speaker significantly. Firstly, total laryngectomy patients often face challenges in making their speech intelligible, especially in noisy environments. Excessive background noise can mask their already limited vocal output, making it difficult for listeners to understand them. By reducing the additional noise present in the environment, speech clarity and intelligibility can be improved, allowing patients to communicate more effectively. Secondly, speaking on the phone can be particularly challenging for individuals after laryngectomy [96]. Background noise, distortions, and limited vocal output can make it difficult for the listener to comprehend the speech. Unwanted noise can be minimized by implementing noise-reduction techniques, enabling clearer and more understandable phone conversations for laryngectomy patients.

Minimal Pareto–NMF optimization impact on speech benefits perfect TEP speakers more, as the spoken segments are largely unaltered and rely solely on the speaker's ability to speak clearly. Patients who have trouble articulating with a TEP could potentially benefit more from Pareto–NMF optimization combined with a speech enhancement model that addresses unvoiced segments, aperiodicity, and phonatory breaks that are more frequent in less experienced alaryngeal speakers.

A typical laryngeal cancer patient eligible for total laryngectomy and TEP rehabilitation is between 50 and 70 years of age and rarely has significant comorbidities [97,98]. After successful treatment, it is reasonable to expect at least a 40% 5-year survival rate. The combination of these conditions leads to a rather specific problem—a large group of patients that are functionally able to return to completely normal life or even the workforce but are held back by their speech disability. Alaryngeal speech enhancement techniques can help mitigate this problem and to allow complete rehabilitation and reintegration for patients after total laryngectomy.

6. Conclusions

Speech after surgical treatment for laryngeal cancer tends to suffer from aperiodicity, phonatory breaks, and additive noise [90]. These findings become more common as more laryngeal structures are removed. However, the adaptive capabilities of patients can result in vastly different acoustical outcomes despite undergoing identical surgery. This is reflected in the relatively high standard deviation observed when evaluating the ASVI of original and optimized speech samples. With this in mind, studies on acoustic speech after laryngeal oncosurgery should be carried out with a greater number of recordings.

Author Contributions: Conceptualization, V.U. and R.M.; Data curation, K.P.; Formal analysis, R.M., R.D., A.K., K.P., N.U.-S. and V.U.; Funding acquisition, V.U.; Investigation, K.P. and N.U.-S.; Methodology, K.P. and V.U.; Project administration, R.M. and V.U.; Resources, R.D., K.P. and V.U.; Software, A.K.; Supervision, R.M.; Validation, R.M., R.D. and K.P.; Visualization, R.D. and K.P.; Writing—original draft, R.M.; Writing—review and editing, R.M., K.P. and R.D. All authors have read and agreed to the published version of the manuscript.

Funding: This project received funding from the European Regional Development Fund (project no. 13.1.1-LMT-K-718-05-0027) under a grant agreement from the Research Council of Lithuania (LMTLT). This project was funded as a measure by the European Union in response to the COVID-19 pandemic.

Institutional Review Board Statement: This study was approved by the Kaunas Regional Ethics Committee for Biomedical Research (2022-04-20 No. BE-2-49).

Informed Consent Statement: Informed consent was obtained from all subjects involved in the study.

Data Availability Statement: The data presented in this study are available in this article.

Acknowledgments: The authors acknowledge the use of artificial intelligence tools for grammar checking and language improvement.

Conflicts of Interest: The authors declare no conflict of interest.

Abbreviations

The following abbreviations are used in this manuscript:

NMF	non-negative matrix factorization
UA-SPEECH	sound dataset
GMM	Gaussian mixture model
SVM	support vector machine
AGMM	adjusted Gaussian mixture model
DSP	digital signal processing
AI	Artificial Intelligence
LMS	least mean square
SNR	signal-to-noise ratio
MSE	mean square error
PSNR	peak signal-to-noise ratio
LPC	linear predictive coding
CNN	convolutional neural network
RNN	recurrent neural network
GAN	generative adversarial network
TEP	tracheoesophageal prosthesis
Prob0	probability of healthy speech
Prob1	probability of speech with a single vocal fold
Prob2	probability of tracheoesophageal speech
AVE	average voicing evidence
ASVI	acoustic substitution voicing index

References

1. Steuer, C.E.; El-Deiry, M.; Parks, J.R.; Higgins, K.A.; Saba, N.F. An update on larynx cancer. *CA Cancer J. Clin.* **2016**, *67*, 31–50. [CrossRef] [PubMed]
2. Groome, P.A.; O'Sullivan, B.; Irish, J.C.; Rothwell, D.M.; Schulze, K.; Warde, P.R.; Schneider, K.M.; Mackenzie, R.G.; Hodson, D.I.; Hammond, J.A.; et al. Management and Outcome Differences in Supraglottic Cancer Between Ontario, Canada, and the Surveillance, Epidemiology, and End Results Areas of the United States. *J. Clin. Oncol.* **2003**, *21*, 496–505. [CrossRef] [PubMed]
3. Groome, P.; Schulze, K.; Keller, S.; Mackillop, W.; O'Sullivan, B.; Irish, J.; Bissett, R.; Dixon, P.; Eapen, L.; Gulavita, S.; et al. Explaining Socioeconomic Status Effects in Laryngeal Cancer. *Clin. Oncol.* **2006**, *18*, 283–292. [CrossRef]
4. Hoffman, H.T.; Porter, K.; Karnell, L.H.; Cooper, J.S.; Weber, R.S.; Langer, C.J.; Ang, K.K.; Gay, G.; Stewart, A.; Robinson, R.A. Laryngeal Cancer in the United States: Changes in Demographics, Patterns of Care, and Survival. *Laryngoscope* **2006**, *116*, 1–13. [CrossRef] [PubMed]

5. Caudell, J.J.; Gillison, M.L.; Maghami, E.; Spencer, S.; Pfister, D.G.; Adkins, D.; Birkeland, A.C.; Brizel, D.M.; Busse, P.M.; Cmelak, A.J.; et al. NCCN Guidelines® Insights: Head and Neck Cancers, Version 1.2022. *J. Natl. Compr. Cancer Netw.* **2022**, *20*, 224–234. [CrossRef]
6. Allegra, E.; Mantia, I.L.; Bianco, M.R.; Drago, G.D.; Fosse, M.C.L.; Azzolina, A.; Grillo, C.; Saita, V. Verbal performance of total laryngectomized patients rehabilitated with esophageal speech and tracheoesophageal speech: Impacts on patient quality of life. *Psychol. Res. Behav. Manag.* **2019**, *12*, 675–681. [CrossRef]
7. van Sluis, K.E.; van der Molen, L.; van Son, R.J.J.H.; Hilgers, F.J.M.; Bhairosing, P.A.; van den Brekel, M.W.M. Objective and subjective voice outcomes after total laryngectomy: A systematic review. *Eur. Arch. Oto-Rhino-Laryngol.* **2017**, *275*, 11–26. [CrossRef]
8. Chakravarty, P.D.; McMurran, A.E.L.; Banigo, A.; Shakeel, M.; Ah-See, K.W. Primary versus secondary tracheoesophageal puncture: Systematic review and meta-analysis. *J. Laryngol. Otol.* **2017**, *132*, 14–21. [CrossRef]
9. Hurren, A.; Miller, N. Voice outcomes post total laryngectomy. *Curr. Opin. Otolaryngol. Head Neck Surg.* **2017**, *25*, 205–210. [CrossRef]
10. Kotby, M.; Hegazi, M.; Kamal, I.; el Dien, N.G.; Nassar, J. Aerodynamics of the Pseudo-Glottis. *Folia Phoniatr. Logop.* **2009**, *61*, 24–28. [CrossRef]
11. Brook, I.; Goodman, J.F. Tracheoesophageal Voice Prosthesis Use and Maintenance in Laryngectomees. *Int. Arch. Otorhinolaryngol.* **2020**, *24*, e535–e538. [CrossRef] [PubMed]
12. de Coul, B.M.R.O.; Hilgers, F.J.M.; Balm, A.J.M.; Tan, I.B.; van den Hoogen, F.J.A.; van Tinteren, H. A Decade of Postlaryngectomy Vocal Rehabilitation in 318 Patients. *Arch. Otolaryngol. Head Neck Surg.* **2000**, *126*, 1320. [CrossRef] [PubMed]
13. Dejonckere, P.H.; Bradley, P.; Clemente, P.; Cornut, G.; Crevier-Buchman, L.; Friedrich, G.; Heyning, P.V.D.; Remacle, M.; Woisard, V. A basic protocol for functional assessment of voice pathology, especially for investigating the efficacy of (phonosurgical) treatments and evaluating new assessment techniques. *Eur. Arch. Oto-Rhino-Laryngol.* **2001**, *258*, 77–82. [CrossRef] [PubMed]
14. Semple, C.; Parahoo, K.; Norman, A.; McCaughan, E.; Humphris, G.; Mills, M. Psychosocial interventions for patients with head and neck cancer. *Cochrane Database Syst. Rev.* **2013**. [CrossRef] [PubMed]
15. Uscher-Pines, L.; Sousa, J.; Raja, P.; Mehrotra, A.; Barnett, M.L.; Huskamp, H.A. Suddenly Becoming a "Virtual Doctor": Experiences of Psychiatrists Transitioning to Telemedicine During the COVID-19 Pandemic. *Psychiatr. Serv.* **2020**, *71*, 1143–1150. [CrossRef]
16. Bohnenkamp, T.A. Postlaryngectomy Respiratory System and Speech Breathing. In *Clinical Care and Rehabilitation in Head and Neck Cancer*; Springer International Publishing: Berlin/Heidelberg, Germany, 2019; pp. 103–117. [CrossRef]
17. Qian, Z.; Niu, H.; Wang, L.; Kobayashi, K.; Zhang, S.; Toda, T. Mandarin Electro-Laryngeal Speech Enhancement based on Statistical Voice Conversion and Manual Tone Control. In Proceedings of the 2021 Asia-Pacific Signal and Information Processing Association Annual Summit and Conference (APSIPA ASC), Tokyo, Japan, 14–17 December 2021; pp. 546–552.
18. Dinh, T.; Kain, A.; Samlan, R.; Cao, B.; Wang, J. Increasing the Intelligibility and Naturalness of Alaryngeal Speech Using Voice Conversion and Synthetic Fundamental Frequency. *Proc. Interspeech* **2020**, *2020*, 4781–4785. [CrossRef]
19. Graham, M.S. Strategies for Excelling With Alaryngeal Speech Methods. *Perspect. Voice Voice Disord.* **2006**, *16*, 25–32. [CrossRef]
20. Kabir, R.; Greenblatt, A.; Panetta, K.; Agaian, S. Enhancement of alaryngeal speech utilizing spectral subtraction and minimum statistics. In Proceedings of the 2008 International Conference on Machine Learning and Cybernetics, Kunming, China, 12–15 July 2008; Volume 7, pp. 3704–3709. [CrossRef]
21. Garg, A.; Sahu, O.P. Enhancement of speech signal using diminished empirical mean curve decomposition-based adaptive Wiener filtering. *Pattern Anal. Appl.* **2019**, *23*, 179–198. [CrossRef]
22. Wang, Q.; Du, X.; Gu, W. A Source-Filter Model-Based Unvoiced Speech Detector for Speech Coding. In Proceedings of the 2nd International Conference on Computer Science and Electronics Engineering (ICCSEE 2013), Hangzhou, China, 22–23 March 2013; Atlantis Press: Dordrecht, The Netherlands, 2013. [CrossRef]
23. Huq, M.; Maskeliunas, R. Speech Enhancement Using Generative Adversarial Network (GAN). In *Hybrid Intelligent Systems*; Springer International Publishing: Berlin/Heidelberg, Germany, 2022; pp. 273–282. [CrossRef]
24. Sack, A.; Jiang, W.; Perlmutter, M.; Salanevich, P.; Needell, D. On Audio Enhancement via Online Non-Negative Matrix Factorization. In Proceedings of the 2022 56th Annual Conference on Information Sciences and Systems (CISS), Princeton, NJ, USA, 9–11 March 2022; pp. 287–291. [CrossRef]
25. Wang, D.; Cui, J.; Wang, J.; Tan, H.; Xu, M. Convex Hull Convolutive Non-negative Matrix Factorization Based Speech Enhancement For Multimedia Communication. In Proceedings of the 2022 6th International Conference on Cryptography, Security and Privacy (CSP), Tianjin, China, 14–16 January 2022; pp. 138–142. [CrossRef]
26. Knollhoff, S.M.; Borrie, S.A.; Barrett, T.S.; Searl, J.P. Listener impressions of alaryngeal communication modalities. *Int. J. Speech-Lang. Pathol.* **2021**, *23*, 540–547. [CrossRef]
27. Mouret, F.; Crevier-Buchman, L.; Pillot-Loiseau, C. Intelligibility of pseudo-whispered speech after total laryngectomy. *Clin. Linguist. Phon.* **2022**, 1–17. [CrossRef]
28. Hui, T.F.; Cox, S.R.; Huang, T.; Chen, W.R.; Ng, M.L. The Effect of Clear Speech on Cantonese Alaryngeal Speakers' Intelligibility. *Folia Phoniatr. Logop.* **2021**, *74*, 103–111. [CrossRef] [PubMed]
29. Aueworakhunanan, T.; Dechongkit, S.; Jeeraumporn, J.; Punkla, W. An Evaluation Pertaining to Esophageal Speech Outcomes in Alaryngeal Patients. *Ramathibodi Med. J.* **2022**, *45*, 16–24. [CrossRef]

30. Cao, B.; Teplansky, K.; Sebkhi, N.; Bhavsar, A.; Inan, O.; Samlan, R.; Mau, T.; Wang, J. Data Augmentation for End-to-end Silent Speech Recognition for Laryngectomees. *Proc. Interspeech* **2022**, *2022*, 3653–3657. [CrossRef]
31. Kent, R.D.; Kim, Y.; mei Chen, L. Oral and Laryngeal Diadochokinesis Across the Life Span: A Scoping Review of Methods, Reference Data, and Clinical Applications. *J. Speech Lang. Hear. Res.* **2022**, *65*, 574–623. [CrossRef]
32. Dahl, K.L.; Bolognone, R.K.; Childes, J.M.; Pryor, R.L.; Graville, D.J.; Palmer, A.D. Characteristics associated with communicative participation after total laryngectomy. *J. Commun. Disord.* **2022**, *96*, 106184. [CrossRef] [PubMed]
33. Roy, N.; Barkmeier-Kraemer, J.; Eadie, T.; Sivasankar, M.P.; Mehta, D.; Paul, D.; Hillman, R. Evidence-Based Clinical Voice Assessment: A Systematic Review. *Am. J. Speech-Lang. Pathol.* **2013**, *22*, 212–226. [CrossRef]
34. Rosdi, F.; Salim, S.S.; Mustafa, M.B. An FPN-based classification method for speech intelligibility detection of children with speech impairments. *Soft Comput.* **2019**, *23*, 2391–2408. [CrossRef]
35. Failla, S.; Al-Zanoon, N.; Smith, N.; Doyle, P.C. The Effects of Contextual Priming and Alaryngeal Speech Mode on Auditory-Perceptual Ratings of Listener Comfort. *J. Voice* **2021**, *35*, 934.e17–934.e23. [CrossRef]
36. Stipancic, K.L.; Tjaden, K. Minimally Detectable Change of Speech Intelligibility in Speakers With Multiple Sclerosis and Parkinson's Disease. *J. Speech Lang. Hear. Res.* **2022**, *65*, 1858–1866. [CrossRef]
37. Malini, S.; Chandrakala, S. Intelligibility assessment of impaired speech using Regularized self-representation based compact supervectors. *Comput. Speech Lang.* **2022**, *74*, 101355. [CrossRef]
38. Albaqshi, H.; Sagheer, A. Dysarthric Speech Recognition using Convolutional Recurrent Neural Networks. *Int. J. Intell. Eng. Syst.* **2020**, *13*, 384–392. [CrossRef]
39. Bessell, N.; Gurd, J.M.; Coleman, J. Dissociation between speech modalities in a case of altered accent with unknown origin. *Clin. Linguist. Phon.* **2020**, *34*, 222–241. [CrossRef] [PubMed]
40. Moon, A.M.; Kim, H.P.; Cook, S.; Blanchard, R.T.; Haley, K.L.; Jacks, A.; Shafer, J.S.; Fried, M.W. Speech patterns and enunciation for encephalopathy determination—A prospective study of hepatic encephalopathy. *Hepatol. Commun.* **2022**, *6*, 2876–2885. [CrossRef] [PubMed]
41. De Cock, E.; Oostra, K.; Bliki, L.; Volkaerts, A.; Hemelsoet, D.; De Herdt, V.; Batens, K. Dysarthria following acute ischemic stroke: Prospective evaluation of characteristics, type and severity. *Int. J. Lang. Commun. Disord.* **2021**, *56*, 549–557. [CrossRef]
42. Rowe, H.P.; Gutz, S.E.; Maffei, M.F.; Tomanek, K.; Green, J.R. Characterizing Dysarthria Diversity for Automatic Speech Recognition: A Tutorial From the Clinical Perspective. *Front. Comput. Sci.* **2022**, *4*, 770210. [CrossRef]
43. Stipancic, K.L.; van Brenk, F.; Kain, A.; Wilding, G.; Tjaden, K. Clear Speech Variants: An Investigation of Intelligibility and Speaker Effort in Speakers With Parkinson's Disease. *Am. J. Speech-Lang. Pathol.* **2022**, *31*, 2789–2805. [CrossRef]
44. Rosdi, F.; Mustafa, M.B.; Salim, S.S.; Mat Zin, N.A. Automatic speech intelligibility detection for speakers with speech impairments: The identification of significant speech features. *Sains Malays.* **2019**, *48*, 2737–2747. [CrossRef]
45. Maskeliūnas, R.; Kulikajevas, A.; Damaševičius, R.; Pribuišis, K.; Ulozaitė-Stanienė, N.; Uloza, V. Lightweight Deep Learning Model for Assessment of Substitution Voicing and Speech after Laryngeal Carcinoma Surgery. *Cancers* **2022**, *14*, 2366. [CrossRef]
46. Kim, H.; Jeon, J.; Han, Y.J.; Joo, Y.; Lee, J.; Lee, S.; Im, S. Convolutional Neural Network Classifies Pathological Voice Change in Laryngeal Cancer with High Accuracy. *J. Clin. Med.* **2020**, *9*, 3415. [CrossRef]
47. Feng, Y.; Chen, F.; Ma, J.; Wang, L.; Peng, G. Production of Mandarin consonant aspiration and monophthongs in children with Autism Spectrum Disorder. *Clin. Linguist. Phon.* **2022**. [CrossRef]
48. Vieira, S.T.; Rosa, R.L.; Rodrguez, D.Z. A speech quality classifier based on tree-cnn algorithm that considers network degradations. *J. Commun. Softw. Syst.* **2020**, *16*, 180–187. [CrossRef]
49. Poncelet, J.; Renkens, V.; Van hamme, H. Low resource end-to-end spoken language understanding with capsule networks. *Comput. Speech Lang.* **2021**, *66*, 101142. [CrossRef]
50. Cave, R.; Bloch, S. The use of speech recognition technology by people living with amyotrophic lateral sclerosis: A scoping review. *Disabil. Rehabil. Assist. Technol.* **2021**. [CrossRef] [PubMed]
51. Schultz, B.G.; Tarigoppula, V.S.A.; Noffs, G.; Rojas, S.; van der Walt, A.; Grayden, D.B.; Vogel, A.P. Automatic speech recognition in neurodegenerative disease. *Int. J. Speech Technol.* **2021**, *24*, 771–779. [CrossRef]
52. Gupta, S.; Patil, A.T.; Purohit, M.; Parmar, M.; Patel, M.; Patil, H.A.; Guido, R.C. Residual Neural Network precisely quantifies dysarthria severity-level based on short-duration speech segments. *Neural Netw.* **2021**, *139*, 105–117. [CrossRef]
53. Latha, M.; Shivakumar, M.; Manjula, G.; Hemakumar, M.; Kumar, M.K. Deep Learning-Based Acoustic Feature Representations for Dysarthric Speech Recognition. *SN Comput. Sci.* **2023**, *4*, 272. [CrossRef]
54. Vishnika Veni, S.; Chandrakala, S. Investigation of DNN-HMM and Lattice Free Maximum Mutual Information Approaches for Impaired Speech Recognition. *IEEE Access* **2021**, *9*, 168840–168849.
55. Chandrakala, S.; Malini, S.; Veni, S.V. Histogram of States Based Assistive System for Speech Impairment Due to Neurological Disorders. *IEEE Trans. Neural Syst. Rehabil. Eng.* **2021**, *29*, 2425–2434. [CrossRef]
56. Srinivasan, M.; Shanmuganathan, C.; Gupta, S.M.K.; Sikkandar, M.Y. Multi-view representation based speech assisted system for people with neurological disorders. *J. Ambient. Intell. Humaniz. Comput.* **2021**. [CrossRef]
57. Chandrakala, S.; Malini, S.; Jayalakshmi, S.L. Bag of Models Based Embeddings for Assessment of Neurological Disorders Using Speech Intelligibility. *IEEE Trans. Emerg. Top. Comput.* **2021**, *9*, 1265–1275. [CrossRef]
58. Fu, J.; Yang, S.; He, F.; He, L.; Li, Y.; Zhang, J.; Xiong, X. Sch-net: A deep learning architecture for automatic detection of schizophrenia. *BioMed. Eng. Online* **2021**, *20*, 75. [CrossRef] [PubMed]

59. Marini, M.; Vanello, N.; Fanucci, L. Optimising speaker-dependent feature extraction parameters to improve automatic speech recognition performance for people with dysarthria. *Sensors* **2021**, *21*, 6460. [CrossRef] [PubMed]
60. Mathew, L.R.; Gopakumar, K. Evaluation of speech enhancement algorithms applied to electrolaryngeal speech degraded by noise. *Appl. Acoust.* **2021**, *174*, 107771. [CrossRef]
61. Ishikawa, K.; Boyce, S.; Kelchner, L.; Powell, M.G.; Schieve, H.; de Alarcon, A.; Khosla, S. The Effect of Background Noise on Intelligibility of Dysphonic Speech. *J. Speech Lang. Hear. Res.* **2017**, *60*, 1919–1929. [CrossRef] [PubMed]
62. Dhivya, R.; Justin, J. Performance Evaluation of a Speech Enhancement Technique Using Wavelets. In *Proceedings of the International Conference on Soft Computing Systems;* Springer: New Delhi, India, 2015; pp. 637–646. [CrossRef]
63. Jaiswal, R.K.; Yeduri, S.R.; Cenkeramaddi, L.R. Single-channel speech enhancement using implicit Wiener filter for high-quality speech communication. *Int. J. Speech Technol.* **2022**, *25*, 745–758. [CrossRef]
64. Pauline, S.H.; Dhanalakshmi, S.; Kumar, R.; Narayanamoorthi, R. Noise reduction in speech signal of Parkinson's Disease (PD) patients using optimal variable stage cascaded adaptive filter configuration. *Biomed. Signal Process. Control* **2022**, *77*, 103802. [CrossRef]
65. Doi, H.; Toda, T.; Nakamura, K.; Saruwatari, H.; Shikano, K. Alaryngeal Speech Enhancement Based on One-to-Many Eigenvoice Conversion. *IEEE/ACM Trans. Audio Speech Lang. Process.* **2014**, *22*, 172–183. [CrossRef]
66. Pauline, S.H.; Dhanalakshmi, S. A low-cost automatic switched adaptive filtering technique for denoising impaired speech signals. *Multidimens. Syst. Signal Process.* **2022**, *33*, 1387–1408. [CrossRef]
67. Pandey, P.; Bhandarkar, S.; Bachher, G.; Lehana, P. Enhancement of alaryngeal speech using spectral subtraction. In Proceedings of the 2002 14th International Conference on Digital Signal Processing Proceedings. DSP 2002 (Cat. No.02TH8628), Santorini, Greece, 1–3 July 2002; Volume 2, pp. 591–594. [CrossRef]
68. Azarnoush, H.; Mir, F.; Agaian, S.; Jamshidi, M.; Shadaram, M. Alaryngeal Speech Enhancement Using Minimum Statistics Approach to Spectral Subtraction. In Proceedings of the 2007 IEEE International Conference on System of Systems Engineering, San Antonio, TX, USA, 16–18 April 2007; pp. 1–5. [CrossRef]
69. Wei, Y.; Li, C.; Li, T.; Zeng, Y. Whispered Speech Enhancement Based on Improved Mel Frequency Scale and Modified Compensated Phase Spectrum. *Circuits Syst. Signal Process.* **2019**, *38*, 5839–5860. [CrossRef]
70. Mollaei, F.; Shiller, D.M.; Baum, S.R.; Gracco, V.L. The Relationship Between Speech Perceptual Discrimination and Speech Production in Parkinson's Disease. *J. Speech Lang. Hear. Res.* **2019**, *62*, 4256–4268. [CrossRef]
71. Giri, M.; Rayavarapu, N. Improving the intelligibility of dysarthric speech using a time domain pitch synchronous-based approach. *Int. J. Electr. Comput. Eng.* **2023**, *13*, 4041–4051. [CrossRef]
72. Ishaq, R.; Shahid, M.; Lövström, B.; Zapirain, B.G.; Claesson, I. Modulation frequency domain adaptive gain equalizer using convex optimization. In Proceedings of the 2012 6th International Conference on Signal Processing and Communication Systems, Gold Coast, QLD, Australia, 12–14 December 2012; pp. 1–5. [CrossRef]
73. Vijayan, K.; Murty, K.S.R. Prosody Modification Using Allpass Residual of Speech Signals. *Proc. Interspeech* **2016**, *2016*, 1069–1073. [CrossRef]
74. Bhangale, K.B.; Kothandaraman, M. Survey of Deep Learning Paradigms for Speech Processing. *Wirel. Pers. Commun.* **2022**, *125*, 1913–1949. [CrossRef]
75. Kobayashi, K.; Toda, T. Implementation of low-latency electrolaryngeal speech enhancement based on multi-task CLDNN. In Proceedings of the 2020 28th European Signal Processing Conference (EUSIPCO), Amsterdam, The Netherlands, 18–21 January 2021; pp. 396–400. [CrossRef]
76. Saleem, N.; Khattak, M.I.; Alqahtani, S.A.; Jan, A.; Hussain, I.; Khan, M.N.; Dahshan, M. U-Shaped Low-Complexity Type-2 Fuzzy LSTM Neural Network for Speech Enhancement. *IEEE Access* **2023**, *11*, 20814–20826. [CrossRef]
77. Huq, M. Enhancement of Alaryngeal Speech using Generative Adversarial Network (GAN). In Proceedings of the 2021 IEEE/ACS 18th International Conference on Computer Systems and Applications (AICCSA), Tangier, Morocco, 30 November–3 December 2021; pp. 1–2. [CrossRef]
78. Pascual, S.; Bonafonte, A.; Serrà, J.; Gonzalez, J.A. Whispered-to-voiced Alaryngeal Speech Conversion with Generative Adversarial Networks. *arXiv* **2018**, arXiv:1808.10687.
79. Pascual, S.; Serrà, J.; Bonafonte, A. Towards Generalized Speech Enhancement with Generative Adversarial Networks. *arXiv* **2019**, arXiv:1904.03418.
80. Amarjouf, M.; Bahja, F.; Di-Martino, J.; Chami, M.; Ibn-Elhaj, E.H. Predicted Phase Using Deep Neural Networks to Enhance Esophageal Speech. In *Lecture Notes on Data Engineering and Communications Technologies*; Springer Nature: Cham, Switzerland, 2023; pp. 68–76. [CrossRef]
81. Subramanian, A.S.; Wang, X.; Baskar, M.K.; Watanabe, S.; Taniguchi, T.; Tran, D.; Fujita, Y. Speech Enhancement Using End-to-End Speech Recognition Objectives. In Proceedings of the 2019 IEEE Workshop on Applications of Signal Processing to Audio and Acoustics (WASPAA), New Paltz, NY, USA, 20–23 October 2019; pp. 234–238. [CrossRef]
82. Muthusamy, H.; Polat, K.; Yaacob, S. Improved Emotion Recognition Using Gaussian Mixture Model and Extreme Learning Machine in Speech and Glottal Signals. *Math. Probl. Eng.* **2015**, *2015*, 394083. [CrossRef]
83. Li, M.; Wang, L.; Xu, Z.; Cai, D. Mandarin electrolaryngeal voice conversion with combination of Gaussian mixture model and non-negative matrix factorization. In Proceedings of the 2017 Asia-Pacific Signal and Information Processing Association Annual Summit and Conference (APSIPA ASC), Kuala Lumpur, Malaysia, 12–15 December 2017; pp. 1360–1363. [CrossRef]

84. Xu, T.; Feng, K.; Ge, Y.; Zhang, X.; Tao, Z. Identification of vocal nodules and laryngitis by Gauss mixture model. In Proceedings of the 2017 4th International Conference on Systems and Informatics (ICSAI), Hangzhou, China, 11–13 November 2017; pp. 1098–1102. [CrossRef]
85. Areiza-Laverde, H.J.; Castro-Ospina, A.E.; Peluffo-Ordóñez, D.H. Voice Pathology Detection Using Artificial Neural Networks and Support Vector Machines Powered by a Multicriteria Optimization Algorithm. In *Communications in Computer and Information Science*; Springer International Publishing: Berlin/Heidelberg, Germany, 2018; pp. 148–159. [CrossRef]
86. Das, N.; Chakraborty, S.; Chaki, J.; Padhy, N.; Dey, N. Fundamentals, present and future perspectives of speech enhancement. *Int. J. Speech Technol.* **2020**, *24*, 883–901. [CrossRef]
87. Lee, S.H.; Kim, M.; Seo, H.G.; Oh, B.M.; Lee, G.; Leigh, J.H. Assessment of Dysarthria Using One-Word Speech Recognition with Hidden Markov Models. *J. Korean Med. Sci.* **2019**, *34*, e108. [CrossRef]
88. van Sluis, K.E.; van Son, R.J.J.H.; van der Molen, L.; MCGuinness, A.J.; Palme, C.E.; Novakovic, D.; Stone, D.; Natsis, L.; Charters, E.; Jones, K.; et al. Multidimensional evaluation of voice outcomes following total laryngectomy: A prospective multicenter cohort study. *Eur. Arch. Oto-Rhino-Laryngol.* **2020**, *278*, 1209–1222. [CrossRef]
89. Succo, G.; Peretti, G.; Piazza, C.; Remacle, M.; Eckel, H.E.; Chevalier, D.; Simo, R.; Hantzakos, A.G.; Rizzotto, G.; Lucioni, M.; et al. Open partial horizontal laryngectomies: A proposal for classification by the working committee on nomenclature of the European Laryngological Society. *Eur. Arch. Oto-Rhino-Laryngol.* **2014**, *271*, 2489–2496. [CrossRef] [PubMed]
90. Dejonckere, P.H.; Moerman, M.B.J.; Martens, J.P.; Schoentgen, J.; Manfredi, C. Voicing quantification is more relevant than period perturbation in substitution voices: An advanced acoustical study. *Eur. Arch. Oto-Rhino-Laryngol.* **2012**, *269*, 1205–1212. [CrossRef] [PubMed]
91. Maskeliūnas, R.; Damaševičius, R.; Kulikajevas, A.; Padervinskis, E.; Pribuišis, K.; Uloza, V. A Hybrid U-Lossian Deep Learning Network for Screening and Evaluating Parkinson's Disease. *Appl. Sci.* **2022**, *12*, 11601. [CrossRef]
92. Moerman, M.; Martens, J.P.; Dejonckere, P. Multidimensional assessment of strongly irregular voices such as in substitution voicing and spasmodic dysphonia: A compilation of own research. *Logop. Phoniatr. Vocology* **2014**, *40*, 24–29. [CrossRef]
93. Uloza, V.; Maskeliunas, R.; Pribuisis, K.; Vaitkus, S.; Kulikajevas, A.; Damasevicius, R. An Artificial Intelligence-Based Algorithm for the Assessment of Substitution Voicing. *Appl. Sci.* **2022**, *12*, 9748. [CrossRef]
94. Campbell, I. Chi-squared and Fisher–Irwin tests of two-by-two tables with small sample recommendations. *Stat. Med.* **2007**, *26*, 3661–3675. [CrossRef]
95. Schindler, A.; Mozzanica, F.; Ginocchio, D.; Invernizzi, A.; Peri, A.; Ottaviani, F. Voice-related quality of life in patients after total and partial laryngectomy. *Auris Nasus Larynx* **2012**, *39*, 77–83. [CrossRef]
96. Teruya, N.; Sunagawa, Y.; Toyosato, T.; Yokota, T. Association between Daily Life Difficulties and Acceptance of Disability in Cancer Survivors after Total Laryngectomy: A Cross-Sectional Survey. *Asia-Pac. J. Oncol. Nurs.* **2019**, *6*, 170–176. [CrossRef]
97. Lin, Z.; Lin, H.; Chen, Y.; Xu, Y.; Chen, X.; Fan, H.; Wu, X.; Ke, X.; Lin, C. Long-term survival trend after primary total laryngectomy for patients with locally advanced laryngeal carcinoma. *J. Cancer* **2021**, *12*, 1220–1230. [CrossRef]
98. Birkeland, A.C.; Beesley, L.; Bellile, E.; Rosko, A.J.; Hoesli, R.; Chinn, S.B.; Shuman, A.G.; Prince, M.E.; Wolf, G.T.; Bradford, C.R.; et al. Predictors of survival after total laryngectomy for recurrent/persistent laryngeal squamous cell carcinoma. *Head Neck* **2017**, *39*, 2512–2518. [CrossRef]

cancers

MDPI

Communication

Statin Medication Improves Five-Year Survival Rates in Patients with Head and Neck Cancer: A Retrospective Case-Control Study of about 100,000 Patients

Jonas Wüster [1], Max Heiland [1], Susanne Nahles [1], Robert Preissner [2,†] and Saskia Preissner [1,*,†]

1 Department of Oral and Maxillofacial Surgery, Charité—Universitätsmedizin Berlin, Corporate Member of Freie Universität Berlin, Humboldt-Universität zu Berlin, and Berlin Institute of Health, Augustenburger Platz 1, 13353 Berlin, Germany; jonas.wuester@charite.de (J.W.)

2 Institute of Physiology and Science-IT, Charité—Universitätsmedizin Berlin, Corporate Member of Freie Universität Berlin, Humboldt-Universität zu Berlin, and Berlin Institute of Health, Philippstr. 12, 10115 Berlin, Germany; robert.preissner@charite.de

* Correspondence: saskia.preissner@charite.de; Tel.: +49-30-450-655-208

† The authors contributed equally to this work.

Simple Summary: Usually: statins are prescribed to lower cholesterol levels. Besides, various studies showed that statins have beneficial effects on cancer prevention and treatment. We investigated the effect of statin medication in patients with head and neck cancer in a real-world cohort from a federated network of more than 80 healthcare organizations. We created two cohorts diagnosed with head and neck cancer, with similar age, sex, and risk factors like alcohol and nicotine. Cohort I received statins and cohort II did not. Both cohorts contained about 50,000 patients. We performed a survival analysis and found five-year survival was to be significantly higher for cohort I and a lower risk of death, respectively. As our analysis was conducted retrospectively, the results need further clinical research to be confirmed.

Abstract: Introduction: The overall survival among head and neck cancer patients is still low, even in a time of new therapy regimes. Regarding cancer patients' survival, statin use has already proven to be associated with favorable survival outcomes. Our objective was to investigate the influence of statin medication on the overall survival of head and neck cancer patients. Methods: Retrospective clinical data of patients diagnosed with head and neck cancer (International Classification of Diseases codes: C00–C14) were retrieved from a real-world evidence database. The initial cohort was divided into patients with statin medication, who were assigned to building cohort I, and subjects without statin medication, who were assigned to cohort II, both matched by age, gender, and risk factors (nicotine and alcohol abuse/dependence). Subsequently, Kaplan–Meier and risk analyses were performed, and odds and hazard ratios were calculated. Results: After matching, each cohort contained 48,626 patients (cohort I = females: 15,409; (31.7%), males 33,212 (68.3%); mean age ± standard deviation (SD) at diagnosis 66.3 ± 11.4 years; cohort II = females: 15,432; (31.7%), males 33,187 (68.2%); mean age ± standard deviation (SD) at diagnosis 66.4 ± 11.5 years). Five-year survival was found to be significantly higher for cohort I, with 75.19%, respectively 70.48% for cohort II. These findings were correlated significantly with a risk of death of 15.9% (cohort I) and 17.2% (cohort II); the odds ratio was 0.91 (95% CI: 0.881–0.942) and the hazard ratio 0.80 (0.777–0.827). Conclusions: The results indicate that the five-year survival of head and neck cancer patients is significantly improved by statin medication. As this study was conducted retrospectively, our data must be interpreted with caution, especially since other potential influencing factors and the initial tumor stage were not available.

Keywords: statins; head and neck cancer; HNSCC; OSCC; survival; real-world data

1. Introduction

Head and neck cancers (HNC) are the seventh-most-common tumors worldwide, including all epithelial malignancies of the oral cavity, pharynx (subdivision into naso-, oro-, and hypopharynx), larynx, nasal cavity, paranasal sinus, and salivary glands [1–3]. Apart from HNC related to heavy tobacco and/or alcohol consumption [2,4], HPV-associated HNC has increased, especially HPV-positive oropharyngeal squamous cell cancer (OPSCC) among younger people [5]. Lately, due to improved radiotherapy, the introduction of concurrent radio-sensitizing systemic therapy and definitive radiotherapy/chemoradiotherapy, the survival of patients with HNC, particularly in HPV-positive OPSCC patients, has increased noticeably [2,5].

With their lipid-lowering characteristics, statins are often used to reduce cholesterol blood levels in heart disease(s) and stroke prevention [6,7]. This effect is achieved through competitive inhibition of the enzyme, 3-hydroxy-3-methylglutaryl-coenzyme A reductase (HMG-CoA reductase; HMGCR), the key enzyme of the cholesterol synthesis pathway [7]. The structural similarity between the acid form of statins and HMG-CoA as the natural substrate of HMGCR allows the inhibition of this process [7]. Normally, the conversion of 3-hydroxy-3-methylglutaryl-coenzyme A (HMG-CoA) into mevalonate is catalyzed by HMGCR [7]. Decreasing mevalonate levels result in a higher expression of low-density lipoprotein (LDL) receptors on the cell surface and consequently, in an increased LDL catabolism [7,8]. In addition, (clinical) data have revealed that some statins are capable of inhibiting the synthesis of LDL in the liver through the prevention of very-low-density lipoprotein (VLDL) synthesis. Furthermore, some statins increase the level of high-density lipoprotein (HDL) [7,9]. Regarding the influence of statins on cancer in general, recent data suggest suppression of tumor growth, metastasis, and induction of apoptosis for statins [10–12]. Moreover, metabolic modulation in tumors has been found to be induced by statins through inhibition of monocarboxylate transporter function [13]. Furthermore, chemopreventive effects on different solid tumors have been detected, which are probably achieved via arresting cell cycle progression, inducing apoptosis, inhibiting angiogenesis, and immunomodulation [11]. Additionally, statins may disrupt the crosstalk of cancer cells and the tumor microenvironment, which inhibits tumor progression [14,15]. Various studies have examined the in vitro effect of statins on head and neck cancer squamous cell carcinomas (HNSCC); here, statins have proven to be (dose-dependent) cytotoxic to HNSCC cells and to have reduced cell viability to less than 50% in HNSCC cell lines [16–20]. Recent in vitro studies suggest that cell cycle regulation and apoptosis follow persistence in the G0/G1 phase of HNSCC cells [21,22]. Clinical data on the influence of statins in cancer patients exist, e.g., for pancreatic cancer [23], lung cancer [24], and gynecological cancer [15], but data for statin use and the potential influence in HNC patients' survival are still rare. Only a few clinical studies have focused on statin use and the potential influence on survival outcomes in HNC. Patients with hyperlipidemia and statin use at the time of diagnosis showed improved overall and cancer-specific survival compared to patients with hyperlipidemia and not taking a statin, as well as patients with hyperlipidemia and no statin use [25]. For HPV-negative HNSCC, Lebo et al. showed that patients with statins had better overall and disease-specific survival than those who were not taking a statin at or before cancer diagnosis [26,27]. Getz et al. confirmed the potential beneficial effect of statin medication on overall survival for patients suffering from HNSCC [28]. Here, a subdivision was made to examine the effect of statins on HPV-negative and HPV-positive tumors separately, revealing new findings: a protective association between statin use and disease-specific death and recurrence that was restricted to HPV-positive patients [28].

Aiming to add further insights to the relationship between statins and HNC, this study investigates the impact of statin medication in HNC patients on the clinical outcome (five-year survival) in a large case-control study. In this context, the TriNetX Global Health Research Network (TriNetX, Cambridge, MA, USA), a real-world database, was selected to gain data on this subject.

2. Materials and Methods

2.1. Ethics Statement

By the local legislation and institutional requirements, no ethical review/approval was required, due to the retrospective nature of the study and the de-identification of the data. Likewise, written informed consent was not required following the national legislation and the institutional requirements.

2.2. Data Acquisition, Inclusion and Exclusion Criteria, and Patient Matching

The TriNetX Global Health Research Network provides access to medical records from more than 80 healthcare organizations (HCOs) in 30 countries, enabling the collection and exchange of longitudinal clinical data between contract research institutes and pharmaceutical companies. At the time of data acquisition, electronic medical records of more than 250 million individuals were collected and available for statistical analysis, as implemented in previous studies [29,30]. The TriNetX database was searched for individuals who were diagnosed with HNC (International Classification of Diseases (ICD)-10 codes C00–C14 5 to 20 years before the access date (27 January 2023)). To be included, patients' medical records had to cover at least five years (1825 days) of follow-up after visiting the HCO for an inpatient encounter. Medical records older than 20 years were not included. Patients with statin medication were assigned to cohort I (subjects with ICD-10 codes C00–C14 and medication of Rosuvastatin, Simvastatin, Fluvastatin, Pravastatin, Lovastatin, Atorvastatin, and Pitavastatin). Further, cohort II was formed of subjects who were diagnosed with ICD-10 codes C00–C14 and no history of statin medication. As in previous studies, one-to-one matching was performed for age, gender, and tobacco and/or alcohol abuse (ICD-10: Z87.891, F10.1, or F10.2) to receive randomized conditions as closely as possible by obtaining cohorts with similar covariate distributions [29,30].

2.3. Data Analysis

The primary outcome was defined as "death" with subsequent calculation of Kaplan–Meier survival analysis, Cox proportional hazards regression, risk ratios (RR), odds ratios (OR), and hazard ratios (HR) for each cohort. Data analysis was limited to a period of 5 years after the first HNC diagnosis, as patients are regarded as healed in case of absence/no recurrence of HNC or metastases within the defined period. Statistical analysis was performed using the log-rank test, whereby the probability level for statistical significance was set at 5% ($p = 0.05$). Before matching, 136,755 patients were assigned to cohort II. Subsequently, with one-to-one matching, the same number of patients as in cohort I (n = 48,626 patients) were assigned to cohort II (Figure 1).

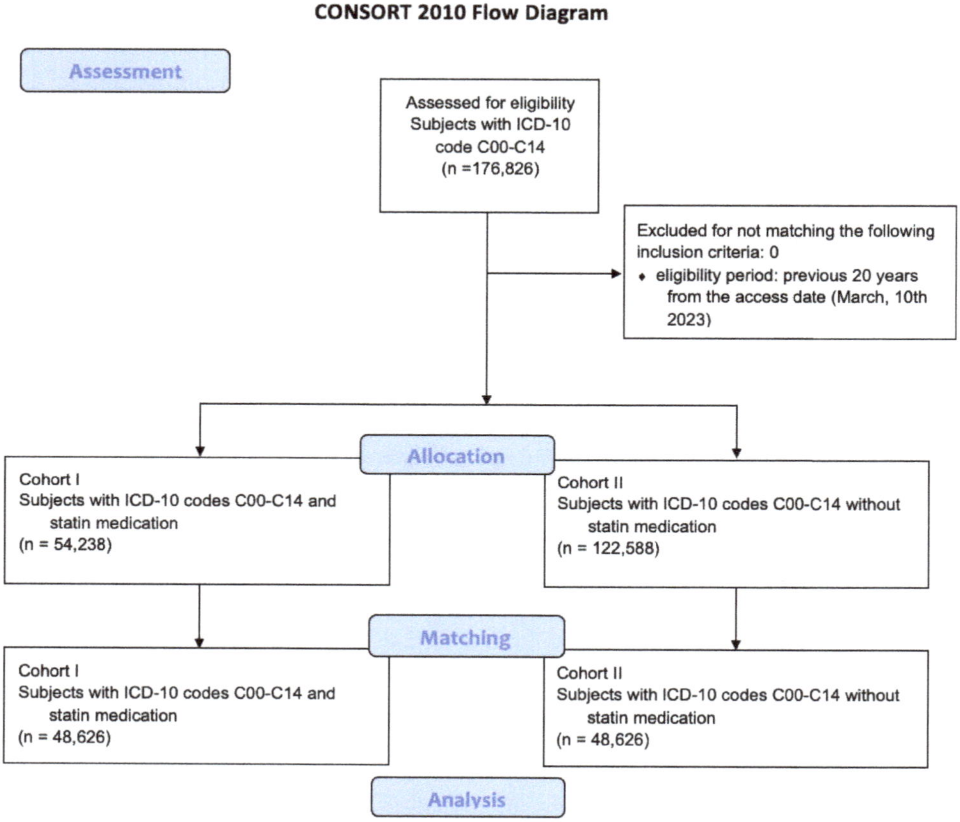

Figure 1. Modified CONSORT flowchart.

3. Results

3.1. Assessment, Allocation, and Matching

Overall, 176,826 patients from 73 HCOs met the inclusion criteria (ICD-10 codes C00-C14) and could be retrieved from the database. Firstly, cohort I was defined by the use of statins, which led to a cohort of 54,238 patients (females: 16,966 (31.3%), males 7309 (68.7%), mean age ± standard deviation (SD) 67.7 ± 11.2 years). All patients who met the inclusion criteria and had no history of statin medication were assigned to cohort II, resulting in a cohort of 122,588 patients (females: 37,309 (33.0%), males 82,100 (67.0%), mean age 58.5 ± 16.7 years). Subsequently, using propensity score matching, 48,626 patients were assigned to each cohort, which led to cohorts as follows:

Cohort I with 15,409 (31.7%) females, 33,212 (68.3%) males and a mean age at diagnosis of 66.3 ± 11.4 years. Within the cohort, I, 5710 patients (11.7%) with ICD-10 code Z87.891, 2088 patients (4.3%) with ICD-10 code F10.1, and 1689 patients (3.5%) with ICD-10 code F10.2 were found.

Cohort II with 15,432 (31.7%) females, 33,187 (68.2%) males and a mean age of 66.4 ± 11.5 years. Here, 5596 patients (11.5%) with ICD-10 code Z87.891, 2047 patients (4.2%) with ICD-10 code F10.1, and 1658 patients (3.4%) with ICD-10 code F10.2 were found. The patient characteristics of cohort I and cohort II, before and after matching, are listed in Table 1.

Table 1. Characteristics of cohort I and cohort II, before and after matching for age, gender, tobacco use, and alcohol abuse. Note that some patients have indeterminate gender.

	Before Matching				After Matching			
Patients (n)	**Cohort I**	**Cohort II**	***p*-Value**	**Standardized Mean Difference**	**Cohort I**	**Cohort II**	***p*-Value**	**Standardized Mean Difference**
Total	54,238	122,588	<0.001	0.582	48,626	48,626	0.189	0.008
Female	16,966 (31.3%)	37,309 (33.0%)	<0.001	0.038	15,409 (31.7%)	15,432 (31.7%)	0.874	0.001
Male	37,309 (68.7%)	82,100 (67.0%)	<0.001	0.038	33,212 (68.3%)	33,187 (68.2%)	0.863	0.001
Mean age at diagnosis (years)	66.7	58.5			66.3	66.4		
Standard deviation	11.2	16.7			11.4	11.5		
ICD-10 Z87.891	11,307 (20.8%)	5935 (4.8%)	<0.001	0.0492	5710 (11.7%)	5596 (11.5%)	0.254	0.007
ICD-10 F10.1	2839 (5.2%)	2935 (2.4%)	<0.001	0.149	2088 (4.3%)	2.047 (4.2%)	0.515	0.004
ICD-10 F10.2	2348 (4.3%)	2520 (2.1%)	<0.001	0.129	1689 (3.5%)	1658 (3.4%)	0.586	0.003

3.2. Patient Survival

During the five-year observation period after the initial diagnosis of HNC, 7719 patients in cohort I and 8344 patients in cohort II died. These findings correlate with a risk of death of 15.9% (cohort I) and 17.2% (cohort II). The survival probability at the end of the time window was 75.19% for cohort I and 70.48% for cohort II, as seen in Figure 2. The related risk ratio (RR) was 0.925 (95% confidence interval (CI): 0.899–0.952), and the odds ratio (OR) and hazard ratio (HR) were 0.991 (95% CI: 0.881–0.942) and 0.801 (95% CI: 0.777–0.827) (Figure 3).

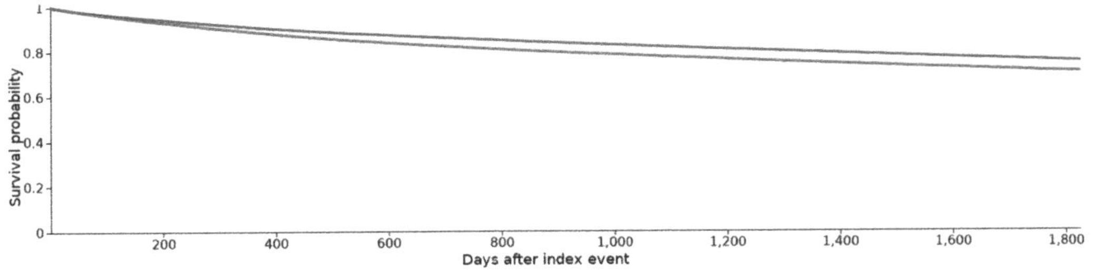

Figure 2. Kaplan–Meier survival curves for both cohorts. Cohort I (ICD-10 codes C00-C14 and statin medication; purple) and cohort II (ICD-10 codes C00-C14 without statin medication; green).

Cohort	Patients in Cohort	Patients with Outcome	Risk
ICD C00-C14 with statins	48,626	7719	15.9%
ICD C00-C14 without statins	48,626	8344	17.2%

Risk Difference	Risk Difference 95% CI	z	p	Risk Ratio	Risk Ratio 95% CI	Odds Ratio	Odds Ratio 95% CI
1.3%	(−1.8%; −0.8%)	−5.397	0.000	0.925	(0.899; 0.952)	0.911	(0.881; 0.942)

Figure 3. Risk of death, risk ratios, and odds ratio of cohort I (ICD codes C00–C14 with statin use) and cohort II (ICD codes C00–C14 without statin use).

4. Discussion

The present study investigated the relationship between statin medication on the five-year survival rate in HNC patients. To the best of the authors' knowledge, this study was the first to address this question by evaluating data retrospectively in larger cohorts. Our data indicate considerable benefits regarding the survival probability for HNC patients with statin medication compared to HNC patients without statin medication.

Recently, a growing interest in statins has arisen since statin use and its beneficial influence on cancer survival outcomes have been evaluated in previous studies [31–33]. In this context, most studies have revealed higher survival rates for patients with statin use, regardless of the cancer type [31–35]. Our retrospective study focused on patients with pre-diagnostic statin use that continued during the post-diagnostic stage, which makes the study comparable to the study design of most other studies [36,37] that have dealt with the influence of statins on cancer. Nevertheless, other findings suggest that statin use even after cancer diagnosis seems to be related to reducing overall and cancer-specific mortality [38], or even reveal that statin users after diagnosis had higher overall survival than those before diagnosis and current users [24]. Since this observation refers to patients with lung cancer, further studies might investigate whether the date of statin exposure and the influence on survival also applies to HNC patients. Besides statins, another effective cholesterol inhibitor has come into focus: ezetimibe, which is recommended in the current guidelines and increasingly used for the treatment of hypercholesterinemia, alone or in combination with statins, in the prevention of cardiovascular disease events [39–41]. Ezetimibe achieves its cholesterol-lowering effect by blocking the sterol transporter Niemann–Pick C1-Like 1 (NPC1L1), a key regulator of intestinal cholesterol uptake [39,42]. The latest in vitro and in vivo studies have shown that ezetimibe is capable of inhibiting prostate cancer [43] and pancreatic cancer, and protects against colitis-associated tumorigenesis [44]. Other cholesterol-lowering drugs, such as proprotein convertase subtilisin/kexin type 9 (PCSK9) inhibitors, seem to potentiate immune checkpoint therapy in cancer patients [45] and might even be used as a potential future therapeutic target in personalized cancer medicine [46]. Nevertheless, available studies still lack data about rarely used cholesterol-lowering medication. Therefore, further studies are required to investigate the influence of such medication on the survival of HNC patients.

Regarding HNC, our findings provide first clinical data on statin use and the prognostic value in HNC in a large cohort, and lead to the conclusion that statin use in HNC patients correlates with higher five-year survival. These findings support previous studies on the relationship between statin use and HNC [25–28]. In 2018, the first connection of statin use and improved overall and disease-specific survival in HPV-negative HNSCC patients, when compared to those who were not taking a statin at or before cancer diagnosis, was shown [27]. Getz et al. confirmed these findings for statin use and improved HNSCC overall survival and further compared the influence of statin medication on the outcome of

HPV-negative and -positive HNSCC. Here, an inverse association between statin use and cancer-specific death was seen only in the HPV-positive cohort, which might be of interest in further studies. Since our study did not merely focus on HNSCC, but also on all HNC, the HPV-status might be negligible.

Additionally, our data support the results of various in vitro studies on the effect of statins on HNSCC cells [21,22,47] and allow translation into a clinical context. However, the obtained results need to be cautiously interpreted, as limitations of this study exist. Specifically, the TriNetX database was used to search for subjects with diagnoses (ICD-10 codes C00–C14), which presupposes the correct classification of the malignant neoplasia in the head and neck. Moreover, patients suffering from different subtypes, or even rare entities of HNC might be included in this study, leading to a certain risk of confounder bias. Furthermore, staging following the Union for International Cancer Control (UICC), clinical, histological, and molecular features, as well as the applied therapy have not been considered, despite the well-known influence on the probability of patients' survival [48–52]. Statins were regarded as one group, despite different potencies and dosages. Information about the duration of statin therapy was not available but in general, statins are administered on a long-term basis. Even though one-to-one matching was performed, a certain risk of confounder bias remained since no detailed data on tobacco use (total pack years), alcohol abuse (consumed alcohol units), race [53], secondary diagnosis [54,55], and HPV status [56,57] were available.

Nevertheless, due to the large cohorts of 48,626 patients for each group and by matching, these differences should have been levelled out to a certain extent. In addition, the quality of all data retrieved from the TriNetX database can be considered as high, as the database meets the strict requirements of the National COVID Cohort Collaborative N3C. Therefore, the beneficial effect of statin use on the survival of HNC patients presented in this study might lead to further research on this topic—and if the presented results could be confirmed, HNC treatment might benefit from the chemopreventive effect of statins.

5. Conclusions

Pre-diagnostic statin medication in HNC patients correlates with a higher survival probability after five years (75.19%) when compared to patients without statin use (70.48%). Accordingly, the risk of death was lower in patients with statin use (15.9% vs. 17.2%). Further research is required to confirm these findings, which might lead to new supplementary treatment options in HNC therapy.

Author Contributions: Conceptualization, S.P. and R.P.; methodology, S.P. and R.P.; software, S.P. and R.P.; validation, S.P., R.P. and J.W.; formal analysis, J.W. and S.N.; investigation, M.H., S.P. and J.W.; resources, S.P., M.H. and R.P.; data curation, J.W., S.N. and S.P.; writing—original draft preparation, J.W.; writing—review and editing, S.P., R.P., S.N. and M.H.; visualization, J.W. and S.P.; supervision, R.P. and M.H.; project administration, R.P.; funding acquisition, R.P. and M.H. All authors have read and agreed to the published version of the manuscript.

Funding: This research received no external funding.

Institutional Review Board Statement: Not applicable.

Informed Consent Statement: Not applicable.

Data Availability Statement: Original data is available upon request.

Conflicts of Interest: The authors declare no conflict of interest.

References

1. Moura, A.C.; Assad, D.X.; Amorim Dos Santos, J.; Porto de Toledo, I.; Barra, G.B.; Castilho, R.M.; Squarize, C.H.; Guerra, E.N.S. Worldwide prevalence of PI3K-AKT-mTOR pathway mutations in head and neck cancer: A systematic review and meta-analysis. *Crit. Rev. Oncol. Hematol.* **2021**, *160*, 103284. [CrossRef]
2. Chow, L.Q.M. Head and Neck Cancer. *N. Engl. J. Med.* **2020**, *382*, 60–72. [CrossRef] [PubMed]

3. Bray, F.; Ferlay, J.; Soerjomataram, I.; Siegel, R.L.; Torre, L.A.; Jemal, A. Global cancer statistics 2018: GLOBOCAN estimates of incidence and mortality worldwide for 36 cancers in 185 countries. *CA Cancer J. Clin.* **2018**, *68*, 394–424. [CrossRef] [PubMed]
4. Fitzmaurice, C.; Allen, C.; Barber, R.M.; Barregard, L.; Bhutta, Z.A.; Brenner, H.; Dicker, D.J.; Chimed-Orchir, O.; Dandona, R.; Dandona, L.; et al. Global, Regional, and National Cancer Incidence, Mortality, Years of Life Lost, Years Lived With Disability, and Disability-Adjusted Life-years for 32 Cancer Groups, 1990 to 2015: A Systematic Analysis for the Global Burden of Disease Study. *JAMA Oncol.* **2017**, *3*, 524–548. [CrossRef]
5. Chaturvedi, A.K.; Engels, E.A.; Anderson, W.F.; Gillison, M.L. Incidence trends for human papillomavirus-related and-unrelated oral squamous cell carcinomas in the United States. *J. Clin. Oncol.* **2008**, *26*, 612–619. [CrossRef] [PubMed]
6. Yang, J.; Li, C.; Shen, Y.; Zhou, H.; Shao, Y.; Zhu, W.; Chen, Y. Impact of statin use on cancer-specific mortality and recurrence: A meta-analysis of 60 observational studies. *Medicine* **2020**, *99*, 19596. [CrossRef] [PubMed]
7. Matusewicz, L.; Meissner, J.; Toporkiewicz, M.; Sikorski, A.F. The effect of statins on cancer cells—Review. *Tumour Biol.* **2015**, *36*, 4889–4904. [CrossRef]
8. Brown, M.S.; Faust, J.R.; Goldstein, J.L.; Kaneko, I.; Endo, A. Induction of 3-hydroxy-3-methylglutaryl coenzyme A reductase activity in human fibroblasts incubated with compactin (ML-236B), a competitive inhibitor of the reductase. *J. Biol. Chem.* **1978**, *253*, 1121–1128. [CrossRef]
9. Manzoni, M.; Rollini, M. Biosynthesis and biotechnological production of statins by filamentous fungi and application of these cholesterol-lowering drugs. *Appl. Microbiol. Biotechnol.* **2002**, *58*, 555–564. [CrossRef]
10. Liu, H.; Liang, S.L.; Kumar, S.; Weyman, C.M.; Liu, W.; Zhou, A. Statins induce apoptosis in ovarian cancer cells through activation of JNK and enhancement of Bim expression. *Cancer Chemother. Pharm.* **2009**, *63*, 997–1005. [CrossRef]
11. Cheung, K.S.; Chan, E.W.; Wong, A.Y.S.; Chen, L.; Seto, W.K.; Wong, I.C.K.; Leung, W.K. Statins Were Associated with a Reduced Gastric Cancer Risk in Patients with Eradicated Helicobacter Pylori Infection: A Territory-Wide Propensity Score Matched Study. *Cancer Epidemiol. Biomark. Prev.* **2020**, *29*, 493–499. [CrossRef] [PubMed]
12. Hoque, A.; Chen, H.; Xu, X.C. Statin induces apoptosis and cell growth arrest in prostate cancer cells. *Cancer Epidemiol. Biomark. Prev.* **2008**, *17*, 88–94. [CrossRef] [PubMed]
13. Mehibel, M.; Ortiz-Martinez, F.; Voelxen, N.; Boyers, A.; Chadwick, A.; Telfer, B.A.; Mueller-Klieser, W.; West, C.M.; Critchlow, S.E.; Williams, K.J.; et al. Statin-induced metabolic reprogramming in head and neck cancer: A biomarker for targeting monocarboxylate transporters. *Sci. Rep.* **2018**, *8*, 16804. [CrossRef] [PubMed]
14. Galland, S.; Martin, P.; Fregni, G.; Letovanec, I.; Stamenkovic, I. Attenuation of the pro-inflammatory signature of lung cancer-derived mesenchymal stromal cells by statins. *Cancer Lett.* **2020**, *484*, 50–64. [CrossRef]
15. Wang, K.H.; Liu, C.H.; Ding, D.C. Statins as Repurposed Drugs in Gynecological Cancer: A Review. *Int. J. Mol. Sci.* **2022**, *23*, 13937. [CrossRef]
16. Ma, L.; Niknejad, N.; Gorn-Hondermann, I.; Dayekh, K.; Dimitroulakos, J. Lovastatin induces multiple stress pathways including LKB1/AMPK activation that regulate its cytotoxic effects in squamous cell carcinoma cells. *PLoS ONE* **2012**, *7*, e46055. [CrossRef]
17. Dimitroulakos, J.; Marhin, W.H.; Tokunaga, J.; Irish, J.; Gullane, P.; Penn, L.Z.; Kamel-Reid, S. Microarray and biochemical analysis of lovastatin-induced apoptosis of squamous cell carcinomas. *Neoplasia* **2002**, *4*, 337–346. [CrossRef]
18. Niknejad, N.; Morley, M.; Dimitroulakos, J. Activation of the integrated stress response regulates lovastatin-induced apoptosis. *J. Biol. Chem.* **2007**, *282*, 29748–29756. [CrossRef]
19. Takeda, I.; Maruya, S.; Shirasaki, T.; Mizukami, H.; Takahata, T.; Myers, J.N.; Kakehata, S.; Yagihashi, S.; Shinkawa, H. Simvastatin inactivates beta1-integrin and extracellular signal-related kinase signaling and inhibits cell proliferation in head and neck squamous cell carcinoma cells. *Cancer Sci.* **2007**, *98*, 890–899. [CrossRef]
20. Wang, W.; Le, W.; Cho, D.Y.; Hwang, P.H.; Upadhyay, D. Novel effects of statins in enhancing efficacy of chemotherapy in vitro in nasopharyngeal carcinoma. *Int. Forum Allergy Rhinol.* **2011**, *1*, 284–289. [CrossRef]
21. Gabryś, D.; Dörfler, A.; Yaromina, A.; Hessel, F.; Krause, M.; Oertel, R.; Baumann, M. Effects of lovastatin alone or combined with irradiation on tumor cells in vitro and in vivo. *Strahlenther Onkol.* **2008**, *184*, 48–53. [CrossRef]
22. Mantha, A.J.; Hanson, J.E.; Goss, G.; Lagarde, A.E.; Lorimer, I.A.; Dimitroulakos, J. Targeting the mevalonate pathway inhibits the function of the epidermal growth factor receptor. *Clin. Cancer Res.* **2005**, *11*, 2398–2407. [CrossRef]
23. Zhang, Y.; Liang, M.; Sun, C.; Qu, G.; Shi, T.; Min, M.; Wu, Y.; Sun, Y. Statin Use and Risk of Pancreatic Cancer: An Updated Meta-analysis of 26 Studies. *Pancreas* **2019**, *48*, 142–150. [CrossRef] [PubMed]
24. Chen, Y.; Li, X.; Zhang, R.; Xia, Y.; Shao, Z.; Mei, Z. Effects of statin exposure and lung cancer survival: A meta-analysis of observational studies. *Pharm. Res.* **2019**, *141*, 357–365. [CrossRef] [PubMed]
25. Gupta, A.; Stokes, W.; Eguchi, M.; Hararah, M.; Amini, A.; Mueller, A.; Morgan, R.; Bradley, C.; Raben, D.; McDermott, J.; et al. Statin use associated with improved overall and cancer specific survival in patients with head and neck cancer. *Oral Oncol.* **2019**, *90*, 54–66. [CrossRef]
26. Bourguillon, R.O.; Stokes, W.A.; Dorth, J.; Schmitt, N.C. Repurposing Statin Drugs to Decrease Toxicity and Improve Survival Outcomes in Head and Neck Cancer. *OTO Open* **2021**, *5*, 2473974X211065715. [CrossRef] [PubMed]
27. Lebo, N.L.; Griffiths, R.; Hall, S.; Dimitroulakos, J.; Johnson-Obaseki, S. Effect of statin use on oncologic outcomes in head and neck squamous cell carcinoma. *Head Neck* **2018**, *40*, 1697–1706. [CrossRef] [PubMed]
28. Getz, K.R.; Bellile, E.; Zarins, K.R.; Rullman, C.; Chinn, S.B.; Taylor, J.M.G.; Rozek, L.S.; Wolf, G.T.; Mondul, A.M. Statin use and head and neck squamous cell carcinoma outcomes. *Int. J. Cancer* **2021**, *148*, 2440–2448. [CrossRef]

29. Heym, M.; Heiland, M.; Preissner, R.; Huebel, C.; Nahles, S.; Schmidt-Westhausen, A.M.; Preissner, S.; Hertel, M. The risk of oral squamous cell carcinoma in patients with and without somatoform disorders including bruxism: A retrospective evaluation of 309,278 individuals. *Front. Oncol.* **2022**, *12*, 1080492. [CrossRef]
30. Hertel, M.; Hagedorn, L.; Schmidt-Westhausen, A.M.; Dommisch, H.; Heiland, M.; Preissner, R.; Preissner, S. Comparison of five-year survival rates among patients with oral squamous cell carcinoma with and without association with syphilis: A retrospective case-control study. *BMC Cancer* **2022**, *22*, 454. [CrossRef]
31. Zhao, G.; Ji, Y.; Ye, Q.; Ye, X.; Wo, G.; Chen, X.; Shao, X.; Tang, J. Effect of statins use on risk and prognosis of breast cancer: A meta-analysis. *Anticancer Drugs* **2022**, *33*, e507–e518. [CrossRef] [PubMed]
32. Zhong, S.; Zhang, X.; Chen, L.; Ma, T.; Tang, J.; Zhao, J. Statin use and mortality in cancer patients: Systematic review and meta-analysis of observational studies. *Cancer Treat Rev.* **2015**, *41*, 554–567. [CrossRef] [PubMed]
33. Li, Y.; He, X.; Ding, Y.; Chen, H.; Sun, L. Statin uses and mortality in colorectal cancer patients: An updated systematic review and meta-analysis. *Cancer Med.* **2019**, *8*, 3305–3313. [CrossRef]
34. Raval, A.D.; Thakker, D.; Negi, H.; Vyas, A.; Kaur, H.; Salkini, M.W. Association between statins and clinical outcomes among men with prostate cancer: A systematic review and meta-analysis. *Prostate Cancer Prostatic Dis.* **2016**, *19*, 151–162. [CrossRef]
35. Gray, R.T.; Coleman, H.G.; Hughes, C.; Murray, L.J.; Cardwell, C.R. Statin use and survival in colorectal cancer: Results from a population-based cohort study and an updated systematic review and meta-analysis. *Cancer Epidemiol.* **2016**, *45*, 71–81. [CrossRef] [PubMed]
36. Nayan, M.; Punjani, N.; Juurlink, D.N.; Finelli, A.; Austin, P.C.; Kulkarni, G.S.; Uleryk, E.; Hamilton, R.J. Statin use and kidney cancer survival outcomes: A systematic review and meta-analysis. *Cancer Treat Rev.* **2017**, *52*, 105–116. [CrossRef]
37. Wang, J.; Li, X. Impact of statin use on the risk and prognosis of hepatocellular carcinoma: A meta-analysis. *Eur. J. Gastroenterol. Hepatol.* **2021**, *33*, 1603–1609. [CrossRef]
38. Cai, H.; Zhang, G.; Wang, Z.; Luo, Z.; Zhou, X. Relationship between the use of statins and patient survival in colorectal cancer: A systematic review and meta-analysis. *PLoS ONE* **2015**, *10*, e0126944. [CrossRef]
39. Gu, J.; Zhu, N.; Li, H.F.; Zhang, C.J.; Gong, Y.Z.; Liao, D.F.; Qin, L. Ezetimibe and Cancer: Is There a Connection? *Front. Pharm.* **2022**, *13*, 831657. [CrossRef]
40. Ouchi, Y.; Sasaki, J.; Arai, H.; Yokote, K.; Harada, K.; Katayama, Y.; Urabe, T.; Uchida, Y.; Hayashi, M.; Yokota, N.; et al. Ezetimibe Lipid-Lowering Trial on Prevention of Atherosclerotic Cardiovascular Disease in 75 or Older (EWTOPIA 75): A Randomized, Controlled Trial. *Circulation* **2019**, *140*, 992–1003. [CrossRef]
41. Mourikis, P.; Zako, S.; Dannenberg, L.; Nia, A.M.; Heinen, Y.; Busch, L.; Richter, H.; Hohlfeld, T.; Zeus, T.; Kelm, M.; et al. Lipid lowering therapy in cardiovascular disease: From myth to molecular reality. *Pharmacol. Ther.* **2020**, *213*, 107592. [CrossRef] [PubMed]
42. Luo, J.; Yang, H.; Song, B.L. Mechanisms and regulation of cholesterol homeostasis. *Nat. Rev. Mol. Cell Biol.* **2020**, *21*, 225–245. [CrossRef] [PubMed]
43. Solomon, K.R.; Pelton, K.; Boucher, K.; Joo, J.; Tully, C.; Zurakowski, D.; Schaffner, C.P.; Kim, J.; Freeman, M.R. Ezetimibe is an inhibitor of tumor angiogenesis. *Am. J. Pathol.* **2009**, *174*, 1017–1026. [CrossRef]
44. He, J.; Shin, H.; Wei, X.; Kadegowda, A.K.; Chen, R.; Xie, S.K. NPC1L1 knockout protects against colitis-associated tumorigenesis in mice. *BMC Cancer* **2015**, *15*, 189. [CrossRef]
45. Liu, X.; Bao, X.; Hu, M.; Chang, H.; Jiao, M.; Cheng, J.; Xie, L.; Huang, Q.; Li, F.; Li, C.Y. Inhibition of PCSK9 potentiates immune checkpoint therapy for cancer. *Nature* **2020**, *588*, 693–698. [CrossRef] [PubMed]
46. Bhattacharya, A.; Chowdhury, A.; Chaudhury, K.; Shukla, P.C. Proprotein convertase subtilisin/kexin type 9 (PCSK9): A potential multifaceted player in cancer. *Biochim. Biophys. Acta Rev. Cancer* **2021**, *1876*, 188581. [CrossRef] [PubMed]
47. Pavan, L.M.; Rêgo, D.F.; Elias, S.T.; De Luca Canto, G.; Guerra, E.N. In vitro Anti-Tumor Effects of Statins on Head and Neck Squamous Cell Carcinoma: A Systematic Review. *PLoS ONE* **2015**, *10*, e0130476. [CrossRef]
48. Winquist, E.; Agbassi, C.; Meyers, B.M.; Yoo, J.; Chan, K.K.W. Systemic therapy in the curative treatment of head and neck squamous cell cancer: A systematic review. *J. Otolaryngol. Head Neck Surg.* **2017**, *46*, 29. [CrossRef]
49. Wushou, A.; Hou, J.; Zhao, Y.J.; Miao, X.C. Postoperative adjuvant radiotherapy improves loco-regional recurrence of head and neck mucosal melanoma. *J. Cranio-Maxillo-Facial Surg.* **2015**, *43*, 553–558. [CrossRef]
50. Habib, A. Management of advanced hypopharyngeal carcinoma: Systematic review of survival following surgical and non-surgical treatments. *J. Laryngol. Otol.* **2018**, *132*, 385–400. [CrossRef]
51. Reiersen, D.A.; Pahilan, M.E.; Devaiah, A.K. Meta-analysis of treatment outcomes for sinonasal undifferentiated carcinoma. *Otolaryngol. Head Neck Surg.* **2012**, *147*, 7–14. [CrossRef] [PubMed]
52. Sahovaler, A.; Krishnan, R.J.; Yeh, D.H.; Zhou, Q.; Palma, D.; Fung, K.; Yoo, J.; Nichols, A.; MacNeil, S.D. Outcomes of Cutaneous Squamous Cell Carcinoma in the Head and Neck Region With Regional Lymph Node Metastasis: A Systematic Review and Meta-analysis. *JAMA Otolaryngol. Head Neck Surg.* **2019**, *145*, 352–360. [CrossRef]
53. Russo, D.P.; Tham, T.; Bardash, Y.; Kraus, D. The effect of race in head and neck cancer: A meta-analysis controlling for socioeconomic status. *Am. J. Otolaryngol.* **2020**, *41*, 102624. [CrossRef] [PubMed]
54. Takenaka, Y.; Takemoto, N.; Oya, R.; Inohara, H. Prognostic impact of sarcopenia in patients with head and neck cancer treated with surgery or radiation: A meta-analysis. *PLoS ONE* **2021**, *16*, e0259288. [CrossRef] [PubMed]

55. Van der Elst, S.; Bardash, Y.; Wotman, M.; Kraus, D.; Tham, T. The prognostic impact of depression or depressive symptoms on patients with head and neck cancer: A systematic review and meta-analysis. *Head Neck* **2021**, *43*, 3608–3617. [CrossRef] [PubMed]
56. O'Rorke, M.A.; Ellison, M.V.; Murray, L.J.; Moran, M.; James, J.; Anderson, L.A. Human papillomavirus related head and neck cancer survival: A systematic review and meta-analysis. *Oral Oncol.* **2012**, *48*, 1191–1201. [CrossRef]
57. Koyanagi, Y.N.; Matsuo, K.; Ito, H.; Wakai, K.; Nagata, C.; Nakayama, T.; Sadakane, A.; Tanaka, K.; Tamakoshi, A.; Sugawara, Y.; et al. Cigarette smoking and the risk of head and neck cancer in the Japanese population: A systematic review and meta-analysis. *Jpn. J. Clin. Oncol.* **2016**, *46*, 580–595. [CrossRef]

cancers

MDPI

Article

Predicting Lymph Node Metastasis Status from Primary Muscle-Invasive Bladder Cancer Histology Slides Using Deep Learning: A Retrospective Multicenter Study

Qingyuan Zheng [1,2,†], Jun Jian [1,2,†], Jingsong Wang [1,2], Kai Wang [3], Junjie Fan [4,5], Huazhen Xu [6], Xinmiao Ni [1,2], Song Yang [1,2], Jingping Yuan [7], Jiejun Wu [1,2], Panpan Jiao [1,2], Rui Yang [1,2], Zhiyuan Chen [1,2], Xiuheng Liu [1,2,*] and Lei Wang [1,2,*]

1 Department of Urology, Renmin Hospital of Wuhan University, Wuhan 430060, China; zqy710890394@whu.edu.cn (Q.Z.)
2 Institute of Urologic Disease, Renmin Hospital of Wuhan University, Wuhan 430060, China
3 Department of Urology, People's Hospital of Hanchuan City, Xiaogan 432300, China
4 University of Chinese Academy of Sciences, Beijing 100049, China
5 Trusted Computing and Information Assurance Laboratory, Institute of Software, Chinese Academy of Sciences, Beijing 100190, China
6 Department of Pharmacology, School of Basic Medical Sciences, Wuhan University, Wuhan 430072, China
7 Department of Pathology, Renmin Hospital of Wuhan University, Wuhan 430060, China
* Correspondence: drliuxh@hotmail.com (X.L.); drwanglei@whu.edu.cn (L.W.)
† These authors contributed equally to this work.

Simple Summary: Accurate prediction of lymph node metastasis (LNM) status in patients with muscle-invasive bladder cancer (MIBC) before radical cystectomy can guide the use of neoadjuvant chemotherapy and the extent of pelvic lymph node dissection. However, there are no reliable tools available for achieving this goal. Data-driven deep-learning techniques have been widely used in disease diagnosis, prognosis assessment, and treatment response prediction by identifying subtle patterns in digitized histopathological images. In this study, we developed a weakly-supervised model based on multiple instance learning and attention mechanism for predicting LNM status in MIBC patients, demonstrating decent performance in three independent cohorts. The visualization technique revealed that the stroma surrounding the tumor with lymphocytic inflammation seemed to be the critical feature for predicting LNM. This deep learning-based study provides a non-invasive and low-cost preoperative prediction tool for identifying MIBC patients with a high risk of LNM.

Abstract: Background: Accurate prediction of lymph node metastasis (LNM) status in patients with muscle-invasive bladder cancer (MIBC) before radical cystectomy can guide the use of neoadjuvant chemotherapy and the extent of pelvic lymph node dissection. We aimed to develop and validate a weakly-supervised deep learning model to predict LNM status from digitized histopathological slides in MIBC. Methods: We trained a multiple instance learning model with an attention mechanism (namely SBLNP) from a cohort of 323 patients in the TCGA cohort. In parallel, we collected corresponding clinical information to construct a logistic regression model. Subsequently, the score predicted by the SBLNP was incorporated into the logistic regression model. In total, 417 WSIs from 139 patients in the RHWU cohort and 230 WSIs from 78 patients in the PHHC cohort were used as independent external validation sets. Results: In the TCGA cohort, the SBLNP achieved an AUROC of 0.811 (95% confidence interval [CI], 0.771–0.855), the clinical classifier achieved an AUROC of 0.697 (95% CI, 0.661–0.728) and the combined classifier yielded an improvement to 0.864 (95% CI, 0.827–0.906). Encouragingly, the SBLNP still maintained high performance in the RHWU cohort and PHHC cohort, with an AUROC of 0.762 (95% CI, 0.725–0.801) and 0.746 (95% CI, 0.687–0.799), respectively. Moreover, the interpretability of SBLNP identified stroma with lymphocytic inflammation as a key feature of predicting LNM presence. Conclusions: Our proposed weakly-supervised deep learning model can predict the LNM status of MIBC patients from routine WSIs, demonstrating decent generalization performance and holding promise for clinical implementation.

Keywords: muscle-invasive bladder cancer; lymph node metastasis; deep learning; whole slide image; new predictive biomarker

1. Introduction

Bladder cancer is the most commonly diagnosed urological malignancy worldwide, with approximately 573,278 new cases and 212,536 deaths in 2020 [1]. Based on the depth of invasion, bladder cancer can be classified into non-muscle invasive bladder cancer and muscle-invasive bladder cancer (MIBC) [2]. Generally, MIBC has a poorer prognosis and a higher recurrence rate, requiring more aggressive diagnosis and treatment [3]. Transurethral resection of bladder tumor (TURBT) with histopathological examination is the gold standard for diagnosis and staging in clinical practice [4]. For patients diagnosed with localized MIBC, guidelines recommend radical cystectomy (RC) and pelvic lymph node dissection (PLND) as the standard treatment [5]. Although RC achieves negative surgical margins in the vast majority of patients, the disease recurrence rate remains high at approximately 50%, suggesting the presence of extravesical tumor deposits at the time of surgical resection [6,7]. To reduce postoperative recurrence and decrease the burden of micrometastases, cisplatin-based neoadjuvant chemotherapy (NAC) regimens have been used for management, but the resulting systemic toxicity reactions and potentially fatal surgical delays associated with NAC cannot be ignored [8]. Therefore, it is necessary to identify MIBC patients who may benefit from NAC while turning to other treatment strategies for non-responsive patients [9]. Unfortunately, there are still no reliable tools available to achieve this goal and avoid the risks of under- or overtreatment [10].

Accurately predicting the risk of tumor spread to regional lymph nodes in MIBC is crucial for making effective treatment decisions, such as determining the extent of PLND and the use of NAC, as the presence of LNM is associated with disease recurrence and significantly higher cancer-related mortality [11]. The possibility of positive lymph nodes is typically assessed through preoperative imaging, with contrast-enhanced CT being the mainstay of preoperative lymph node staging. However, a large proportion of patients may have lymph node involvement that is not apparent on imaging, with a sensitivity of only 33–46% [12,13]. Traditional histopathological evaluation [14] and biomarkers [15,16] are currently suboptimal in predicting LNM status, limited by high intra- and inter-observer variability, and have yet to be applied in clinical practice. Thus, there is an urgent need to find a new approach that can accurately and objectively determine the LNM status to optimize treatment decisions for MIBC patients.

Deep learning, a technique in the field of artificial intelligence (AI) that can identify subtle patterns in complex pathological images, has broad applications in computational pathology [17]. In bladder cancer, AI-based methods can be used to detect histological patterns such as malignant tumor potential [18], tumor stroma ratio [19], and tumor-infiltrating lymphocytes [20], and have been used to predict molecular subtypes [21] and overall survival [22,23]. In breast cancer [24], colorectal cancer [25–27], and prostate cancer [28], deep learning has successfully predicted the LNM status from primary tumor specimens. To our knowledge, only one study [29] has shown the potential of deep learning to predict LNM status from digital hematoxylin and eosin (H&E)-stained slides in primary bladder cancer. However, this study used only a single public dataset, which is susceptible to bias and may not be applicable to clinical practice. In addition to being a potentially clinically useful tool, interpretable deep learning should also provide quantitative evidence for the association of histopathological features. For example, in previous studies, deep learning has been used to identify tumor heterogeneity and vascular infiltration as negative prognostic features for MIBC [22]. Furthermore, the time-consuming and labor-intensive high-quality pixel-level image annotation is also a major challenge for current AI, which seriously hinders the development of AI in pathology [30].

Hence, in this study, we developed a weakly-supervised deep learning model to predict LNM status from routine H&E-stained slides of primary MIBC and attempted to identify new histopathological features. We validated the effectiveness and robustness of the deep learning model in three independent cohorts and compared it with the logistic regression model constructed from clinical data. Finally, we evaluated the combined classifier consisting of deep learning and clinical data.

2. Materials and Methods

2.1. Patient Cohorts

In this multicenter study, we retrospectively collected three independent cohorts to improve the generalization of the model for achieving clinical utility. We utilized the publicly available cohort of patients from The Cancer Genome Atlas (TCGA), a large international multicenter study that included patients with stage I–IV bladder cancer from 1999 to 2013 and consisted of 457 whole slide images (WSIs) from 386 cases. In the Renmin Hospital of Wuhan University (RHWU; Wuhan, China) cohort, we continuously collected 548 candidate patients from 2017 to 2023 with corresponding formalin-fixed and paraffin-embedded tumor tissue blocks (resected by surgery). Additionally, tumor tissue blocks and clinical data from 364 candidate patients were collected from 2014 and 2022 at People's Hospital of Hanchuan City (PHHC; Hanchuan, China). Only cases with a definitive pathological diagnosis of MIBC, available pathological images or blocks, known LNM status, and clinical data regarding age, gender, T stage, lymphovascular invasion, histologic grade, and without NAC were included in all cohorts. The patient recruitment pathway is shown in Figure 1.

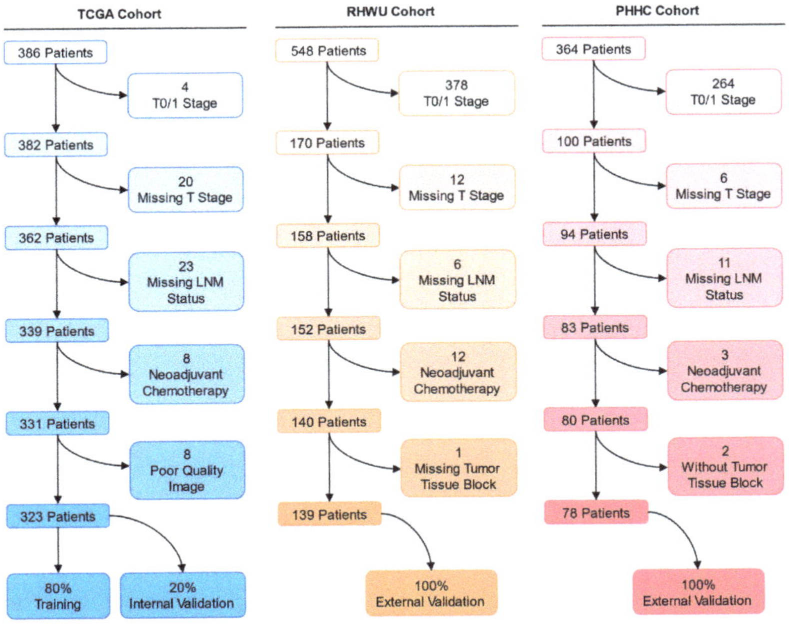

Figure 1. Description of pathways to recruit patients from the TCGA, RHWU, and PHHC cohorts. LNM, lymph node metastasis; TCGA, The Cancer Genome Atlas; RHWU, Renmin Hospital of Wuhan University; PHHC, People's Hospital of Hanchuan City.

2.2. Image Preprocessing

For the RHWU and PHHC cohorts, we obtained formalin-fixed and paraffin-embedded tumor tissue blocks from each patient and then prepared H&E-stained slides. Subsequently, all slides were scanned into WSIs at 20× magnification (0.5 μm per pixel) using a digital scanner (KF-PRO-020, KFBIO Co., Ltd., Ningbo, China) and carefully reviewed by a pathologist. In principle, each patient in the RHWU and PHHC cohorts had 1 to 4 representative WSIs, while each patient in the TCGA cohort had 1 to 9 representative WSIs. The labels for multiple WSIs of the same patient were consistent.

Considering that the WSIs from the three cohorts have different magnifications, we uniformly loaded the images at 20× magnification and automatically detected the foreground using the Otsu-based method (maximal variance between-class) to segment the tissue regions. After segmentation, we used the openslide-python toolkit (https://openslide.org/, accessed on 7 January 2023) to crop patches with a size of 448 × 448 pixels for each WSI from within the segmented foreground while recording the coordinates of each patch and the corresponding WSI-level information. A color thresholding method was employed to exclude potentially mixed blank images (background pixels exceeding 80%) from all patches. Since the WSIs from the three cohorts exhibited staining differences, we used the structure-preserving color normalization method proposed by Vahadane [31] and Anand [32] to reduce image heterogeneity.

2.3. Feature Extraction and Reduction

Feature extraction is an important component of recognition tasks and can be used to predict performance and reduce computational requirements by utilizing feature selection. We extracted 2048 relevant features for each patch using a ResNet-50 neural network [33] with ImageNet pre-trained weights. With the emergence of novel feature selection methods, it is possible to alleviate the impact of the curse of dimensionality and facilitate the understanding of data [34,35]. To avoid the potential overfitting, long computation time, and heavy memory usage, we used an adaptive encoder for dimensionality reduction, reducing the 2048 dimensions extracted from ResNet-50 to 512 dimensions. This adaptive encoder consisted of a hidden layer architecture with 512 neurons, trained on a total of 64,600 patches (200 patches randomly selected from each WSI) over 100 epochs. After 100 epochs, the mean-squared error loss converged to 0.003.

2.4. Slide-Based Lymph Node Predictor (SBLNP)

SBLNP is an end-to-end weakly-supervised deep learning model, an advanced binary classification network based on multiple instance learning (MIL) and attention mechanism derived from our previously developed diagnostic and prognostic models [22].

Each WSI from three cohorts can be regarded as a bag composed of a large number of instances, which are patches segmented from the WSI. For a positive bag, there must be at least one instance classified as positive by MIL. In contrast, for the negative bag, all instances must be classified as negative. Given a bag, each instance is assigned a probability of being positive and ranked accordingly. If the bag is positive, the instances with a high probability of being positive should be close to 1, whereas if the bag is negative, all instances should be close to 0.

Unlike previous average- or max-pooling aggregation functions, SBLNP uses an attention-based pooling function [36] to construct a WSI-level representation by aggregating patch-level attention scores assigned during training and inference while providing interpretability. We adopted the binary smooth top-1 SVM loss [37] as the loss function for SBLNP, which proved to be more robust to noise and overfitting issues than the widely used cross-entropy classification loss. To train SBLNP, we used a five-fold cross-validation strategy for repeated validation to prevent overfitting. The Adam optimizer with an initial learning rate of 1×10^{-4} and $\ell 2$ weight decay of 1×10^{-5} was used to update the training weights and parameters of SBLNP. The remaining hyperparameters were set to $\beta 1$ of 0.9 and $\beta 2$ of 0.999. We set the maximum epoch during training to 200, and when the loss of SBLNP did not change for 20 consecutive epochs, we used early stopping to stop training and saved the best model for internal and external validation. A simplified layout of the SBLNP is shown in Figure 2.

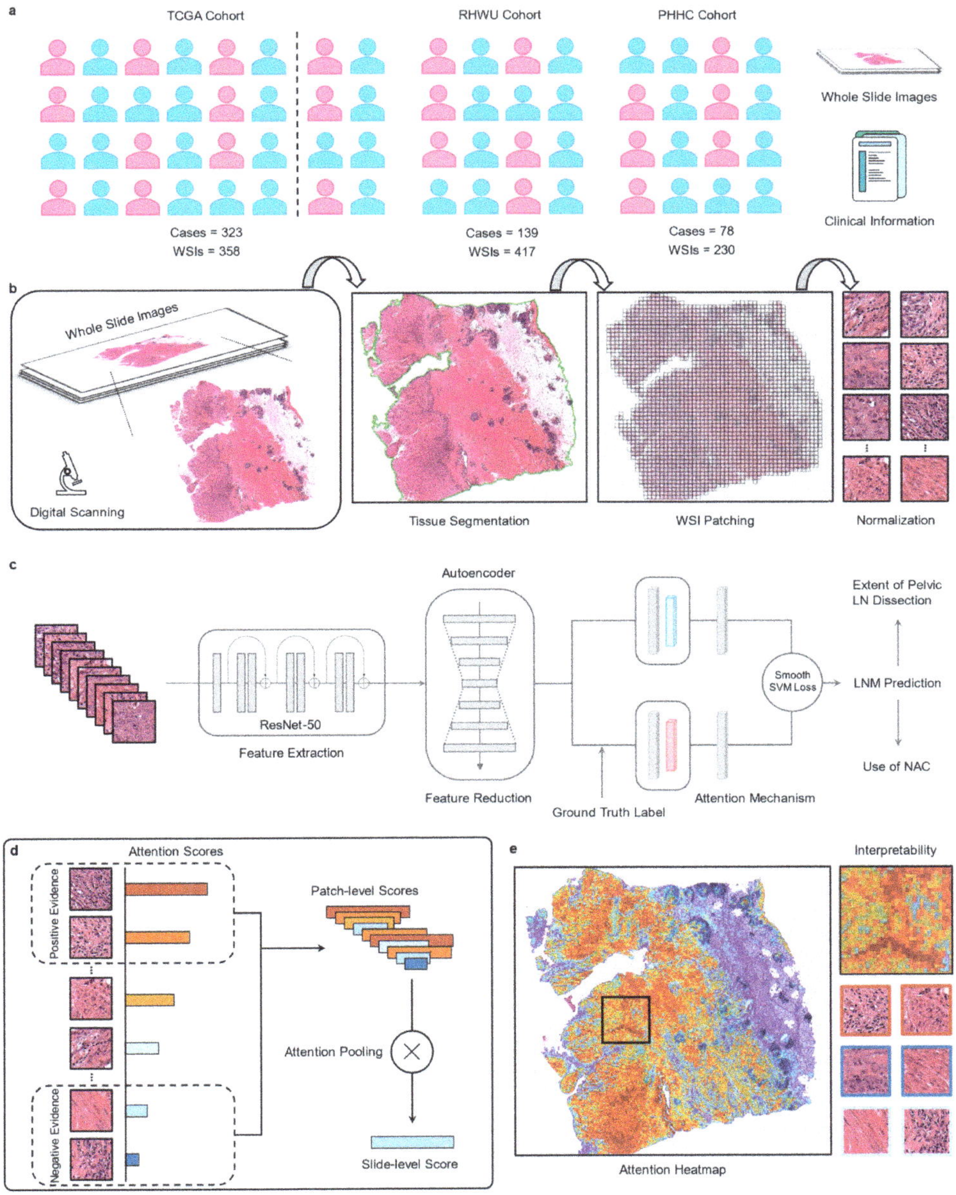

Figure 2. Data and workflow of the deep learning-based model. (**a**) We collected WSIs and clinical information from three cohorts of MIBC patients for the development of a predictive model. (**b**) All WSIs were digitized, then segmented into fixed-size patches, and staining differences were normalized. (**c**) We used the Resnet-50 model to extract the features of all patches and input them into MIL with an attention mechanism for training and validation after dimensionality reduction. (**d**) The attention mechanism assigned scores to each patch and ranked them, and then weighed them through the attention pooling to get the WSI-level scores. (**e**) All patches were visualized as a heatmap to identify the important histological features used for prediction. Red represented strong contributions, while blue represented weak contributions. WSIs, Whole Slide Images.

2.5. Interpreting Predictions via Attention Heatmap

To explain the degree of attention of the SBLNP in different regions of WSI, we saved the attention scores of all patches. These scores represented their importance to the entire WSI and were converted to percentages, normalized, and scaled between 0 and 1. Scores closer to 1 indicated a greater contribution to prediction, while scores closer to 0 indicated a smaller contribution. We then used diverging colormap to convert the normalized scores into RGB colors and mapped them to the original WSI based on the saved spatial position information to generate an attention heatmap, with a transparency value set to 0.6 to facilitate simultaneous visualization of the underlying histological features. Red represented the areas with high attention by the SBLNP (positive evidence), while blue represented low attention (negative evidence).

2.6. Quantification of Histopathological Features

In addition to gaining deeper insights into the histopathological features identified by SBLNP as predictive of LNM status through heatmap visualization, we performed a blinded observer study with a pathologist. We randomly extracted 100 WSIs (LNM-positive:LNM-negative = 1:1) and then selected the 15 top-scoring patches from each WSI and aggregated them together. A total of 1500 patches were obtained from LNM-positive and -negative cases and were reviewed by a pathologist in a blinded manner, with recorded histological features for quantitative comparison.

2.7. Clinical Classifier and Combined Classifier (Clinical Classifier + SBLNP)

For the clinical classifier, we performed logistic regression analyses based on clinical data of patients regarding age, gender, T stage, Lymphovascular invasion (LVI), and histologic grade, which were available in all three cohorts. In addition, we constructed a combined classifier encompassing the above variables and integrating SBLNP scores. The T stage used in this study was the pathological T stage (pT stage) rather than the clinical T stage. The datasets used for both classifiers were consistent with the training and internal/external validation datasets of SBLNP for analysis and comparison, and a five-fold cross-validation strategy was also carried out.

2.8. Statistical Analysis

The performance of three classifiers (Clinical classifier, SBLNP and SBLNP + Clinical classifier) was evaluated by calculating the area under the receiver operating characteristic (AUROC) on internal and external validation sets. The 95% confidence interval (CI) of the internal validation set was obtained by five-fold cross-validation, while the 95% CIs of the external validation sets were calculated from five repeated experiments. Statistical significance was assessed using DeLong's test [38] among the three classifiers. Categorical variables were described as number (percentage), and continuous values were described as the median (extremum). A two-sided p-value less than 0.05 was considered statistically significant.

3. Results

3.1. Patient Characteristics

After the screening, we included 358 WSIs from 323 MIBC patients in the TCGA cohort, 417 WSIs from 139 MIBC patients in the RHWU cohort, and 230 WSIs from 78 MIBC patients in the PHHC cohort. Among these, 80% of the WSIs (n = 286) from the TCGA cohort were used as a training set for model development, and the remaining 20% (n = 72) were used as an internal validation set. The RHWU and PHHC cohorts were used as external validation sets to test the generalization performance of the SBLNP. The detailed data distribution is shown in Supplementary Tables S1 and S2. Table 1 displays the characteristics of the included patients in the three cohorts.

Table 1. Clinical, biological, and pathological characteristics of MIBC patients included in the TCGA, RHWU, and PHHC cohorts.

	TCGA (n = 323)	RHWU (n = 139)	PHHC (n = 78)
Age (years)	69 (34, 90)	66 (26, 87)	70 (45, 90)
Gender			
Female	88 (27.24%)	21 (15.11%)	17 (21.79%)
Male	235 (72.76%)	118 (84.89%)	61 (78.21%)
pT stage			
pT2	98 (30.34%)	67 (48.20%)	30 (38.46%)
pT3	175 (54.18%)	44 (31.65%)	28 (35.90%)
pT4	50 (15.48%)	28 (20.14%)	20 (25.64%)
pM stage			
pM0	146 (45.20%)	104 (74.82%)	57 (73.08%)
pM1	7 (2.17%)	35 (35.18%)	21 (26.92%)
pMx	170 (52.63%)	0 (0%)	0 (0%)
pTNM stage			
Stage II	83 (25.70%)	58 (41.73%)	74 (32.18%)
Stage III	122 (37.77%)	45 (32.37%)	78 (33.91%)
Stage IV	118 (36.53%)	36 (25.90%)	78 (33.91%)
Histologic grade			
High grade	303 (93.81%)	129 (92.81%)	74 (94.87%)
Low grade	18 (5.57%)	10 (7.19%)	4 (5.13%)
Missing	2 (0.62%)	0 (0%)	0 (0%)
LVI			
No	104 (32.20%)	81 (58.27%)	47 (60.26%)
Yes	127 (39.32%)	58 (41.73%)	31 (39.74%)
Missing	92 (28.48%)	0 (0%)	0 (0%)
LN status			
Negative (pN0)	207 (64.09%)	102 (73.38%)	53 (67.95%)
Positive (pN1-3)	116 (35.91%)	37 (26.62%)	25 (32.05%)
LNs examined number	18 (1, 170)	21 (1, 64)	16 (1, 47)
Positive LNs number	2 (1, 97)	2 (1, 20)	3 (1, 31)
Survival status			
Alive	178 (55.11%)	-	-
Dead	145 (44.89%)	-	-
OS time (months)	17.4 (0, 165.6)	-	-

MIBC, Muscle-invasive Bladder Cancer; TCGA, The Cancer Genome Atlas; RHWU, Renmin Hospital of Wuhan University; PHHC, People's Hospital of Hanchuan City; LVI, Lymphovascular Invasion; LN, Lymph Node; OS, overall survival.

3.2. Performance of the SBLNP

The SBLNP achieved an AUROC of 0.811 (95% CI, 0.771–0.855; Table 2, Figure 3) on the internal validation set (TCGA cohort). On the external validation sets (RHWU cohort and PHHC cohort), its predictive performance was robust as it achieved decent AUROCs of 0.762 (95% CI, 0.725–0.801) and 0.746 (95% CI, 0.687–0.799), respectively.

Table 2. The AUROCs of clinical classifier, SBLNP, and combined classifier (Clinical + SBLNP) in internal and external validation sets.

Model	TCGA Cohort	RHWU Cohort	PHHC Cohort
	AUROC (95% CI)	AUROC (95% CI)	AUROC (95% CI)
Clinical	0.697 (0.661, 0.728)	0.657 (0.595, 0.713)	0.683 (0.537, 0.829)
SBLNP	0.811 (0.771, 0.855)	0.762 (0.725, 0.801)	0.746 (0.687, 0.799)
Clinical + SBLNP	0.864 (0.827, 0.906)	0.810 (0.780, 0.844)	0.824 (0.788, 0.861)

CI, Confidence Interval; TCGA, The Cancer Genome Atlas; RHWU, Renmin Hospital of Wuhan University; PHHC, People's Hospital of Hanchuan City; SBLNP, Slide-Based Lymph Node Predictor.

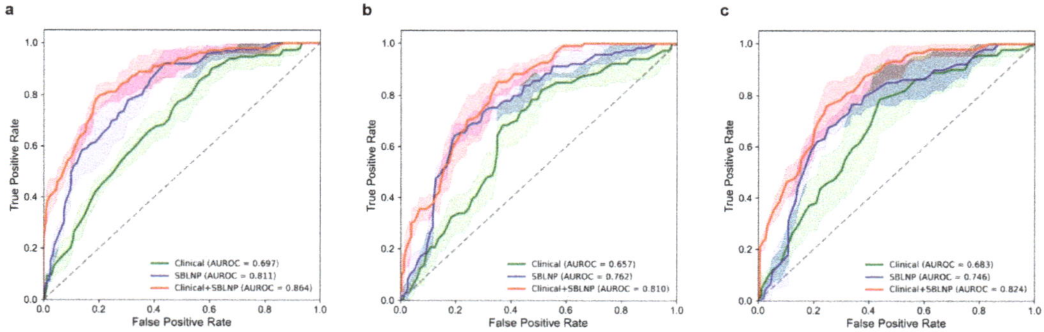

Figure 3. Performance of the clinical classifier, the SBLNP, and the combined classifier in (**a**) the TCGA cohort, (**b**) the RHWU cohort, and (**c**) the PHHC cohort. SBLNP, Slide-Based Lymph Node Predictor.

3.3. Performance of the Clinical Classifier

The clinical classifier purely based on patient information yielded an AUROC of 0.811 (95% CI, 0.661–0.728; Table 2, Figure 3) on the internal validation set (TCGA cohort). In the RHWU cohort and the PHHC cohort, the AUROCs were 0.657 (95% CI, 0.595–0.713) and 0.683 (95% CI, 0.537–0.829), respectively, and their performance was lower than that of the SBLNP.

3.4. Performance of the Combined Classifier (Clinical Classifier + SBLNP)

We achieved the best predictive performance when we incorporated the prediction scores from SBLNP into the logistic regression model. We calculated coefficients and odds ratios (ORs) for each input variable in the logistic regression model to roughly quantify the strength of the association with LNM status (Table 3). The results showed that LVI (ORs = 1.379; $p < 0.001$), pT stage (ORs = 1.113; $p = 0.005$), and SBLNP-based score (ORs = 2.072; $p < 0.001$) were significantly associated with LNM status, among which the SBLNP achieved highest coefficient. The combined classifier yielded an AUROC of 0.864 (95% CI, 0.827–0.906; Table 2, Figure 3) on the internal validation set (TCGA cohort). In the RHWU cohort and the PHHC cohort, the AUROCs of the combined classifier were 0.810 (95% CI, 0.780–0.844) and 0.824 (95% CI, 0.788–0.861), which outperformed the clinical classifier significantly (Delong's test, $p = 0.004$ and $p = 0.021$, respectively; Table 4). Together, the SBLNP is a strong predictor of LNM status in addition to established clinicopathological features.

Table 3. Coefficients, *p* values, and odds ratios with 95% CIs for all variables of the logistic regression model of the combined classifier (Clinical + SBLNP) in the TCGA cohort.

Characteristic	Coefficient	*p* Value	Odds Ratio (95% CI)
Age	0.0034	0.120	1.003 (0.999–1.008)
Gender	0.0591	0.256	1.061 (0.958–1.175)
LVI	0.3211	<0.001	1.379 (1.252–1.518)
pT stage	0.1072	0.005	1.113 (1.033–1.199)
Histologic grade	−0.0808	0.474	0.922 (0.739–1.151)
SBLNP	0.7285	<0.001	2.072 (1.694–2.535)

CI, Confidence Interval; TCGA, The Cancer Genome Atlas; LVI, Lymphovascular Invasion; SBLNP, Slide-Based Lymph Node Predictor.

Table 4. Performance comparisons (DeLong's test) between clinical classifier, SBLNP, and combined classifier (Clinical + SBLNP) in internal and external validation sets.

Comparisons	TCGA Cohort	RHWU Cohort	PHHC Cohort
Clinical vs. SBLNP	$p = 0.028$	$p = 0.632$	$p = 0.703$
Clinical vs. Clinical + SBLNP	$p = 0.001$	$p = 0.004$	$p = 0.021$
SBLNP vs. Clinical + SBLNP	$p = 0.093$	$p = 0.014$	$p = 0.005$

TCGA, The Cancer Genome Atlas; RHWU, Renmin Hospital of Wuhan University; PHHC, People's Hospital of Hanchuan City; SBLNP, Slide-Based Lymph Node Predictor.

3.5. Visualizing Deep Learning-Based Predictions

Next, we intended to use visualization techniques to understand how the deep learning-based model predicted, thereby guiding pathologists to discover potentially relevant recognition patterns. To achieve this goal, the SBLNP with an attention mechanism assigned each patch an attention score, which is used to represent its contribution to the prediction. We then converted the scores into a heatmap to intuitively understand the region of interest of the model. This visualization method allowed us to identify the pathological patterns most associated with LNM-positive or -negative status. As shown in Figure 4, for LNM-positive WSIs, the model visually paid more attention to the stromal region around the tumor; on the contrary, for LNM-negative WSIs, the model focused more on bladder cancer itself. In addition, Figure 5 presented the five top-scoring patches for each of the five LNM-positive and five LNM-negative WSIs in the TCGA cohort. Regarding LNM-positive patches, we observed that the tissue regions yielding high prediction scores were predominantly located in the surrounding non-neoplastic tissue rather than the bladder cancer itself. Some patches contained inflammatory cell infiltration, mainly composed of lymphocytes. Conversely, tumor cells were dominant in patches with high LNM-negative prediction.

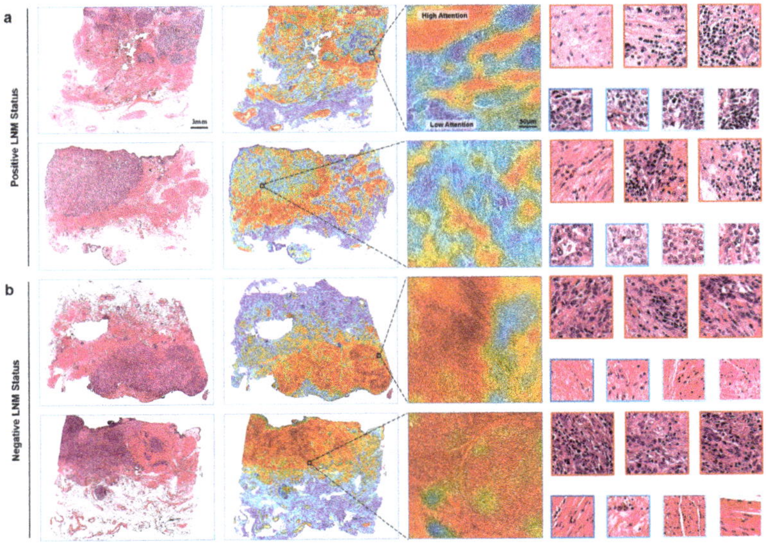

Figure 4. Heatmaps of (**a**) LNM-positive and (**b**) LNM-negative patients from the TCGA cohort predicted correctly by the SBLNP. The attention scores of all patches are calculated by the SBLNP, and an attention heatmap corresponding to each WSI is generated and overlaid on it. Then the local area is further zoomed in to highlight the high- (red) and low-attention (blue) histopathological features. LNM, lymph node metastasis.

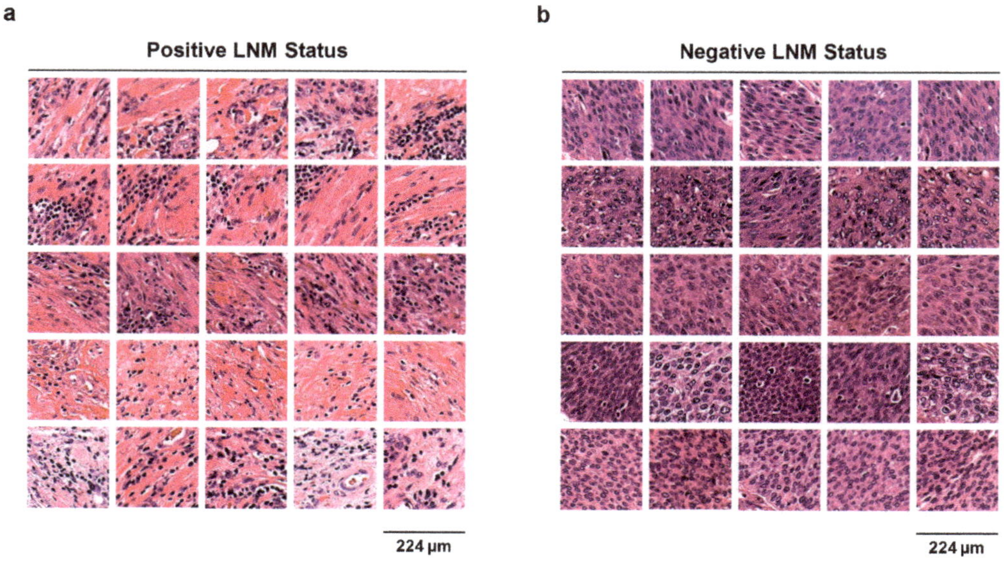

Figure 5. The 5 top-scoring patches of (**a**) the 5 top-scoring LNM-positive and (**b**) 5 top-scoring LNM-negative patients in the TCGA cohort. LNM, lymph node metastasis.

3.6. Quantitative Assessment of Histopathological Features

To further confirm the above findings, we performed a quantitative study of 100 WSIs from LNM-positive and -negative patients. The 15 top-scoring patches were obtained from each WSI, for a total of 1500 patches, and were reviewed by a pathologist blinded to the LNM status in advance. We found that 'immune cells' and 'stroma' were the most abundant tissue classes in LNM-positive patients. Conversely, 'tumor cells' was the most abundant tissue class in LNM-negative patients (Table 5). Surprisingly, most of the LNM-positive patches were predominantly located in the stromal region rather than the tumor region (ratio LNM-positive patches in stroma = 336/750), which was in complete contrast to the LNM-negative results (ratio LNM-negative patches in stroma = 16/750, Chi-squared test, $p < 0.001$). In the LNM-negative group, tumor tissue-related patches accounted for the largest proportion (ratio LNM-negative patches in tumor = 654/750), which also produced the contrary result to the LNM-positive group (ratio LNM-positive patches in tumor = 45/750, Chi-squared test, $p < 0.001$). More precisely, features of the tumor tissue itself do not seem to be too important in the process of predicting LNM-positive status, while the microenvironment around the tumor may need more attention. Finally, we performed a more fine-grained analysis of the "stroma" patches and found that in the LNM-positive group, stroma with lymphocytic inflammation (241/336) outnumbered those without inflammation (95/336) by more than 150%. Conversely, in the LNM-negative group, only 16/750 patches belonged to the stroma, and these patches did not show any inflammatory infiltration.

Table 5. Histopathological quantitative analysis of the 1500 top-scoring patches.

	Positive LNM Status		Negative LNM Status	
Histological Features	***n* Patches**	**% Patches**	***n* Patches**	**% Patches**
Tumor cells	45	6	654	87.2
Normal transitional epithelium	23	3.07	27	3.6
Muscle tissue	82	10.93	24	3.2
Adipose tissue	8	1.07	1	0.13
Immune cells	218	29.06	3	0.4
Necrotic tissue	29	3.87	18	2.4
Stroma	336	44.8	16	2.13
Out of focus	9	1.2	7	0.94

4. Discussion

The presence of LNM in MIBC patients has been shown to be associated with a poorer prognosis, and the 5-year overall survival of LNM-positive patients is significantly lower than that of LNM-negative patients [39–41]. Therefore, predicting the LNM status before RC is crucial for clinical decision-making in MIBC, particularly regarding the extent of PLND and the use of NAC [42,43]. However, the existing tools for predicting LNM status are not satisfactory in terms of accuracy and reliability, with some patients being under or over-staged [13,44,45]. Hence, there is an urgent need to find more tools to accurately predict the LNM status before RC. In this study, we developed a weakly-supervised deep learning model (SBLNP) that can predict the LNM status from digital H&E-stained images of the primary MIBC. Our results demonstrated that SBLNP performed well with AUROC values between 0.7 and 0.8 in three independent cohorts, showing excellent generalization ability. In addition, the results of the clinical classifier confirmed that the LVI and pT stage were strongly associated with the LNM status [46,47], and the combined classifier based on SBLNP and clinicopathologic variables demonstrated satisfactory performance.

Previous studies have shown that cisplatin-based NAC can serve as first-line adjuvant therapy for MIBC and prolong survival, with an absolute increase of 8% in the 5-year survival [48] and from 30% to 36% in the 10-year survival [49]. In addition, the European Association of Urology guidelines recommend NAC for MIBC patients with T2-T4a and cN0M0 before RC [10]. However, NAC has not been widely used in clinical practice, with only 19% of patients receiving NAC before RC [50], mainly due to a lack of response to treatment, the potential for surgical delays, and the risks of over-staging and over-treatment. Moreover, MIBC patients with LNM-positive may benefit from NAC, as the goal of NAC is to target distant metastases (including LNM) rather than control the local region [49,51].

Currently, RC and bilateral PLND are the standard treatment for MIBC patients, but the optimal extent of PLND remains controversial. Previous studies have shown that the extent of LNM in some patients exceeds the region of the standard PLND template [52,53], and a larger dissection area is needed to achieve better regional control and more accurate lymph node staging [4]. Another systematic review indicated that extended PLND may provide more therapeutic benefits than standard PLND [54]. However, the use of extended PLND in clinical practice is limited by the increased surgical difficulty, potential surgical risks, and complications.

In clinical practice, the identification of MIBC patients with a high risk of LNM before RC will aid in determining an appropriate population for NAC and extended PLND. Thus, there is an urgent need for the development of new tools for accurate prediction of LNM status before RC to optimize clinical treatment decisions.

The use of radiomics and genomics to predict the LNM status [55–57] has been shown to achieve good performance. However, the cohort used by these methods is single, the amount of data is small, and the generalization performance of the model still needs to be verified. Despite similar studies based on deep learning in breast cancer [24], colorectal cancer [25–27], and prostate cancer [28], the small training data size, poor interpretability, and time-consuming and labor-intensive manual annotation remain obstacles to their clinical application. Therefore, developing a weakly-supervised or unsupervised model with high interpretability and generalization ability is the starting point of this study. In this study, the integration of clinicopathologic information and SBLNP contributes to the improvement of predictive model performance, indicating that they are not redundant with each other. Our SBLNP model requires only H&E-stained pathology slides as input to obtain predictions related to LNM status, which is cost-effective since such slides are readily available in the surgical setting. Interestingly, based on the interpretability of our model, we found that the stromal region around the tumor may contain histological information related to the LNM status. This also reflects that previous studies may have lost important predictive information by only training the model on the annotated tumor region. Through quantitative analysis and blind evaluation of the 1500 top-scoring patches, we validated the above observations. Specifically, a key predictive feature appears to be the stroma with lymphocytic inflammation around the tumor.

To our knowledge, this is the first study that links inflammatory infiltrate in the stroma of MIBC to the LNM status. Improved tumor microenvironment assessment and intervention are critical to the development of effective therapies for bladder cancer [58]. Further mechanistic studies are needed to validate the predictive patterns of deep learning. Previous studies have shown that tumor-associated inflammation in the tumor microenvironment may be related to the tumor's biological behavior and prognosis and may serve as a potential predictor for LNM [59,60]. Lymphocytes and monocyte-differentiated tumor-associated macrophages are involved in the composition of the tumor microenvironment, and their interaction can promote tumor angiogenesis and invasion [61]. In addition, a large number of cancer-associated fibroblasts (CAFs) in the stroma affect the occurrence of LNM. Recently, in cervical squamous cell carcinoma, CAFs were observed to promote LNM through the destruction of the lymphatic endothelial barrier in cell-level experiments [62]. In gastric cancer, the relationship between interleukin-8, CAFs, and lymphocytes was revealed through cell and animal experiments, explaining the possible mechanism of LNM occurrence [63]. Therefore, further elucidation of these mechanisms may improve our understanding of the ability of deep learning to predict LNM in MIBC.

Despite the advantages of our study, limitations exist. First, our study is retrospective and requires larger multicenter prospective studies to further confirm its clinical value. Second, the variables included in our clinical classifier are not comprehensive enough, and clinical information, including tumor size, location, and tumor budding, needs to be collected. Our combined classifier achieved the best performance; integrating pathological features with clinical key information is another important direction. In addition, the inclusion of LNM-positive and -negative categories in this study is unbalanced, as data with better class balance can help improve performance. Finally, we found that a few artifacts and out-of-focus tissues are still mixed in the training data, and future research needs to further control the quality of the data to exclude possible interfering factors.

5. Conclusions

We developed a weakly-supervised deep learning model for predicting LNM status in MIBC patients. In three independent cohorts, the SBLNP demonstrated decent predictive performance. Interestingly, the SBLNP generated a new biological hypothesis, defining the lymphocytic inflammatory stroma as a key factor for prediction, but further experimental validation is needed. Future efforts are needed to improve SBLNP for early clinical implementation, providing precise guidance for the use of NAC and the extent of PLND in MIBC patients.

Supplementary Materials: The following supporting information can be downloaded at: https://www.mdpi.com/article/10.3390/cancers15113000/s1, Table S1: Dataset distribution of patients and corresponding images in the predictor (SBLNP). Table S2: Dataset distribution of images in the training, internal validation, and external validation sets.

Author Contributions: Conceptualization, X.L. and L.W.; Data curation, K.W., H.X., X.N. and P.J.; Formal analysis, Q.Z., J.J., K.W. and J.Y.; Funding acquisition, Z.C. and X.L.; Investigation, J.W. (Jingsong Wang) and X.N.; Methodology, Q.Z., J.J. and J.F.; Project administration, R.Y., Z.C., X.L. and L.W.; Resources, S.Y.; Software, J.J. and J.F.; Supervision, R.Y., Z.C., X.L. and L.W.; Validation, Q.Z., J.W. (Jingsong Wang), X.N. and S.Y.; Visualization, J.Y. and R.Y.; Writing—original draft, Q.Z., H.X. and J.W. (Jiejun Wu); Writing—review and editing, R.Y., Z.C., X.L. and L.W. All authors have read and agreed to the published version of the manuscript.

Funding: This research was funded by the "Hubei Province Key Research and Development Project, grant number 2020BCB051 to Xiuheng Liu" and "Hubei Province Central Guiding Local Science and Technology Development Project, grant number 2022BGE232 to Zhiyuan Chen".

Institutional Review Board Statement: The study was conducted in accordance with the Declaration of Helsinki and approved by the Ethics Committee of RHWU and PHHC (protocol code WDRY2023-K006, approved February 2023).

Informed Consent Statement: The obtained informed consent was waived.

Data Availability Statement: The datasets of the TCGA cohort for this study can be found in the [The Cancer Genome Atlas Program] [https://portal.gdc.cancer.gov/, accessed on 7 January 2023].

Acknowledgments: We thank our colleagues in the Department of Urology and Pathology, RHWU and PHHC, for their support of this work, as well as all colleagues involved in model development and data collection.

Conflicts of Interest: The authors declare no conflict of interest.

References

1. Sung, H.; Ferlay, J.; Siegel, R.L.; Laversanne, M.; Soerjomataram, I.; Jemal, A.; Bray, F. Global cancer statistics 2020: Globocan estimates of incidence and mortality worldwide for 36 cancers in 185 countries. *CA Cancer J. Clin.* **2021**, *71*, 209–249. [CrossRef]
2. Sanli, O.; Dobruch, J.; Knowles, M.A.; Burger, M.; Alemozaffar, M.; Nielsen, M.E.; Lotan, Y. Bladder cancer. *Nat. Rev. Dis. Primers* **2017**, *3*, 17022. [CrossRef]
3. Patel, V.G.; Oh, W.K.; Galsky, M.D. Treatment of muscle-invasive and advanced bladder cancer in 2020. *CA Cancer J. Clin.* **2020**, *70*, 404–423. [CrossRef]
4. Kamat, A.M.; Hahn, N.M.; Efstathiou, J.A.; Lerner, S.P.; Malmström, P.U.; Choi, W.; Guo, C.C.; Lotan, Y.; Kassouf, W. Bladder cancer. *Lancet* **2016**, *388*, 2796–2810. [CrossRef] [PubMed]
5. Perera, M.; Mcgrath, S.; Sengupta, S.; Crozier, J.; Bolton, D.; Lawrentschuk, N. Pelvic lymph node dissection during radical cystectomy for muscle-invasive bladder cancer. *Nat. Rev. Urol.* **2018**, *15*, 686–692. [CrossRef] [PubMed]
6. Yafi, F.A.; Aprikian, A.G.; Chin, J.L.; Fradet, Y.; Izawa, J.; Estey, E.; Fairey, A.; Rendon, R.; Cagiannos, I.; Lacombe, L.; et al. Contemporary outcomes of 2287 patients with bladder cancer who were treated with radical cystectomy: A canadian multicentre experience. *BJU Int.* **2011**, *108*, 539–545. [CrossRef]
7. Stein, J.P.; Lieskovsky, G.; Cote, R.; Groshen, S.; Feng, A.C.; Boyd, S.; Skinner, E.; Bochner, B.; Thangathurai, D.; Mikhail, M.; et al. Radical cystectomy in the treatment of invasive bladder cancer: Long-term results in 1054 patients. *J. Clin. Oncol.* **2001**, *19*, 666–675. [CrossRef] [PubMed]
8. Lobo, N.; Mount, C.; Omar, K.; Nair, R.; Thurairaja, R.; Khan, M.S. Landmarks in the treatment of muscle-invasive bladder cancer. *Nat. Rev. Urol.* **2017**, *14*, 565–574. [CrossRef]
9. Motterle, G.; Andrews, J.R.; Morlacco, A.; Karnes, R.J. Predicting response to neoadjuvant chemotherapy in bladder cancer. *Eur. Urol. Focus* **2020**, *6*, 642–649. [CrossRef] [PubMed]
10. Witjes, J.A.; Bruins, H.M.; Cathomas, R.; Compérat, E.M.; Cowan, N.C.; Gakis, G.; Hernández, V.; Linares, E.E.; Lorch, A.; Neuzillet, Y.; et al. European association of urology guidelines on muscle-invasive and metastatic bladder cancer: Summary of the 2020 guidelines. *Eur. Urol.* **2021**, *79*, 82–104. [CrossRef]
11. Wagner, J.; Simon, R.; Büchler, J.W.; Kirchhoff, F.; Kehl, V.; Retz, M.; Gschwend, J.E.; Sauter, A.; Horn, T. Both radiographical and pathological lymph node statuses are independent predictors for survival following neoadjuvant chemotherapy and radical cystectomy for ct3/4 or cn+ bladder cancer. *World J. Urol.* **2022**, *41*, 101–107. [CrossRef] [PubMed]
12. Swinnen, G.; Maes, A.; Pottel, H.; Vanneste, A.; Billiet, I.; Lesage, K.; Werbrouck, P. Fdg-pet/ct for the preoperative lymph node staging of invasive bladder cancer. *Eur. Urol.* **2010**, *57*, 641–647. [CrossRef] [PubMed]
13. Lodde, M.; Lacombe, L.; Friede, J.; Morin, F.; Saourine, A.; Fradet, Y. Evaluation of fluorodeoxyglucose positron-emission tomography with computed tomography for staging of urothelial carcinoma. *BJU Int.* **2010**, *106*, 658–663. [CrossRef] [PubMed]
14. Tian, Z.; Meng, L.; Wang, X.; Diao, T.; Hu, M.; Wang, M.; Zhang, Y.; Liu, M. Predictive nomogram and risk factors for lymph node metastasis in bladder cancer. *Front. Oncol.* **2021**, *11*, 690324. [CrossRef]

15. Zhang, C.; Hu, J.; Li, H.; Ma, H.; Othmane, B.; Ren, W.; Yi, Z.; Qiu, D.; Ou, Z.; Chen, J.; et al. Emerging biomarkers for predicting bladder cancer lymph node metastasis. *Front. Oncol.* **2021**, *11*, 648968. [CrossRef]
16. Seiler, R.; Lam, L.L.; Erho, N.; Takhar, M.; Mitra, A.P.; Buerki, C.; Davicioni, E.; Skinner, E.C.; Daneshmand, S.; Black, P.C. Prediction of lymph node metastasis in patients with bladder cancer using whole transcriptome gene expression signatures. *J. Urol.* **2016**, *196*, 1036–1041. [CrossRef]
17. van der Laak, J.; Litjens, G.; Ciompi, F. Deep learning in histopathology: The path to the clinic. *Nat. Med.* **2021**, *27*, 775–784. [CrossRef]
18. Nojima, S.; Terayama, K.; Shimoura, S.; Hijiki, S.; Nonomura, N.; Morii, E.; Okuno, Y.; Fujita, K. A deep learning system to diagnose the malignant potential of urothelial carcinoma cells in cytology specimens. *Cancer Cytopathol.* **2021**, *129*, 984–995. [CrossRef]
19. Zheng, Q.; Jiang, Z.; Ni, X.; Yang, S.; Jiao, P.; Wu, J.; Xiong, L.; Yuan, J.; Wang, J.; Jian, J.; et al. Machine learning quantified tumor-stroma ratio is an independent prognosticator in muscle-invasive bladder cancer. *Int. J. Mol. Sci.* **2023**, *24*, 2746. [CrossRef]
20. Zheng, Q.; Yang, R.; Ni, X.; Yang, S.; Jiao, P.; Wu, J.; Xiong, L.; Wang, J.; Jian, J.; Jiang, Z.; et al. Quantitative assessment of tumor-infiltrating lymphocytes using machine learning predicts survival in muscle-invasive bladder cancer. *J. Clin. Med.* **2022**, *11*, 7081. [CrossRef]
21. Woerl, A.C.; Eckstein, M.; Geiger, J.; Wagner, D.C.; Daher, T.; Stenzel, P.; Fernandez, A.; Hartmann, A.; Wand, M.; Roth, W.; et al. Deep learning predicts molecular subtype of muscle-invasive bladder cancer from conventional histopathological slides. *Eur. Urol.* **2020**, *78*, 256–264. [CrossRef] [PubMed]
22. Zheng, Q.; Yang, R.; Ni, X.; Yang, S.; Xiong, L.; Yan, D.; Xia, L.; Yuan, J.; Wang, J.; Jiao, P.; et al. Accurate diagnosis and survival prediction of bladder cancer using deep learning on histological slides. *Cancers* **2022**, *14*, 5807. [CrossRef]
23. Qaiser, T.; Lee, C.Y.; Vandenberghe, M.; Yeh, J.; Gavrielides, M.A.; Hipp, J.; Scott, M.; Reischl, J. Usability of deep learning and h&e images predict disease outcome-emerging tool to optimize clinical trials. *NPJ Precis. Oncol.* **2022**, *6*, 37.
24. Xu, F.; Zhu, C.; Tang, W.; Wang, Y.; Zhang, Y.; Li, J.; Jiang, H.; Shi, Z.; Liu, J.; Jin, M. Predicting axillary lymph node metastasis in early breast cancer using deep learning on primary tumor biopsy slides. *Front. Oncol.* **2021**, *11*, 759007. [CrossRef]
25. Kiehl, L.; Kuntz, S.; Höhn, J.; Jutzi, T.; Krieghoff-Henning, E.; Kather, J.N.; Holland-Letz, T.; Kopp-Schneider, A.; Chang-Claude, J.; Brobeil, A.; et al. Deep learning can predict lymph node status directly from histology in colorectal cancer. *Eur. J. Cancer* **2021**, *157*, 464–473. [CrossRef] [PubMed]
26. Brockmoeller, S.; Echle, A.; Ghaffari, L.N.; Eiholm, S.; Malmstrøm, M.L.; Plato, K.T.; Levic, K.; Grabsch, H.I.; West, N.P.; Saldanha, O.L.; et al. Deep learning identifies inflamed fat as a risk factor for lymph node metastasis in early colorectal cancer. *J. Pathol.* **2022**, *256*, 269–281. [CrossRef] [PubMed]
27. Song, J.H.; Hong, Y.; Kim, E.R.; Kim, S.H.; Sohn, I. Utility of artificial intelligence with deep learning of hematoxylin and eosin-stained whole slide images to predict lymph node metastasis in t1 colorectal cancer using endoscopically resected specimens; Prediction of lymph node metastasis in t1 colorectal cancer. *J. Gastroenterol.* **2022**, *57*, 654–666.
28. Wessels, F.; Schmitt, M.; Krieghoff-Henning, E.; Jutzi, T.; Worst, T.S.; Waldbillig, F.; Neuberger, M.; Maron, R.C.; Steeg, M.; Gaiser, T.; et al. Deep learning approach to predict lymph node metastasis directly from primary tumour histology in prostate cancer. *BJU Int.* **2021**, *128*, 352–360. [CrossRef]
29. Harmon, S.A.; Sanford, T.H.; Brown, G.T.; Yang, C.; Mehralivand, S.; Jacob, J.M.; Valera, V.A.; Shih, J.H.; Agarwal, P.K.; Choyke, P.L.; et al. Multiresolution application of artificial intelligence in digital pathology for prediction of positive lymph nodes from primary tumors in bladder cancer. *JCO Clin. Cancer Info.* **2020**, *4*, 367–382. [CrossRef]
30. Cheng, J.Y.; Abel, J.T.; Balis, U.; Mcclintock, D.S.; Pantanowitz, L. Challenges in the development, deployment, and regulation of artificial intelligence in anatomic pathology. *Am. J. Pathol.* **2021**, *191*, 1684–1692. [CrossRef]
31. Vahadane, A.; Peng, T.Y.; Albarqouni, S.; Baust, M.; Steiger, K.; Schlitter, A.M.; Sethi, A.; Esposito, I.; Navab, N. Structure-preserved color normalization for histological images. In Proceedings of the IEEE 12th International Symposium on Biomedical Imaging (ISBI), Brooklyn, NY, USA, 16–19 April 2015; pp. 1012–1015.
32. Anand, D.; Ramakrishnan, G.; Sethi, A. Fast GPU-enabled color normalization for digital pathology. In Proceedings of the 2019 International Conference on Systems, Signals and Image Processing (IWSSIP 2019), Osijek, Croatia, 5–7 June 2019; pp. 219–224.
33. He, K.M.; Zhang, X.Y.; Ren, S.Q.; Sun, J. Deep residual learning for image recognition. In Proceedings of the IEEE Conference on Computer Vision and Pattern Recognition (CVPR), Las Vegas, NV, USA, 27–30 June 2016; pp. 770–778.
34. Leng, L.; Li, M.; Kim, C.; Bi, X. Dual-source discrimination power analysis for multi-instance contactless palmprint recognition. *Multimed. Tools Appl.* **2017**, *76*, 333–354. [CrossRef]
35. Leng, L.; Zhang, J. Palmhash code vs. Palmphasor code. *Neurocomputing* **2013**, *108*, 1–12. [CrossRef]
36. Ilse, M.; Tomczak, J.M.; Welling, M. Attention-based deep multiple instance learning. In Proceedings of the 35th International Conference on Machine Learning, Stockholm, Sweden, 10–15 July 2018; Volume 80.
37. Berrada, L.; Zisserman, A.; Kumar, M.P. Smooth loss functions for deep top-k classification. *arXiv* **2018**, arXiv:1802.07595.
38. Delong, E.R.; Delong, D.M.; Clarke-Pearson, D.L. Comparing the areas under two or more correlated receiver operating characteristic curves: A nonparametric approach. *Biometrics* **1988**, *44*, 837–845. [CrossRef] [PubMed]

39. Zehnder, P.; Studer, U.E.; Daneshmand, S.; Birkhäuser, F.D.; Skinner, E.C.; Roth, B.; Miranda, G.; Burkhard, F.C.; Cai, J.; Skinner, D.G.; et al. Outcomes of radical cystectomy with extended lymphadenectomy alone in patients with lymph node-positive bladder cancer who are unfit for or who decline adjuvant chemotherapy. *BJU Int.* **2014**, *113*, 554–560. [CrossRef]
40. Bassi, P.; Ferrante, G.D.; Piazza, N.; Spinadin, R.; Carando, R.; Pappagallo, G.; Pagano, F. Prognostic factors of outcome after radical cystectomy for bladder cancer: A retrospective study of a homogeneous patient cohort. *J. Urol.* **1999**, *161*, 1494–1497. [CrossRef]
41. Abdel-Latif, M.; Abol-Enein, H.; El-Baz, M.; Ghoneim, M.A. Nodal involvement in bladder cancer cases treated with radical cystectomy: Incidence and prognosis. *J. Urol.* **2004**, *172*, 85–89. [CrossRef]
42. Karl, A.; Carroll, P.R.; Gschwend, J.E.; Knüchel, R.; Montorsi, F.; Stief, C.G.; Studer, U.E. The impact of lymphadenectomy and lymph node metastasis on the outcomes of radical cystectomy for bladder cancer. *Eur. Urol.* **2009**, *55*, 826–835. [CrossRef]
43. Darwish, C.; Sparks, A.; Amdur, R.; Reddy, A.; Whalen, M. Trends in treatment strategies and comparison of outcomes in lymph node positive bladder cancer: An analysis of the national cancer database. *Urology* **2020**, *146*, 168–176. [CrossRef]
44. Mckibben, M.J.; Woods, M.E. Preoperative imaging for staging bladder cancer. *Curr. Urol. Rep.* **2015**, *16*, 22. [CrossRef]
45. Baltaci, S.; Resorlu, B.; Yagci, C.; Turkolmez, K.; Gogus, C.; Beduk, Y. Computerized tomography for detecting perivesical infiltration and lymph node metastasis in invasive bladder carcinoma. *Urol. Int.* **2008**, *81*, 399–402. [CrossRef]
46. Shariat, S.F.; Rink, M.; Ehdaie, B.; Xylinas, E.; Babjuk, M.; Merseburger, A.S.; Svatek, R.S.; Cha, E.K.; Tagawa, S.T.; Fajkovic, H.; et al. Pathologic nodal staging score for bladder cancer: A decision tool for adjuvant therapy after radical cystectomy. *Eur. Urol.* **2013**, *63*, 371–378. [CrossRef] [PubMed]
47. Werntz, R.P.; Smith, Z.L.; Packiam, V.T.; Smith, N.; Steinberg, G.D. The impact of lymphovascular invasion on risk of upstaging and lymph node metastasis at the time of radical cystectomy. *Eur. Urol. Focus* **2020**, *6*, 292–297. [CrossRef]
48. Sherif, A.; Holmberg, L.; Rintala, E.; Mestad, O.; Nilsson, J.; Nilsson, S.; Malmström, P.U. Neoadjuvant cisplatinum based combination chemotherapy in patients with invasive bladder cancer: A combined analysis of two nordic studies. *Eur. Urol.* **2004**, *45*, 297–303. [CrossRef]
49. Griffiths, G.; Hall, R.; Sylvester, R.; Raghavan, D.; Parmar, M.K. International phase iii trial assessing neoadjuvant cisplatin, methotrexate, and vinblastine chemotherapy for muscle-invasive bladder cancer: Long-term results of the ba06 30894 trial. *J. Clin. Oncol.* **2011**, *29*, 2171–2177. [PubMed]
50. Hanna, N.; Trinh, Q.D.; Seisen, T.; Vetterlein, M.W.; Sammon, J.; Preston, M.A.; Lipsitz, S.R.; Bellmunt, J.; Menon, M.; Choueiri, T.K.; et al. Effectiveness of neoadjuvant chemotherapy for muscle-invasive bladder cancer in the current real world setting in the usa. *Eur. Urol. Oncol.* **2018**, *1*, 83–90. [CrossRef]
51. Mertens, L.S.; Meijer, R.P.; Meinhardt, W.; van der Poel, H.G.; Bex, A.; Kerst, J.M.; van der Heijden, M.S.; Bergman, A.M.; Horenblas, S.; van Rhijn, B.W. Occult lymph node metastases in patients with carcinoma invading bladder muscle: Incidence after neoadjuvant chemotherapy and cystectomy vs after cystectomy alone. *BJU Int.* **2014**, *114*, 67–74. [CrossRef]
52. Wang, L.; Mudaliar, K.; Mehta, V.; Barkan, G.A.; Quek, M.L.; Flanigan, R.C.; Picken, M.M. Seeking a standard for adequate pathologic lymph node staging in primary bladder carcinoma. *Virchows Arch.* **2014**, *464*, 595–602. [CrossRef]
53. Dorin, R.P.; Daneshmand, S.; Eisenberg, M.S.; Chandrasoma, S.; Cai, J.; Miranda, G.; Nichols, P.W.; Skinner, D.G.; Skinner, E.C. Lymph node dissection technique is more important than lymph node count in identifying nodal metastases in radical cystectomy patients: A comparative mapping study. *Eur. Urol.* **2011**, *60*, 946–952. [CrossRef]
54. Bruins, H.M.; Veskimae, E.; Hernandez, V.; Imamura, M.; Neuberger, M.M.; Dahm, P.; Stewart, F.; Lam, T.B.; N'Dow, J.; van der Heijden, A.G.; et al. The impact of the extent of lymphadenectomy on oncologic outcomes in patients undergoing radical cystectomy for bladder cancer: A systematic review. *Eur. Urol.* **2014**, *66*, 1065–1077. [CrossRef]
55. Wu, S.X.; Huang, J.; Liu, Z.W.; Chen, H.G.; Guo, P.; Cai, Q.Q.; Zheng, J.J.; Qin, H.D.; Zheng, Z.S.; Chen, X.; et al. A genomic-clinicopathologic nomogram for the preoperative prediction of lymph node metastasis in bladder cancer. *Ebiomedicine* **2018**, *31*, 54–65. [CrossRef] [PubMed]
56. Wu, S.; Zheng, J.; Li, Y.; Wu, Z.; Shi, S.; Huang, M.; Yu, H.; Dong, W.; Huang, J.; Lin, T. Development and validation of an mri-based radiomics signature for the preoperative prediction of lymph node metastasis in bladder cancer. *Ebiomedicine* **2018**, *34*, 76–84. [CrossRef]
57. Wu, S.; Zheng, J.; Li, Y.; Yu, H.; Shi, S.; Xie, W.; Liu, H.; Su, Y.; Huang, J.; Lin, T. A radiomics nomogram for the preoperative prediction of lymph node metastasis in bladder cancer. *Clin. Cancer Res.* **2017**, *23*, 6904–6911. [CrossRef] [PubMed]
58. Fontanet, S.; Basile, G.; Baboudjian, M.; Gallioli, A.; Huguet, J.; Territo, A.; Parada, R.; Gavrilov, P.; Aumatell, J.; Sanz, I.; et al. Robot-assisted vs. open radical cystectomy: Systematic review and meta-analysis of randomized controlled trials. *Actas Urol. Esp.* **2023**. [CrossRef] [PubMed]
59. Greten, F.R.; Grivennikov, S.I. Inflammation and cancer: Triggers, mechanisms, and consequences. *Immunity* **2019**, *51*, 27–41. [CrossRef] [PubMed]
60. Dupré, A.; Malik, H.Z. Inflammation and cancer: What a surgical oncologist should know. *EJSO* **2018**, *44*, 566–570. [CrossRef]
61. Chittezhath, M.; Dhillon, M.K.; Lim, J.Y.; Laoui, D.; Shalova, I.N.; Teo, Y.L.; Chen, J.; Kamaraj, R.; Raman, L.; Lum, J.; et al. Molecular profiling reveals a tumor-promoting phenotype of monocytes and macrophages in human cancer progression. *Immunity* **2014**, *41*, 815–829. [CrossRef]

62. Wei, W.F.; Chen, X.J.; Liang, L.J.; Yu, L.; Wu, X.G.; Zhou, C.F.; Wang, Z.C.; Fan, L.S.; Hu, Z.; Liang, L.; et al. Periostin(+) cancer-associated fibroblasts promote lymph node metastasis by impairing the lymphatic endothelial barriers in cervical squamous cell carcinoma. *Mol. Oncol.* **2021**, *15*, 210–227. [CrossRef]
63. Li, X.; Zhai, J.; Shen, Y.; Zhang, T.; Wang, Y.; He, Y.; You, Q.; Shen, L. Tumor-derived il-8 facilitates lymph node metastasis of gastric cancer via pd-1 up-regulation in cd8(+) T cells. *Cancer Immunol. Immunother.* **2022**, *71*, 3057–3070. [CrossRef]

cancers

MDPI

Article

Excitement and Concerns of Young Radiation Oncologists over Automatic Segmentation: A French Perspective

Vincent Bourbonne [1,2,*], Adrien Laville [3], Nicolas Wagneur [2,4], Youssef Ghannam [2,4] and Audrey Larnaudie [2,5]

1 Radiation Oncology Department, University Hospital Brest, 2 Avenue Foch, 29200 Brest, France
2 Société Française des Jeunes Radiothérapeutes Oncologues, 47 Rue de la Colonie, 75013 Paris, France
3 Radiation Oncology Department, University Hospital Amiens-Picardie, 30 Avenue de la Croix Jourdain, 80054 Amiens, France
4 Radiation Oncology Department, Institut de Cancérologie de l'Ouest, Centre Paul Papin, 15 Rue André Bocquel, 49055 Angers, France
5 Radiation Oncology Department, Centre François Baclesse, 3 Avenue du Général Harris, 14000 Caen, France
* Correspondence: vincent.bourbonne@chu-brest.fr; Tel.: +33-298223398; Fax: +33-98223087

Simple Summary: Radiation oncology has known tremendous technological advances in recent years, the latest being brought by artificial intelligence (AI). Applied to segmentation, some concerns were raised by academics regarding the impact on young radiation oncologists' training. To answer those concerns, a survey was conducted by the SFjRO (Société Française des jeunes Radiothérapeutes Oncologues). The survey was mandatory for registration to a dosimetry webinar dedicated to head and neck cancers. A significant time gain was observed for the delineation of organs at risk, with almost 35% of the participants saving between 50–100% of the segmentation time, while only 8.6% experienced such a gain for the delineation of target volumes. The majority of participants suggested that these tools should be integrated into the training so that future radiation oncologists do not neglect the importance of radioanatomy. Fully aware of this risk, up to one-third of them even suggested that AI tools should be reserved for senior physicians only.

Abstract: Introduction: Segmentation of organs at risk (OARs) and target volumes need time and precision but are highly repetitive tasks. Radiation oncology has known tremendous technological advances in recent years, the latest being brought by artificial intelligence (AI). Despite the advantages brought by AI for segmentation, some concerns were raised by academics regarding the impact on young radiation oncologists' training. A survey was thus conducted on young french radiation oncologists (ROs) by the SFjRO (Société Française des jeunes Radiothérapeutes Oncologues). Methodology: The SFjRO organizes regular webinars focusing on anatomical localization, discussing either segmentation or dosimetry. Completion of the survey was mandatory for registration to a dosimetry webinar dedicated to head and neck (H & N) cancers. The survey was generated in accordance with the CHERRIES guidelines. Quantitative data (e.g., time savings and correction needs) were not measured but determined among the propositions. Results: 117 young ROs from 35 different and mostly academic centers participated. Most centers were either already equipped with such solutions or planning to be equipped in the next two years. AI segmentation software was mostly useful for H & N cases. While for the definition of OARs, participants experienced a significant time gain using AI-proposed delineations, with almost 35% of the participants saving between 50–100% of the segmentation time, time gained for target volumes was significantly lower, with only 8.6% experiencing a 50–100% gain. Contours still needed to be thoroughly checked, especially target volumes for some, and edited. The majority of participants suggested that these tools should be integrated into the training so that future radiation oncologists do not neglect the importance of radioanatomy. Fully aware of this risk, up to one-third of them even suggested that AI tools should be reserved for senior physicians only. Conclusions: We believe this survey on automatic segmentation to be the first to focus on the perception of young radiation oncologists. Software developers should focus on enhancing the quality of proposed segmentations, while young radiation oncologists should become more acquainted with these tools.

Keywords: artificial intelligence; automatic segmentation; radiation oncology

1. Introduction

Radiation oncology has known tremendous technological advances in recent years [1–3], the latest being brought by artificial intelligence (AI) [4–7]. AI is taking more and more place in the clinical workflow of patients undergoing radiotherapy (RT), from segmentation to dosimetry planning and prediction modeling of clinical endpoints. Segmentation is a major and time-consuming step, mixing repetitive steps, such as the delineation of organs at risk (OARs), but also experience needing tasks for the delineation of target volumes. Automatic segmentation can use atlas-based methods with single-atlas, multi-atlas, or a hybrid. Deep learning techniques have been recently applied [8]. A strong focus was made on head and neck (H & N) delineation due to its particular long time of contouring, estimated at around 2.7–3 h without AI help [9]. Although the delineation of OARs requires anatomical knowledge, there is a little inter-individual variation in their definition. However, when defining the target volumes (gross tumor volume and clinical target volume), one must adapt to the patient's anatomy as well as the disease characteristics, often using multimodal information and imaging. The lack of reliable and robust data is the main limitation of such tasks.

Some concerns were raised by academics regarding the consequences of young radiation oncologists' training. The impact of automated segmentation tools depends on the contours. For OARs, in addition to the loss of technical skills and dependence on computer tools, the extensive use of automatic segmentation tools could lead to a lack of knowledge of radioanatomy and, therefore, an inability to correct the proposed segmentations resulting in a blind trust. For target volumes, delineation takes into account the international guidelines but also the radiation oncologist's experience and all the patient's characteristics, data that are difficult to learn for an AI tool.

The Société Française des jeunes Radiothérapeutes Oncologues (SFjRO) is a national association reuniting all the residents and young radiation oncologists (ROs) funded in 2002 [10]. Its main goals include radiation oncology (RO) training and working in close collaboration with the french society of Radiation Oncology (SFRO) and the National Board of Oncology Teachers (CNEC). Translational lectures are given several times a year to improve the training of RO residents [11–14]. Concerning delineation topics, national courses are organized regularly in radio-anatomy with around 180–200 attendings (Paris 2009, Paris 2012, Paris 2018). Due to the importance and evolution of contouring guidelines, webinars and online delineation courses are proposed.

Given the broader use of AI segmentation, the radiation oncologist's job and his/her daily tasks are rapidly evolving. As there were only scarce data in the literature concerning young ROs, a survey was thus conducted by the SFjRO. After giving an overview of the participants and the use of segmentation AI tools in France, this article consists of the presentation of the main results, projecting on a possible better integration of AI in radiation oncology training.

2. Methodology—Form

The SFjRO organizes regular webinars focusing on anatomical localization, discussing either segmentation or dosimetry in collaboration with Dline.io (https://dline.io). In November 2022, the SFjRO conducted a dosimetry webinar addressing H & N cancers. A Google form was distributed and mandatory for registration to the webinar. It consisted of 22 questions formulated in French as presented in Supplementary Protocol S1. The SFjRO board is composed of 15 young radiation oncologists with different levels of experience. As a member of the board, Vincent Bourbonne was in charge of the questionnaire. Before choosing the questions, several goals were defined:

- Give an overview of the use of automatic segmentation tools in France;

- Give an overview of the pros and cons of such tools;
- Give insight into the future developments of AI tools for radiation oncologists.

Vincent Bourbonne and a second radiation oncologist (Adrien Laville) designed the questionnaire. Before being released, the questionnaire was internally validated by all co-authors but also the full SFjRO board. All members of the board took the test before its release to assess its readability and consistency. The validation process took three months, from the initial conception of the questionnaire to the final validation. The survey was compliant with the CHERRIES guidelines [15] as detailed in Supplementary Table S1. For completeness, the English translation is hereby presented in Table 1. Quantitative data (e.g., time savings and correction needs) were not measured but determined among the propositions.

Table 1. Submitted Form translated into English.

Question	Choices	
1. I would like to register to the H & N dosimetry webinar	- Yes - No	
2. State your name and surname		
3. State your mail address		
4. State your academic left		
5. State your status	- Resident - Attending - Senior physician	- Foreign Intern - Student - No position
5.1 If Resident a. State your year of training		
5.2 If Attending a. state your year of training	o <2 years o >2 years	
5.3 If senior physician a. State your year of training	o 2–5 years o 5–10 years	o 10–20 years o >20 years
6. In what type of structure do you work?	- University hospital - Academic left specializing in cancer care - General hospital - Private clinic	
7. How many patients per year are treated in your department?	- <800 - 800–1000 - 1000–1500	- 1500–2000 - >2000
8. In your left, who performs the delination of organs at risks (OARs)?	- Dosimetrists and physicists - Mostly residents - Attending or senior physicians mostly - Attending, senior physicians, attendings, physicists and dosimetrists	
9. Is your left equipped with an automatic delination solution?	- Yes - No	
9.1 If your department is equipped with an automatic delineation solution:		
a. How long have artificial intelligence tools for delineation been integrated into clinical routine?	o <1 year o 1–2 years o >2 years	
b. Who has access to these tools in your left?	o All ROs whatever their level of experience o Senior physicians only o Dosimetrists and physicists only o Attending, senior physicians, attendings, physicists and dosimetrists	

Table 1. *Cont.*

Question	Choices
c. What is/are the name(s) of the solution available in your department?	o ART-plan Annotate (Therapanacea) o DLCExpert o RayStation automatic segmentation o Mirada Workflow-Box o Elekta ABAS o SPICE o MIM Maestro o Mvision AI o Limbus AI o Syngo via (Siemens) o Not known
d. What were the motivations for your left to integrate these tools?	o Time saving o Available budget o Improve quality of treatment o Reduce inter-physician variability in contouring o Move towards the international recommendations
e. For which locations do you use these tools?	o Breast o Prostate o Pelvis o Head and Neck o Thorax o Neurology o Abdomen o Metastasis o All localizations
f. Rank the following locations in ascending order of time saved (1: little time saved -> 8: maximum time saved)	o Breast o Prostate o Pelvis o Head and Neck o Thorax o Neurology o Abdomen o Metastasis
g. Using this software saves you time in delineating:	o Macroscopic Tumour volumes (GTV T) o Tumour Target volumes (CTV T) o Macroscopic lymph nodes volumes (GTV N) o Prophylactic lymph nodes volumes (CTV N) o Organs at risk
h. How much time do you expect to save on OARs delineation (including correction)?	o 0% o <25% o 25–50% o 50–75% o 75–100%
i. On average, what percentage of the contours should you correct?	o 0% o <25% o 25–50% o 50–75% o 75–100%
j. Have you ever encountered an error during automatic contouring?	o Yes, laterality error o Yes, aberrant contours (wrong location) o Yes, but only minor and easily correctable errors o No, never
9.2 If your department isn't equipped with an automatic delineation solution:	
a. What are the obstacles to the adoption of such a solution?	o Free answer
b. Have you ever tested/used automatic contouring software?	o Yes o No
c. How soon do you expect artificial intelligence tools for delineation to be integrated into your left?	o Never o <1 year o 1–2 years o >2 years

Table 1. *Cont.*

Question	Choices	
10. Regarding the delineation of organs at risk:		
10.1 Brain: From the following list, what are the 3 organs at risk that must be included in software?	- Brain - Brainstem - Lens - Optic nerve - Eye - Optic chiasma	- Hippocampus - Inner ear - Pituitary gland - Hypothalamus - Lacrymal gland
10.2 H & N: From the following list, what are the 3 organs at risk that must be included in software?	- Temporo-mandibular articulation - Mandible - Oral cavity - Parotid - Larynx - Pharyngeal muscles	- Esophagus - Trachea - Spinal cord - Thyroid - Vessels
10.3 Thorax: From the following list, what are the 3 organs at risk that must be included in software?	- Lungs - Heart - Spinal cord - Esophagus	- Thyroid - Cardiac sub-structures - Vessels
10.4 Abdomen: From the following list, what are the 3 organs at risk that must be included in software?	- Spinal cord - Liver - Pancreas - Spleen - Bowel bag	- Small bowel - Large bowel - Kidneys - Vessels
10.5 Pelvis: From the following list, what are the 3 organs at risk that must be included in software?	- Bladder - Rectum - Sigmoid - Anal canal - Small bowel	- Large bowel - Prostate-Seminal vesicles o vagina-uterus - Lumbosacral Vertebrae-Iliac bones - Vessels
10.6 Which interesting OAR(s) have you never seen in automatic segmentation software?	- Free answer	
11. Regarding the delineation of target volumes		
11.1 Does the software at your disposal offer automatic segmentation of target volumes?	- Yes - No	
11.2 If your software allows the definition of target volumes:		
a. What target volumes are proposed?	o Tumour target volume o Nodal target volume o Prophylactic nodal volume	
b. How much time do you expect to save in contouring the target volumes (including correction)?	o 0% o <25% o 25–50%	o 50–75% o 75–100%
c. What are the limitations of segmentation software?	o Speed o Accuracy o Cost o Lack of cross software integration o Lack of completeness of proposed structures o Need for editing o Learning loss o Other:	

Table 1. *Cont.*

Question	Choices
12. Do you think that the use of automatic contouring software improves the quality of the contours?	- Yes - No
12.1 I think that automatic segmentation can improve the quality of the contours: Why?	- Gain in reproducibility - Gain in speed - Gain in accuracy
13. Do you think that the use of automatic contouring software is a danger for the profession of radiation oncologists?	- Yes - No
14. Do you think that the use of automatic contouring software is a danger for the training of young radiation oncologists?	- Yes - No
15. How do you think automatic delineation tools will impact the training of young radiotherapists?	- Free answer
16. Did you receive any training on artificial intelligence during your residency?	- Yes - No
17. In what way (s) do you think the training of radiation oncologists should be adapted?	- Spend less time learning to contour the volumes contoured by the software - Prohibit automatic delineation software at the beginning of the residency - Integrating AI tools into the training - Facilitate personal training on AI (University degree, . . .) - No changes - Other
18. Do you think that automatic delineation tools present an additional risk of error in the workflow?	- Yes - No
19. [Opportunity scale] In your opinion, the integration of artificial intelligence in radiotherapy presents..	- 1 (No opportunity) -> (Very high opportunity)
20. [Menace scale] In your opinion, the integration of artificial intelligence in radiotherapy presents..	- 1 (No menace) -> (Very high menace)
21. [Trust scale] In your opinion, the integration of artificial intelligence in radiotherapy presents..	- 1 (No trust) -> (Very high trust)
22. In a few words, how do you think the radiotherapy specialty will evolve with respect to these artificial intelligence tools?	- Free answer

3. Results

3.1. Participants

A total number of 117 participants registered for the dosimetry webinar, with a high majority of residents (99/117, 84.6%) followed by attendings (11/117, 9.4%). The rest were relatively well distributed between a single student, senior physicians (2/117, 1.7%) and foreign students (3/117, 2.7%). The majority of residents were 3rd-, 4th- or 5th-year residents (28.3%, 24.2% and 30.3%, respectively). First- and second-year residents accounted for 17.1% of the overall participants. All of the eleven attendings had less than 2 years of experience while 85.7% of the senior physicians (6/7) had 2 to 5 years of experience.

The very high majority of participants exercised in academic centers, with 48.7% (57/117) and 47% (55/117) being employed by a university hospital or an academic cancer care facility, respectively. These 35 centers were high-volume centers (on a French base) considering the number of new patients treated per year, with 35.9% of the participants working in a center with >2000 patients per year and 27.4% in centers with 1500–2000 patients per year (Supplementary Figure S1).

For 76.1% of the participants, OARs were mostly delineated by residents, while 60.7% of the centers were equipped with an automatic segmentation solution (71/117). For this subset of participants, the acquisition of the solution was fairly recent, with 40.8% and

33.8% of the participants having less than one year or 1 to 2 years of experience with AI solutions, respectively. Only 25.4% (18/71) were equipped with automatic segmentation software for more than 2 years. The large majority of participants declared that their center was planning to be equipped with such solutions (91.3%), with 52.2% of all participants to be equipped in the next 2 coming years.

Access to the AI software was non-restricted for 45.1% of the participants, with physicians, residents, physicists, and dosimetrists having access to the solution. For 49.3% of the participants, the solution was only available for residents and physicians, while only 4.2% had restricted access for senior physicians only (Supplementary Figure S2).

3.2. *Use of Automatic Segmentation in France*

3.2.1. Overview of AI-Based Segmentation Solutions Used in France

The solution provided by Therapanacea appeared as the most used software (29.5%), followed by Mirada Workflow-Box (16.9%), Raystation automatic segmentation (15.5%) and Limbus AI (15.5%), as presented in Figure 1. Of note, several centers had multiple solutions.

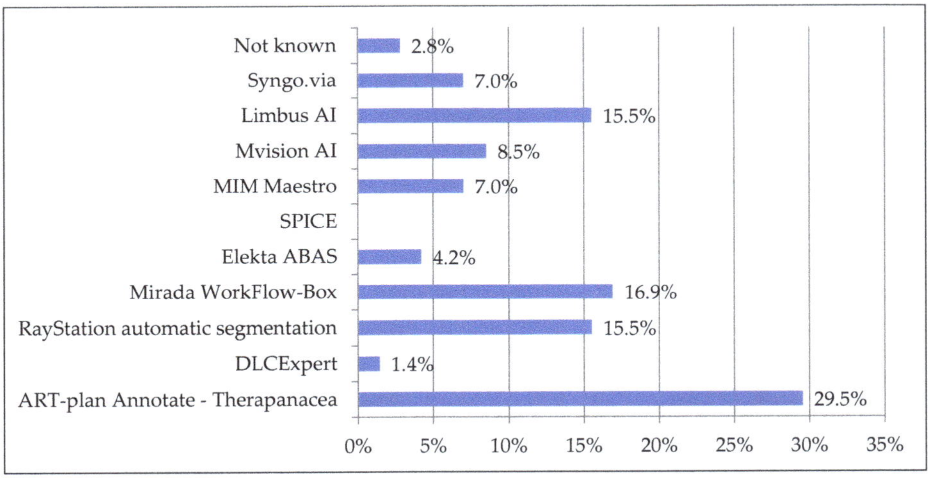

Figure 1. Distribution of automatic segmentation solutions in France, on a participant-by-participant analysis.

Seventy participants (98.6%) declared that time-saving was a motivation for the acquisition of such tools, while 35.2% saw automatic segmentation as a tool to reduce inter-physician variability. Enhancing the quality of treatment planning and leaning towards international guidelines were reasons for only 15.5% and 16.9% of the participants, respectively.

3.2.2. Clinical Use of AI-Based Segmentation Tools

The localizations in which AI tools were mostly used were breast (57.7%) and head and neck (57.7%), closely followed by prostate (49.3%) and thorax (46.5%). Neurological and abdominal localizations were the two indications in which the AI tools were used less (35.2% and 26.8%). Automatic segmentation was also rarely used in palliative settings (19.7%).

Regarding the time saved on a localization-by-localization approach, conflicting results were observed. Breast and metastatic sites were classified as the least time-saving localizations for 22.5% and 28.2% of the participants but also classified as the most time-saving localizations for 23.9% and 28.2% of the participants. When focusing on the moderate to most time-saving localizations (ranked as 6 to 8 on a 1 to 8 scale), H & N appeared as the most time-saving localization (16.4%), followed by breast (15.5%), as seen in Figure 2.

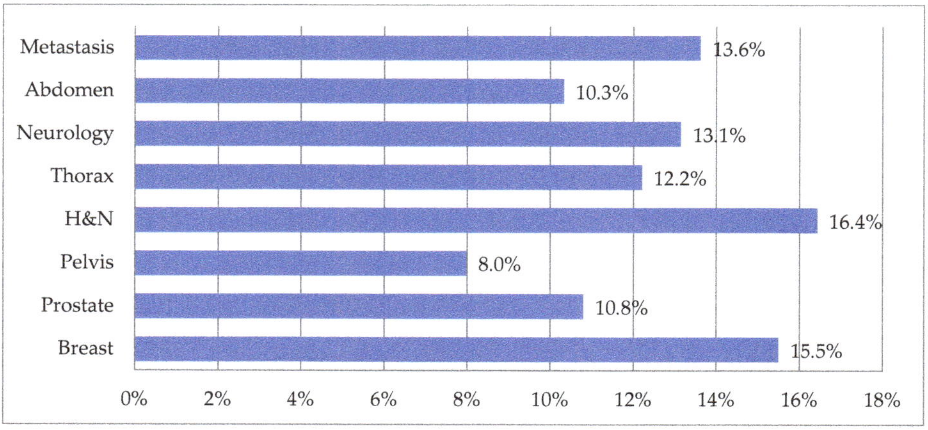

Figure 2. Ranking of localizations based on their time-saving potential—Focus on 6–8 rankings.

Time-saving occurred on the delineation of OARs for 93% of the participants, largely higher than prophylactic lymph node delineation (23.9%). Time gained using AI segmentation tools was estimated to be between 25–50% for 54.9% of the participants, while 31% of them even described a 50–75% time saving, correction included (Figure 3a). The time savings could probably be enhanced given the fact that 38% and 25.4% of the participants, respectively, estimated that 25–50% to 50–75% of the slices needed editing (Figure 3b). Only 26.8% of the participants answered that less than 25% of the slices needed correction.

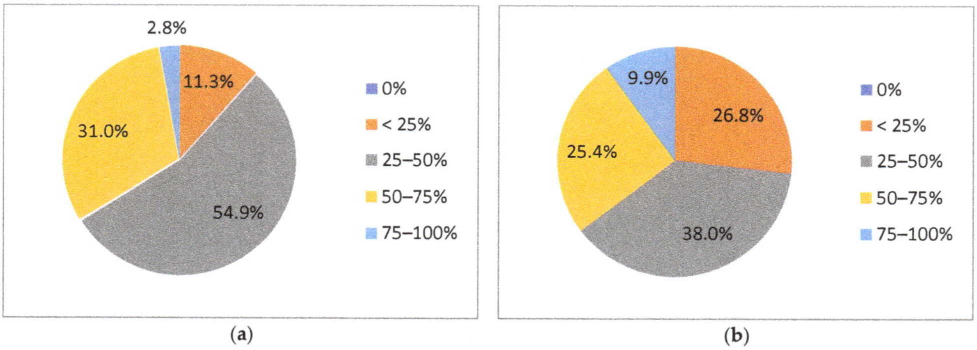

Figure 3. Estimation of time savings (**a**) and correction times (**b**) regarding organs at risk segmentation.

The vast majority of participants noticed small and easily corrected mistakes (62%). Noticeably, up to 11.3% and 40.8% of the participants, respectively, reported laterality errors or aberrant segmentations such as wrong localizations.

3.3. *Definition of Organs at Risk*

Participants were asked to choose three OARs from a proposed list for each localization (brain, H & N, thorax, abdomen and pelvis). The overall list of OARs is detailed in the survey. Regarding the brain, the most important OARs to be integrated were the brain, the brainstem, followed by the eyes. Hypothalamus and pituitary gland were the least important OARs (Supplementary Figure S3).

Regarding the H & N localization, the mandible, parotid glands and spinal cord were the three most important OARs to be integrated, while less than 10% of the participants chose the thyroid gland and the vessels (Supplementary Figure S4). Concerning thoracic irradiation, lungs, heart and spinal cord were the three most important OARs. Noticeably, heart sub-structures were ranked among the three least important OARs with only a 22.2% rate (Supplementary Figure S5).

For abdominal cases, automatic segmentation of the liver, spinal cord and abdominal cavity appeared as the most significant task for participants, closely followed by the kidney. Again, segmentation of the vessels was ranked among the least significant, with a rate of 7.7% (Supplementary Figure S6). Regarding the pelvis localization, the bladder and rectum clearly stood out from other OARs with respective rates of 82.1% and 76.9%, while the first runner-up (sigmoid) was only chosen by 34.2%. The prostate gland for men and the vagina for women were ranked among the five least important OARs (Supplementary Figure S7).

When asked which OARs they would add to currently available structures, the large majority of participants suggested none (88%, 103/117). The anterior interventricular artery and heart sub-structures were the most suggested (3.4%, 4/117).

3.4. *Definition of Target Volumes*

Only 29.9% (35/117) of the participants had an AI solution that proposed the segmentation of target volumes. The large majority of these solutions focused on prophylactic lymph node segmentation (80%), while only 37.1% and 14.3% declared to be proposed with the segmentation of a tumor or invaded lymph node, respectively.

Regarding the segmentation of target volumes, 45.7% of the participants evaluated the time savings to be less than 25%, while 17.1% declared no time gain from AI solutions (Figure 4). When asked about the limitations of AI software for target volumes segmentations, the need for editing (77.1%) and a lack of accuracy (60%) were the two most frequent answers, followed by cost (31.4%) and lack of cross-software integration (20%), as seen in Supplementary Figure S8.

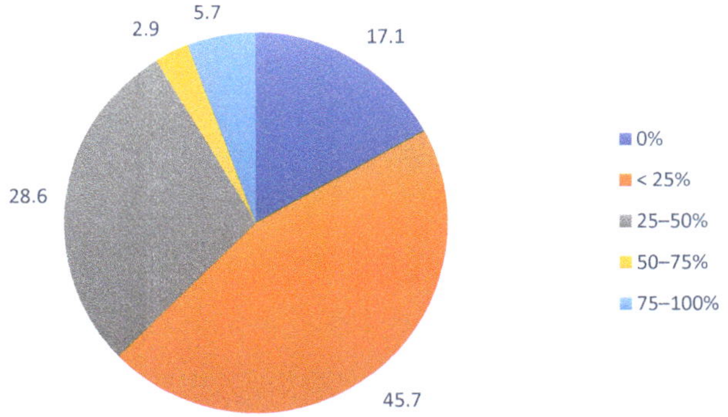

Figure 4. Estimation of time savings regarding target volumes segmentation.

3.4.1. Impact on the Training of Young Radiation Oncologists

Thanks to gains in reproducibility (76.6%) and speed (85.1%), 80.3% of the participants thought that automatic segmentation leads to an improvement in segmentation quality. Only 30.9% of the participants thought that automatic segmentation would improve the accuracy of segmentations.

Despite automatic segmentation not being seen as a menace for the marketplace of radiation oncologists for 88.9% of participants, a small majority (53.8%) thought that it could negatively impact the academic training of young radiation oncologists (Figure 5). AI was not integrated into the training of young ROs for 79.5% of them, in contrast to 69.2% and 56.4% of the participants asking for AI tools to be taught directly during ROs training or through university degrees, respectively. Almost a third of participants (30.8%) would limit access to AI solutions during training.

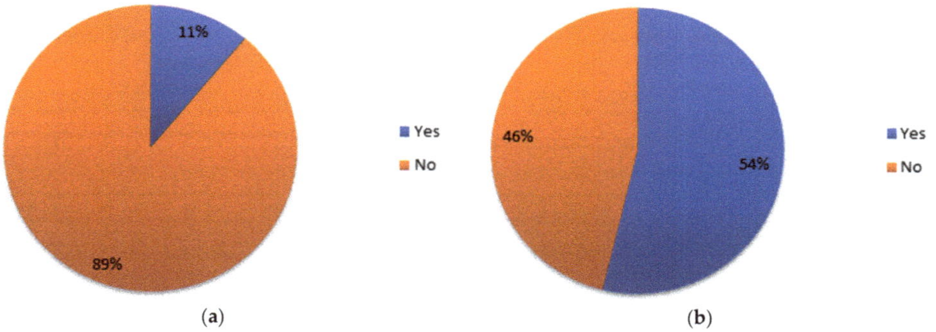

Figure 5. Estimation of automatic segmentation solutions being a menace for radiation oncologists (**a**) and young radiation oncologists training (**b**).

3.4.2. Overall Thoughts of Young Radiation Oncologists on AI Segmentation Solutions

Young ROs were asked to evaluate AI segmentation solutions based on three different scales: opportunity, menace and confidence. The scales ranged from 1 to 5. For instance, on the opportunity scale, a 1 would mean that the participant felt that the AI solution had no opportunity, while a 5 would mean a very high opportunity. Such solutions were ranked as high to very high opportunities for a large majority of participants (86.3%), with no serious menace for 64.9%. The level of confidence was classified as moderate. (3/5) for 51.3%, while only 6% of the participants had very high confidence in AI-proposed segmentations (Figure 6).

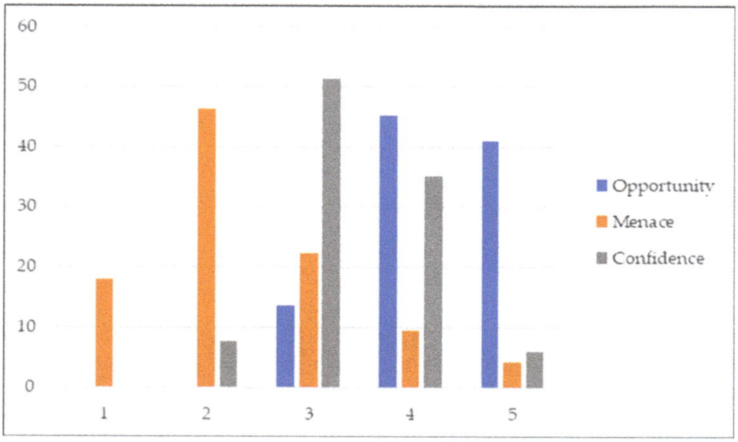

Figure 6. Evaluation of AI segmentation solutions per menace, opportunity and confidence scales.

4. Discussion

As stated, artificial intelligence profoundly modified the exercise of radiation oncologists. With numerous companies and research teams being involved in this field [16–20], the viewpoint of future clinicians was needed.

With 117 participants representing 35 different and mostly academic centers, this survey is, to our knowledge, the first to focus on young radiation oncologists and their view on AI segmentation tools. Most centers were either already equipped with such solutions or planning to be equipped in the next two years. The growing part of radiation treatment encourages the need for time-saving tools. This survey brings an interesting insight into the views of young ROs but also the challenges that AI tools represent and still face.

AI segmentation software was mostly used for H & N cases, closely followed by breast localizations. Delineation of H & N tumors can be challenging and long for young ROs due to the multiplicity of OAR [21–23], explaining the importance of AI segmentation. Caution must be taken as some structures must be delineated using MRI or specific contrast. Breast tumors remain the first cancer treated in radiation service with a high number of patients. Breast and H & N cases were ranked as the most time-saving localizations for approximately 25% of the participants, with a similar number of participants ranking these localizations as the least time-saving. The different levels of performance, according to the tool as well as the users' expectations, could explain these conflicting results.

Recent dosimetry criteria incite the delineation of more OARs, such as cardiac substructure [24–26]. Regular implementation of these "new" OARs might be important in the next years and taken into account for AI segmentation tools. While for the definition of OARs, participants experienced a significant time gain using AI-proposed delineations, with almost 35% of the participants saving between 50–100% of the segmentation time, time gained for target volumes was significantly lower with only 8.6% experiencing such a 50–100% gain. The need for time-saving solutions is high in the field of RT. The efforts should focus on the target volumes' delineation [18,27]. The next years of RT will be marked by new innovations, such as the broader use of adaptative RT [28] and personalized ultra-fractionated stereotactic adaptive radiation therapy (PULSAR) [29]. Brachytherapy could also benefit from automatic delineation before each fraction [30].

Target volumes usually remain more complex, sometimes not well delimitated and with margin depending on anatomic barriers and the natural history of the disease. These characteristics lead to a more difficult automatic realization. Automatic segmentation has two main strengths: speed and reproducibility, but software developers should focus on enhancing the quality. Contours still need to be thoroughly checked and edited, especially target volumes. Concordance with current recommendations must be assessed, as guidelines and consensus can evolve rapidly. Some discordance concerning delineation can be described. These limitations should be known by young ROs.

As suggested by participants, AI segmentation could have a negative impact on the training of young ROs. The majority of them suggested that such tools should be integrated into the training so that future radiation oncologists do not neglect the importance of radioanatomy. Implementation of such tools should follow ESTRO guidelines [31], and centers should share their user experience [32]. AI is not currently implemented in the French oncology radiotherapy cursus. University diplomas or master's are proposed in parallel. Fully aware of this risk, up to one-third of them even suggested that AI tools should be reserved for senior physicians only, accepting a longer delineation time for the student. On the other hand, automatic segmentation would leave ROs more time for an accurate review of the proposed segmentation, a more precise definition of target volumes and a dosimetric plans assessment.

Several limitations of our survey should be acknowledged. Its length possibly limited the participation rate. Being mandatory for the registration to an H & N dosimetry webinar, answers to the survey are possibly skewed with a selection bias. However, with 117 individual participants, the population represents approximately 50% of the target population. By definition, results were oriented by the propositions made available to the participants. Although it facilitates the quantitative analysis of the data, this may limit the findings.

5. Conclusions

We believe this survey on automatic segmentation to be the first to focus on the perception of young radiation oncologists. Software developers should focus on enhancing the quality of proposed segmentations, especially for target volumes, while young radiation oncologists should become more acquainted with these tools and fully apprehend their strengths and weaknesses.

Supplementary Materials: The following are available online at https://www.mdpi.com/article/10.3390/cancers15072040/s1, Supplementary Protocol S1: Form in French with the corresponding English translation; Supplementary Table S1: Checklist for Reporting Results of Internet E-Surveys (CHERRIES); Supplementary Figure S1: Number of new patients per year, on a participant-by-participant analysis; Supplementary Figure S2: Access to automatic segmentation solutions, on a participant-by-participant analysis; Supplementary Figure S3: Ranking of OARs based on their importance—Brain localization; Supplementary Figure S4: Ranking of OARs based on their importance—Head and neck localization; Supplementary Figure S5: Ranking of OARs based on their importance—Thorax localization; Supplementary Figure S6: Ranking of OARs based on their importance—Abdomen localization; Supplementary Figure S7: Ranking of OARs based on their importance—Pelvis localization; Supplementary Figure S8: Limitations of automatic segmentation software regarding target volumes segmentation.

Author Contributions: Conceptualization, V.B. and A.L. (Audrey Larnaudie); data curation, V.B., A.L. (Adrien Laville) and A.L. (Audrey Larnaudie); methodology, V.B., A.L. (Adrien Laville), N.W., Y.G. and A.L. (Audrey Larnaudie); supervision, V.B., Y.G. and A.L. (Audrey Larnaudie); validation, V.B.; writing—original draft, V.B.; writing—review and editing, V.B., A.L. (Adrien Laville), N.W., Y.G. and A.L. (Audrey Larnaudie). All authors have read and agreed to the published version of the manuscript.

Funding: This research received no external funding.

Institutional Review Board Statement: Not applicable.

Informed Consent Statement: Not applicable.

Data Availability Statement: Data available upon request due to restrictions, e.g., privacy or ethical.

Conflicts of Interest: The authors declare no conflict of interest.

References

1. Garibaldi, C.; Jereczek-Fossa, B.A.; Marvaso, G.; Dicuonzo, S.; Rojas, D.P.; Cattani, F.; Starzyńska, A.; Ciardo, D.; Surgo, A.; Leonardi, M.C.; et al. Recent Advances in Radiation Oncology. *Ecancermedicalscience* **2017**, *11*, 785. [CrossRef]
2. Lopez Guerra, J.L.; Isa, N.; Kim, M.M.; Bourgier, C.; Marsiglia, H. New Perspectives in Radiation Oncology: Young Radiation Oncologist Point of View and Challenges. *Rep. Pract. Oncol. Radiother.* **2012**, *17*, 251–254. [CrossRef]
3. Fiorino, C.; Guckemberger, M.; Schwarz, M.; van der Heide, U.A.; Heijmen, B. Technology-driven Research for Radiotherapy Innovation. *Mol. Oncol.* **2020**, *14*, 1500–1513. [CrossRef] [PubMed]
4. Huynh, E.; Hosny, A.; Guthier, C.; Bitterman, D.S.; Petit, S.F.; Haas-Kogan, D.A.; Kann, B.; Aerts, H.J.W.L.; Mak, R.H. Artificial Intelligence in Radiation Oncology. *Nat. Rev. Clin. Oncol.* **2020**, *17*, 771–781. [CrossRef] [PubMed]
5. Deig, C.R.; Kanwar, A.; Thompson, R.F. Artificial Intelligence in Radiation Oncology. *Hematol. Oncol. Clin. N. Am.* **2019**, *33*, 1095–1104. [CrossRef]
6. Netherton, T.J.; Cardenas, C.E.; Rhee, D.J.; Court, L.E.; Beadle, B.M. The Emergence of Artificial Intelligence within Radiation Oncology Treatment Planning. *Oncology* **2021**, *99*, 124–134. [CrossRef]
7. Rattan, R.; Kataria, T.; Banerjee, S.; Goyal, S.; Gupta, D.; Pandita, A.; Bisht, S.; Narang, K.; Mishra, S.R. Artificial Intelligence in Oncology, Its Scope and Future Prospects with Specific Reference to Radiation Oncology. *BJR Open* **2019**, *1*, 20180031. [CrossRef]
8. Isensee, F.; Jaeger, P.F.; Kohl, S.A.A.; Petersen, J.; Maier-Hein, K.H. NnU-Net: A Self-Configuring Method for Deep Learning-Based Biomedical Image Segmentation. *Nat. Methods* **2021**, *18*, 203–211. [CrossRef]
9. Kosmin, M.; Ledsam, J.; Romera-Paredes, B.; Mendes, R.; Moinuddin, S.; de Souza, D.; Gunn, L.; Kelly, C.; Hughes, C.O.; Karthikesalingam, A.; et al. Rapid Advances in Auto-Segmentation of Organs at Risk and Target Volumes in Head and Neck Cancer. *Radiother. Oncol. J. Eur. Soc. Ther. Radiol. Oncol.* **2019**, *135*, 130–140. [CrossRef] [PubMed]
10. Bibault, J.-E.; Fumagalli, I.; Diaz, O.; Faivre, J.-C.; Leroy, T.; Pichon, B.; Riou, O.; Thureau, S.; Rivera, S. The French Society of Young Radiation Oncologists: History, Goals and Perspective. *Rep. Pract. Oncol. Radiother. J. Greatpoland Cancer Cent. Pozn. Pol. Soc. Radiat. Oncol.* **2012**, *17*, 255–258. [CrossRef]
11. Blanchard, P.; Truchot, D.; Albiges-Sauvin, L.; Dewas, S.; Pointreau, Y.; Rodrigues, M.; Xhaard, A.; Loriot, Y.; Giraud, P.; Soria, J.C.; et al. Prevalence and Causes of Burnout amongst Oncology Residents: A Comprehensive Nationwide Cross-Sectional Study. *Eur. J. Cancer* **2010**, *46*, 2708–2715. [CrossRef]
12. Fumagalli, I.; Faivre, J.-C.; Thureau, S.; Bibault, J.-E.; Diaz, O.; Leroy, T.; Pichon, B.; Riou, O.; Fournier, C.; Hannoun-Lévi, J.-M.; et al. Brachytherapy training: A survey of French radiation oncology residents. *Cancer Radiother. J. Soc. Fr. Radiother. Oncol.* **2014**, *18*, 28–34. [CrossRef]

13. Kissel, M.; Ollivier, L.; Fumagalli, I.; Pommier, P.; Chargari, C.; Blanchard, P.; Peiffert, D.; Hannoun-Levi, J.-M. Resident Training in Brachytherapy in France: A 10-Year Update after the First Survey of SFJRO Members. *J. Contemp. Brachytherapy* **2022**, *14*, 501–511. [CrossRef] [PubMed]
14. Rousseau, A.; Laune, Q.; Ollivier, L.; Naoun, N.; Alexandre, J.; Giraud, P.; Azria, D.; Delaye, M. Formation of French oncology resident: A national survey. *Bull. Cancer* **2022**, *109*, 834–843. [CrossRef]
15. Eysenbach, G. Improving the Quality of Web Surveys: The Checklist for Reporting Results of Internet E-Surveys (CHERRIES). *J. Med. Internet Res.* **2004**, *6*, e132. [CrossRef] [PubMed]
16. Wang, J.; Chen, Y.; Xie, H.; Luo, L.; Tang, Q. Evaluation of Auto-Segmentation for EBRT Planning Structures Using Deep Learning-Based Workflow on Cervical Cancer. *Sci. Rep.* **2022**, *12*, 13650. [CrossRef]
17. Harrison, K.; Pullen, H.; Welsh, C.; Oktay, O.; Alvarez-Valle, J.; Jena, R. Machine Learning for Auto-Segmentation in Radiotherapy Planning. *Clin. Oncol.* **2022**, *34*, 74–88. [CrossRef] [PubMed]
18. Liu, X.; Li, K.-W.; Yang, R.; Geng, L.-S. Review of Deep Learning Based Automatic Segmentation for Lung Cancer Radiotherapy. *Front. Oncol.* **2021**, *11*, 717039. [CrossRef]
19. Liu, Z.; Liu, F.; Chen, W.; Tao, Y.; Liu, X.; Zhang, F.; Shen, J.; Guan, H.; Zhen, H.; Wang, S.; et al. Automatic Segmentation of Clinical Target Volume and Organs-at-Risk for Breast Conservative Radiotherapy Using a Convolutional Neural Network. *Cancer Manag. Res.* **2021**, *13*, 8209–8217. [CrossRef]
20. Lin, H.; Xiao, H.; Dong, L.; Teo, K.B.-K.; Zou, W.; Cai, J.; Li, T. Deep Learning for Automatic Target Volume Segmentation in Radiation Therapy: A Review. *Quant. Imaging Med. Surg.* **2021**, *11*, 4847–4858. [CrossRef]
21. Brouwer, C.L.; Steenbakkers, R.J.H.M.; Bourhis, J.; Budach, W.; Grau, C.; Grégoire, V.; van Herk, M.; Lee, A.; Maingon, P.; Nutting, C.; et al. CT-Based Delineation of Organs at Risk in the Head and Neck Region: DAHANCA, EORTC, GORTEC, HKNPCSG, NCIC CTG, NCRI, NRG Oncology and TROG Consensus Guidelines. *Radiother. Oncol.* **2015**, *117*, 83–90. [CrossRef] [PubMed]
22. Biau, J.; Dunet, V.; Lapeyre, M.; Simon, C.; Ozsahin, M.; Grégoire, V.; Bourhis, J. Practical Clinical Guidelines for Contouring the Trigeminal Nerve (V) and Its Branches in Head and Neck Cancers. *Radiother. Oncol.* **2019**, *131*, 192–201. [CrossRef]
23. Gawryszuk, A.; Bijl, H.P.; Holwerda, M.; Halmos, G.B.; Wedman, J.; Witjes, M.J.H.; van der Vliet, A.M.; Dorgelo, B.; Langendijk, J.A. Functional Swallowing Units (FSUs) as Organs-at-Risk for Radiotherapy. PART 2: Advanced Delineation Guidelines for FSUs. *Radiother. Oncol.* **2019**, *130*, 68–74. [CrossRef] [PubMed]
24. Duane, F.; Aznar, M.C.; Bartlett, F.; Cutter, D.J.; Darby, S.C.; Jagsi, R.; Lorenzen, E.L.; McArdle, O.; McGale, P.; Myerson, S.; et al. A Cardiac Contouring Atlas for Radiotherapy. *Radiother. Oncol. J. Eur. Soc. Ther. Radiol. Oncol.* **2017**, *122*, 416–422. [CrossRef] [PubMed]
25. Loap, P.; Servois, V.; Dhonneur, G.; Kirov, K.; Fourquet, A.; Kirova, Y. A Radiation Therapy Contouring Atlas for Cardiac Conduction Node Delineation. *Pract. Radiat. Oncol.* **2021**, *11*, e434–e437. [CrossRef] [PubMed]
26. Socha, J.; Rygielska, A.; Uzięblo-Życzkowska, B.; Chałubińska-Fendler, J.; Jurek, A.; Maciorowska, M.; Mielniczuk, M.; Pawłowski, P.; Tyc-Szczepaniak, D.; Krzesiński, P.; et al. Contouring Cardiac Substructures on Average Intensity Projection 4D-CT for Lung Cancer Radiotherapy: A Proposal of a Heart Valve Contouring Atlas. *Radiother. Oncol. J. Eur. Soc. Ther. Radiol. Oncol.* **2022**, *167*, 261–268. [CrossRef]
27. Kalantar, R.; Lin, G.; Winfield, J.M.; Messiou, C.; Lalondrelle, S.; Blackledge, M.D.; Koh, D.-M. Automatic Segmentation of Pelvic Cancers Using Deep Learning: State-of-the-Art Approaches and Challenges. *Diagnostics* **2021**, *11*, 1964. [CrossRef] [PubMed]
28. Ghose, S.; Holloway, L.; Lim, K.; Chan, P.; Veera, J.; Vinod, S.K.; Liney, G.; Greer, P.B.; Dowling, J. A Review of Segmentation and Deformable Registration Methods Applied to Adaptive Cervical Cancer Radiation Therapy Treatment Planning. *Artif. Intell. Med.* **2015**, *64*, 75–87. [CrossRef] [PubMed]
29. Moore, C.; Hsu, C.-C.; Chen, W.-M.; Chen, B.P.C.; Han, C.; Story, M.; Aguilera, T.; Pop, L.M.; Hannan, R.; Fu, Y.-X.; et al. Personalized Ultrafractionated Stereotactic Adaptive Radiotherapy (PULSAR) in Preclinical Models Enhances Single-Agent Immune Checkpoint Blockade. *Int. J. Radiat. Oncol. Biol. Phys.* **2021**, *110*, 1306–1316. [CrossRef]
30. Lucia, F.; Miranda, O.; Schick, U.; Bourbonne, V.; Duvergé, L. Dose Escalation by Brachytherapy for Gynecological Cancers. *Cancer Radiother. J. Soc. Fr. Radiother. Oncol.* **2022**, *26*, 905–910. [CrossRef]
31. Vandewinckele, L.; Claessens, M.; Dinkla, A.; Brouwer, C.; Crijns, W.; Verellen, D.; van Elmpt, W. Overview of Artificial Intelligence-Based Applications in Radiotherapy: Recommendations for Implementation and Quality Assurance. *Radiother. Oncol. J. Eur. Soc. Ther. Radiol. Oncol.* **2020**, *153*, 55–66. [CrossRef] [PubMed]
32. Robert, C.; Munoz, A.; Moreau, D.; Mazurier, J.; Sidorski, G.; Gasnier, A.; Beldjoudi, G.; Grégoire, V.; Deutsch, E.; Meyer, P.; et al. Clinical Implementation of Deep-Learning Based Auto-Contouring Tools-Experience of Three French Radiotherapy Centers. *Cancer Radiother. J. Soc. Fr. Radiother. Oncol.* **2021**, *25*, 607–616. [CrossRef] [PubMed]

cancers

MDPI

Review

Automatic Segmentation with Deep Learning in Radiotherapy

Lars Johannes Isaksson [1,2], Paul Summers [3], Federico Mastroleo [1,4], Giulia Marvaso [1,*], Giulia Corrao [1], Maria Giulia Vincini [1], Mattia Zaffaroni [1], Francesco Ceci [2,5], Giuseppe Petralia [2,6], Roberto Orecchia [7] and Barbara Alicja Jereczek-Fossa [1,2]

1 Division of Radiation Oncology, IEO European Institute of Oncology IRCCS, 20141 Milan, Italy; larsjohannes.isaksson@ieo.it (L.J.I.); federico.mastroleo@ieo.it (F.M.); giulia.corrao@ieo.it (G.C.); mariagiulia.vincini@ieo.it (M.G.V.); mattia.zaffaroni@ieo.it (M.Z.); barbara.jereczek@ieo.it (B.A.J.-F.)
2 Department of Oncology and Hemato-Oncology, University of Milan, 20141 Milan, Italy; francesco.ceci@ieo.it (F.C.); giuseppe.petralia@ieo.it (G.P.)
3 Division of Radiology, IEO European Institute of Oncology IRCCS, 20141 Milan, Italy; paul.summers@ieo.it
4 Department of Translational Medicine, University of Piemonte Orientale (UPO), 20188 Novara, Italy
5 Division of Nuclear Medicine, IEO European Institute of Oncology IRCCS, 20141 Milan, Italy
6 Precision Imaging and Research Unit, Department of Medical Imaging and Radiation Sciences, IEO European Institute of Oncology IRCCS, 20141 Milan, Italy
7 Scientific Directorate, IEO European Institute of Oncology IRCCS, 20141 Milan, Italy; roberto.orecchia@ieo.it
* Correspondence: giulia.marvaso@ieo.it

Simple Summary: Automatic segmentation of organs and other regions of interest is a promising approach for reducing the workload of doctors in radiotherapeutic planning, but it can be hard for doctors and researchers to keep up with current developments. This review evaluates 807 papers and reveals trends, commonalities, and gaps in the existing corpus. A set of recommendations for conducting effective segmentation studies is also provided.

Abstract: This review provides a formal overview of current automatic segmentation studies that use deep learning in radiotherapy. It covers 807 published papers and includes multiple cancer sites, image types (CT/MRI/PET), and segmentation methods. We collect key statistics about the papers to uncover commonalities, trends, and methods, and identify areas where more research might be needed. Moreover, we analyzed the corpus by posing explicit questions aimed at providing high-quality and actionable insights, including: "What should researchers think about when starting a segmentation study?", "How can research practices in medical image segmentation be improved?", "What is missing from the current corpus?", and more. This allowed us to provide practical guidelines on how to conduct a good segmentation study in today's competitive environment that will be useful for future research within the field, regardless of the specific radiotherapeutic subfield. To aid in our analysis, we used the large language model ChatGPT to condense information.

Keywords: radiotherapy; segmentation; automatic; deep learning; artificial intelligence; artificial neural networks

1. Introduction

Radiotherapy (RT) represents an important treatment modality for cancer patients that uses high-dose ionizing radiation for curative or palliative purposes. When RT is prescribed, accurate delineation of the tumors, target volumes, and organs at risk (OARs) is crucial for effective treatment planning and reducing the risk of radiation-induced toxicity. However, manual segmentation of these structures, which is the current standard of care, is time-consuming and prone to inter- and intra-observer variability [1–7], which can contribute to suboptimal treatment outcomes. Moreover, the task is repetitive and tiresome, which makes the process tedious for doctors, who typically prefer to devote their time elsewhere. Thus, there is a significant need for good automatic segmentation methods that can be incorporated into clinical practice to improve current workflows and outcomes.

The repetitive nature of the segmentation process makes it a prime candidate for automation with modern machine learning methods, which excel in performing monotonous information-based tasks quickly. Recent years have seen deep learning (DL)-based autosegmentation methods gain significant attention in the field of radiotherapy (see results below). These methods typically employ convolutional neural networks (CNNs) to automatically learn relevant features from medical images which helps them segment the structures accurately. The increasing interest in DL-based automatic segmentation is driven by its success over traditional methods such as atlases, active contours, or region-growing, particularly as demonstrated in online segmentation challenges like BraTS [8], KiTS [9], AMOS [10], and PROMISE [11]. The advantages of DL-based methods include improved accuracy, reproducibility, speed, observer variability, and efficiency, which are all crucial factors in radiotherapy treatment planning. But despite the many advantages, several limitations exist, most notably the requirement for large, annotated training datasets, which can be time-consuming and resource-intensive to collect. Another limitation is the potential for overfitting and related generalization issues, which can lead to erroneous segmentation results when the model encounters atypical samples [12,13]. Some notable developments such as transfer learning [14], data augmentation [15], and ensemble models [16] may aid in overcoming these limitations. Transfer learning has shown promise in reducing the amount of required training data, while data augmentation techniques can increase the diversity of the training dataset at hand. Ensemble models can be used to improve both segmentation accuracy and robustness by combining multiple models into a better performing ensemble (e.g., using models with different architectures or training parameters).

The problem setting for automatic segmentation varies greatly, partly because RT is applied to treat various types of cancer located in many different body regions, including the brain, breast, prostate, lung, and others. Multiple different image types, including magnetic resonance imaging (MRI), computed tomography (CT), and positron emission tomography (PET), are all frequently utilized to visualize the tumor and surrounding normal tissues in the treatment planning process. Each imaging modality excels at depicting different information, which means that they are used to varying extents in different cancer sites. However, most DL models are modality agnostic, meaning that they can be adequately applied to different image types provided that they have been trained on similar images. Therefore, much can be learned from observing advances in adjacent fields, even for researchers working exclusively on a single cancer site or image modality. Another important source of variability relies on the different pathological conditions and physical characteristics of the patients. Automatic segmentation is further complicated by the fact that imaging protocols may vary between institutions or even according to who performs the examination. Therefore, developing robust and versatile automatic segmentation methods that can handle different cancer sites and imaging modalities is essential for their success in radiotherapy treatment planning and execution.

The aim of this review is to analyze the current state of the field of medical image segmentation with deep learning for RT and attempt to answer questions about general trends and needs. We are particularly interested in the datasets, images, cancer sites, and limitations. Our intention is to help identify areas where more research might be needed, to illuminate common flaws, and to guide new research in the field. To do this, we pose explicit questions aimed at providing concrete overviews of the common trends and methods. The analysis we put forward helped us distill a set of four key points that we believe can be useful in designing new studies and maximizing the impact of future work in the field.

2. Related Work

Many reviews have been published on automatic segmentation methods for specific regions of interest [17–26], image modalities [17,20,24,27,28], and methods [29–40]. However, none of these thoroughly cover all three aspects to provide a holistic overview of the state of the field. Moreover, previous reviews tend to focus on quantitative analysis of a relatively limited set of papers, or the different methods and models applied within them.

Our contribution to this work is three-fold. First, we gathered a very large set of 807 papers and collected statistics to provide a comprehensive overview of the field of medical image segmentation in radiotherapy. Second, we highlight a novel way to leverage modern large language models (LLMs) like ChatGPT for condensing large bodies of information. Third, we pose explicit questions for the analysis to provide a valuable resource for researchers seeking actionable insights.

3. Data Collection

To collect relevant academic papers in the field of automatic segmentation with deep learning in radiotherapy, we searched the Scopus and PubMed databases using the following query and collected all unique results:

- Title: "segmenting" or "*segmentation";
- Title, abstract, or keywords: "CT", "MRI", "PET", "DWI", or "*medical image*";
- Title, abstract, or keywords: "deep learning" or "artificial neural network*";
- Title, abstract, or keywords: "radiotherapy";
- Document type: article or conference proceeding;
- Language: English.

All review articles and unrelated papers were removed from the dataset. The relevant metadata (including abstract, publication date, URL, and citation information) were collected for all remaining publications using both web-scraping tools and manual annotations.

As a data mining tool, we utilized the large language model ChatGPT (v3.5-turbo, Mar 14 version, OpenAI [41]). This model is designed to respond to arbitrary natural language queries by producing text outputs. The model was asked to answer the following questions about the abstract of each paper (the answers can be found online in the Supplementary Material):

- Is the paper a review article? (Yes/No).
- How many patients were used in the study? Only answer with a number.
- What type of images were used in the study? Choose from MRI/PET/CT/DWI/Ultrasound/Other.
- Did the paper use images from multiple sources or multiple organs? (Yes/No).
- Is the paper about organ or tumor segmentation? Choose from Organ/Tumor/Both.
- Did the paper propose a novel segmentation method or deep learning architecture? (Yes/No).
- Was the code made public? (Yes/No).
- Was the data made public? (Yes/No).
- What is the key takeaway of the paper? Answer in one sentence.

The responses were then reviewed such that the answers were correct and consistent. To instruct the language model to answer properly, we gave it the following system prompt (this prompt acts as a form of base instruction that the model takes into account when answering the users' queries):

> *"You will be asked to read a scientific paper and then answer questions about it. The paper is about automatic segmentation with deep learning in radiotherapy. Please prioritize correctness in your answers. If you don't know the answer, respond with 'I don't know.'"*

4. Analysis

4.1. Statistics

Statistics about the publication year, number of included patients, target site, imaging modality (MRI/CT/PET/Ultrasound), and segmentation type (organ/tumor) were collected and plotted. To gauge the extent of research conducted on various topics of interest, we scanned the abstracts and GPT responses for the appearance of certain keywords relating to each topic. These topics included: transfer learning or pretraining, self-supervised or semi-supervised or contrastive learning, cross-validation, transformers, publicly available data, and open-sourcing code.

4.2. Region-Specific Analysis

All papers related to each body region (head and neck, brain, prostate, lung, cervix and uterus, liver, heart, stomach and colon, kidney, breast, pancreas, spleen, and skin) were also isolated and analyzed separately to uncover what research patterns and trends are common within the different cancer sites. This includes the images used, the organs and structures segmented, the methods employed, and the most common results and conclusions mentioned in the abstracts.

4.3. Subjective Analysis

To support and encourage further research in the field, we attempted to distill more actionable material from the collected papers by posing and discussing explicit questions aimed at providing more guidance. The questions were:

- What is missing from the current corpus?
- What should researchers think about when starting a segmentation study?
- How can research practices in medical image segmentation be improved?
- Do authors agree on conclusions, and is it possible to spot trends in the employed methods?

5. Results

5.1. Statistics

A flowchart of the paper and data collection process is shown in Figure 1. A total of 905 unique papers matched the query. After removing review articles and unrelated papers (e.g., papers in foreign languages or papers we were unable to access), 807 remained. The number of studies published per year is plotted in Figure 2. The field has been growing steadily since its mainstream adoption around 2013 (not counting five early adopters in 1999 [42], 2006 [43], 2008 [44], and 2010 [45,46]), accumulating a total of 225 publications in 2022 alone. The five most common cancer sites were: head and neck (H and N; 198 papers), brain (130 papers), prostate (117 papers), lung (107 papers), and cervix (101 papers; see Figure 3). The H and N area further stands out as having the most structures of interest for segmentation (e.g., larynx, pharynx, parotid glands, esophagus, masseter, thorax, etc.). Less frequently studied cancer sites included: the skin (6 papers), spleen (12 papers), pancreas (30 papers), breast (30 papers), and kidney (32 papers). In Figure 4, the number of publications per imaging modality and segmentation type is plotted. Roughly 58% of the publications (457 papers) studied CT images, 33% studied MRI (254 papers, of which 22 were specific to DWI), 8% studied PET images (64 papers), and 22 (3%) studied ultrasound images. The majority of the studies focused on organ segmentation (415 papers, or 56%) rather than tumor segmentation (260 studies, or 35%), with only about 9% (68 studies) focusing on both. A spreadsheet of the included studies along with abstracts, the generated answers, one-sentence summaries, and corresponding metadata can be found in Supplementary Table S1.

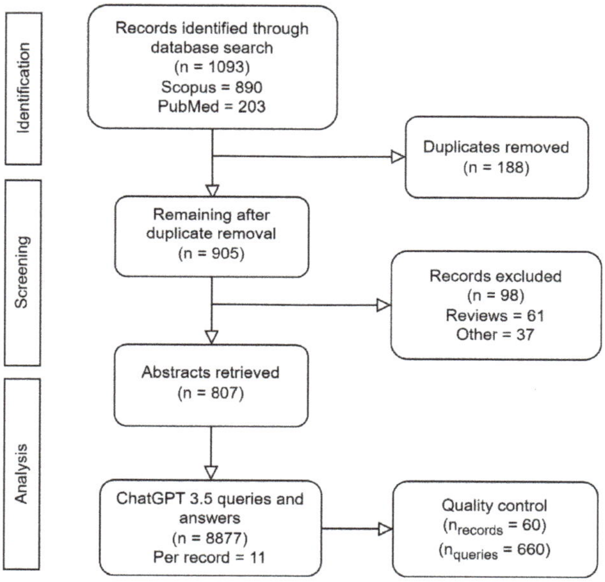

Figure 1. Flowchart of the paper selection and analysis process.

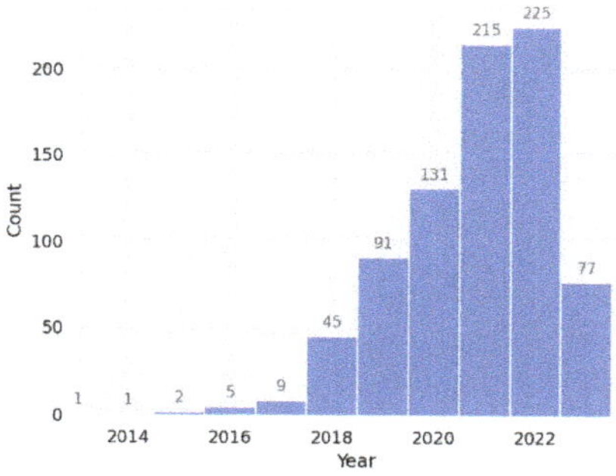

Figure 2. Number of deep learning medical image segmentation studies published per year. Not pictured: five papers published between 1999 and 2012.

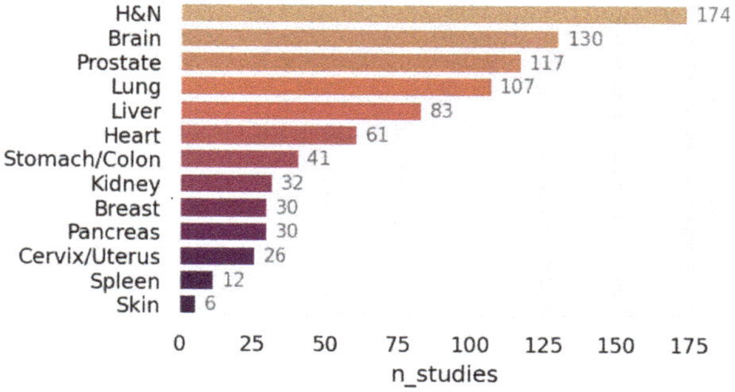

Figure 3. The total number of published studies per cancer site.

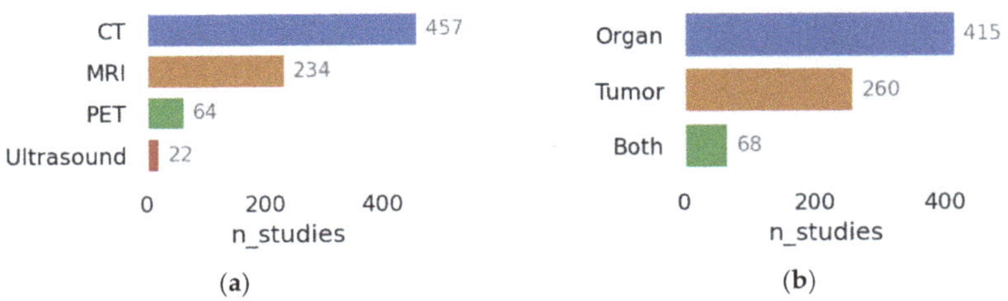

Figure 4. The total number of published studies organized by (**a**) image type and (**b**) segmentation type.

The combined studies yielded a median and mean patient count of 128 and 363, respectively (in cases where a study used multiple datasets, we used the total sum of patients). A graph showing the distribution of sample sizes is shown in Figure 5. Only 407 papers disclosed the sample size in the abstract. Of these, roughly 40% had fewer than 100 patients, and 42% were in the 100–500 patients range. The three cancer regions with the largest cohorts, as measured by median sample size (see Figure 6), were the brain (250 patients), spleen (215 patients), and lung (144 patients). The sites with the smallest cohorts were the heart (66 patients), liver (72 patients), and H and N (87 patients). Notably, heart and H and N also had the studies with the second and third largest sample sizes (6535 [47] and 6000 [48] patients, respectively)—not too far off from the largest sample size of 9032 [49].

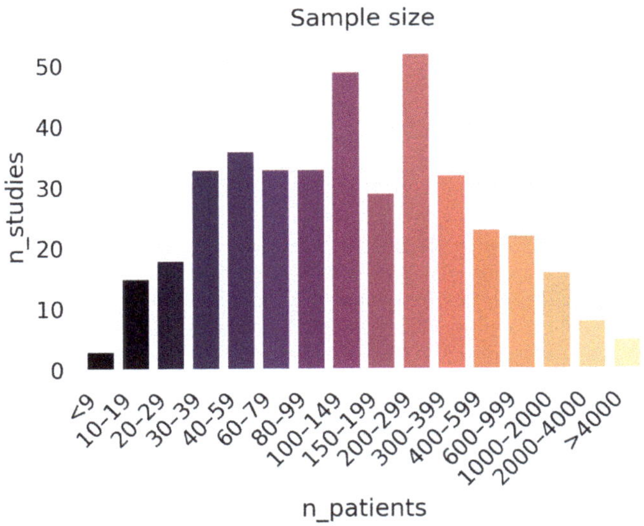

Figure 5. Distribution of the number of patients included in the studies (if a study used multiple datasets, their sizes were added together).

When asked whether the study proposes a novel deep learning model or architecture, the language model responded "Yes" for 550 studies (70%) and "No" for only 232 studies (see Figure 7), revealing a strong tendency to introduce new methods.

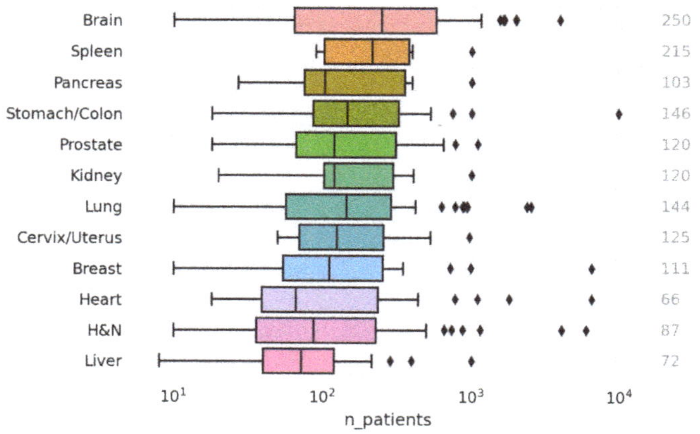

Figure 6. Distribution of dataset sizes per body region. The numbers to the right indicate the median sample size. Note the log scale on the *x*-axis.

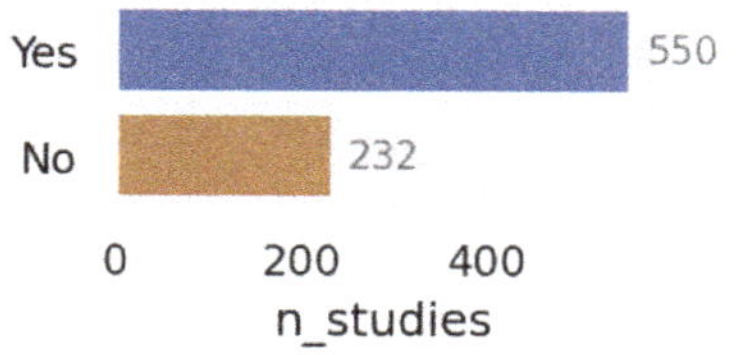

Figure 7. The number of yes and no responses when asked: "Did the paper propose a novel segmentation method or deep learning architecture? (Yes/No)". The number of studies proposing novel models/architectures shows that the vast majority of papers focus on developing new methods.

5.2. Region-Specific Analysis

5.2.1. Head and Neck

Within the head and neck region, 48 studies specifically concerned segmentation of the tumors while 59 segmented the pharynx, 41 segmented the esophagus, 32 segmented the parotid gland, 8 segmented the larynx, and 3 segmented the masseter. The most common architecture by far was a standard 3D U-net, but a notable fraction also employed GAN architectures while a few used 2D networks. A total of 64 papers used data from multiple sources or organs. In all papers, deep learning segmentation was superior to the competing method. Even though the head and neck region is one of the most studied body regions, it is one of the regions suffering the most from small data sets (median sample size 87).

5.2.2. Brain

In the brain, the vast majority (94 out of 130) of studies focused on tumor segmentation. Only a handful focused on specific structures like the brain stem, pituitary gland, cerebellum, etc. Papers published regarding brain segmentation appeared to propose novel segmentation methods to a larger extent compared to the other regions; only 39 papers do not make specific mention of a new contribution. The 3D U-net was again the most common architecture, but many alternative approaches exist. Only 31 papers tested their methods on multiple datasets or organs. Apart from 27 studies that were inconclusive, all papers concluded that deep learning was superior to the alternative approach.

5.2.3. Prostate

For the prostate, only 19 out of 117 studies focused on tumor segmentation while the majority focused on segmentation of the whole prostate. Many studies also performed segmentation of surrounding organs like the bladder (68 studies) and rectum (57 studies). Although the majority of papers focused on 3D networks, 12 papers also tested 2D models. Only 30 papers tested their methods on multiple datasets or organs. All but 5 out of the 117 studies concluded that deep learning performed better than other methods.

5.2.4. Lung

The papers studying lung segmentation were dominated by 3D U-net type architectures, with a handful of 2D hybrid networks. Out of the 107 papers, roughly 80 proposed new architectures and 49 focused on tumor segmentation. A total of 9 papers used MRI images, 14 used PET, and 89 used CT images. All but one lung segmentation study that compared deep learning with other approaches concluded that the performance of deep learning was superior.

5.2.5. Liver

Almost all studies of the liver analyzed CT images, but 11 also analyzed MRI images, 5 analyzed PET images, and 1 analyzed ultrasound images. A total of 49 papers studied the segmentation of tumors (20 of which studied segmentation of both tumors and organs); almost 60% of the 83 papers. Only 19 papers did not propose a new method or architecture, but 36 used images from multiple sources or organs. All but four papers concluded that deep learning was better than the alternative approach.

5.2.6. Heart

For the heart, 53 out of 61 papers studied CT images while 2, 4, and 1 paper studied PET, MRI, and ultrasound images, respectively. Only 12 papers studied tumor segmentation, meaning that most papers focused on segmenting the heart and its various substructures. About 42 papers proposed a novel method or architecture while 18 did not. Two papers were inconclusive as to whether deep learning performed better than the competing approach and fifty-eight studies concluded that deep learning was better.

5.2.7. Colon

Among the papers studying the colon, 41 focused on CT images and 12 focused on MRI images. Only a total of 12 out of 54 studies focused on tumor segmentation. Roughly two-thirds (41) of the papers proposed novel methods or architectures and 26 used images from multiple sources or organs. Most studies appeared to use fairly standard 3D U-net-type architectures. In total, 52 papers concluded that deep learning was superior (two studies were inconclusive).

5.2.8. Kidney

Among the kidney studies, 3 out of 32 papers studied tumor segmentation only, while 4 papers studied both rumor and organ segmentation. Four studies used MRI images and twenty-four studies used CT images. Sixteen papers tested their methods on multiple datasets or organs. All but seven studies proposed novel methods and architectures and all but one study (which was inconclusive) concluded that deep learning was superior to alternative approaches.

5.2.9. Breast

Within the breast studies, 14 used CT images, 8 used MRI images, and 5 used ultrasound images. Eleven out of the thirty studies focused on tumor segmentation, while four focused on both tumor and organ segmentation. Nine papers tested their methods on multiple datasets or organs. Twenty-two (22) studies proposed novel methods or architectures and all but two inconclusive studies concluded that deep learning outperformed alternative methods.

5.2.10. Pancreas

In studies of the pancreas, 21 papers used CT images and 8 used MRI. Seven out of the thirty papers focused on tumor segmentation and only five did not explicitly propose new methods or deep learning architectures. More than half (18 papers) used data from multiple organs. All studies (except for two that were inconclusive) showed that deep learning outperformed conventional approaches.

5.2.11. Cervix

Among the 26 studies of the cervix and uterus, 15 used CT images, 1 used PET images, 7 used MRI images, and 1 used ultrasound. Thirteen papers focused on tumor segmentation, seven on organ segmentation, and six on both. A total of nine papers did not propose any new methods or architectures. All studies concluded that deep learning was superior to competing approaches.

5.2.12. Spleen

Of the twelve papers studying the spleen, eight used CT images, and two used MRI images. Eight papers specifically mention developing new deep learning architectures or methods. None of them were specifically testing methods for automatic tumor segmentation, but most (nine papers) used data from multiple organs to test their methods. In total, all papers concluded that deep learning was superior to the alternative, apart from one study that was inconclusive.

5.2.13. Skin

In studies of the skin, three papers used ultrasound images, one used MRI images, one used dermoscopic images, and one used photographs of the skin. All six papers explicitly examined the segmentations of tumors, while half of them proposed novel methods. Five studies concluded that deep learning was superior to the alternative approaches.

5.3. Subjective Analysis

5.3.1. What Is Missing from the Current Corpus?

- Benchmark datasets: At present, direct comparisons of results remain unfeasible since very few studies use the same data. Specifically, only 92 studies employed data sourced from at least one of the following datasets: UK Biobank, BraTS, KiTS, HECKTOR, OASIS, or PROMISE. Moreover, there is a very strong preference for novelty over replication in the current corpus. This prevents researchers from knowing how their model fares against other models without having to implement them themselves (often from scratch), which in itself is often not possible due to insufficient details having been given in the publications of other groups. Efforts to publish high-quality benchmarks, analogous to the CIFAR10 and ImageNet datasets in general computer vision, are much more likely to yield high-impact results, especially since the literature is dominated by presentations of novel "state of the art" models. It is possible that this overabundance is a direct consequence of the lack of benchmarks, possibly convincing researchers that minor improvements on very small datasets result in a state-of-the-art model (while, in reality, it may just be the result of statistical variations).
- Open sourcing and making code available: Out of 807 papers, only three made code of their models available; an abysmal number compared to numbers in related research disciplines. Open-sourcing code is a great way to promote research and enable other researchers to benchmark their models and implement strong baselines, ultimately driving the field forward. If there are privacy objections to open-sourcing, a good compromise is to publish the code without the model weights.
- More research on, e.g., spleen and pancreas: As seen clearly in Figure 3, relatively few papers have been published on the spleen and pancreas compared to, e.g., H and N or lung cancer. It might be worthwhile for institutions to put more effort into collecting data in these areas so models and methods can be tested in a wider variety of settings.

- Evaluation of alternative training techniques: Computer vision is a rapidly evolving field with successful novel paradigms being introduced relatively frequently. Some notable training strategies appear to be less studied in the field of medical image segmentation. In particular, only 48 papers made use of transfer learning or pretraining, only 21 papers studied self-supervised, semi-supervised, or contrastive learning, and only 11 papers explicitly studied transformer-based architectures. It is possible that segmenting medical images could be more amenable to these methods than what is currently being realized.

5.3.2. What Should Researchers Consider When Starting a Segmentation Study?

- Collect more (high-quality) data: An alarming number of studies use very small datasets: 163 studies used fewer than 100 patients. While this can be good as a proof of concept, it is hard to draw conclusions from such a narrow scope. Furthermore, increasing the number of data samples can often be more effective than developing a stronger training pipeline (e.g., a better model) when it comes to both performance and generalizability.
- Test models on multiple datasets and cancer sites: Diversifying a model by training it on qualitatively different images is a great way to demonstrate the capacity of a model, even if it is intended for a very specific purpose. Moreover, models trained on multiple modalities (e.g., both images and patient data) often show superior performance compared to single-modality training [50–54]. One way to do this is to include images from open sources like the UK Biobank, the Cancer Imaging Archive (TCIA), the BraTS (brain tumor segmentation) dataset, the MM-WHS (Multi-modality whole heart segmentation) dataset, and even The Cancer Genome Atlas (TCGA).
- Evaluate existing models and training techniques over developing new ones: There is a relative overabundance of papers proposing novel deep learning architectures/modules and claiming state-of-the-art performance on rather narrow datasets. It seems exceedingly unlikely that a model trained on just about 50 patients can really be considered state-of-the-art within a certain field. As such, the scientific community should focus more on evaluating existing models and training techniques on larger and more representative datasets and benchmarking them against established baselines.
- Focus on clinical viability over minor improvements in metrics: A limited number of publications assess the practical feasibility of their models, such as subjecting them to downstream applications, investigating their generalizability across different patient populations and clinical scenarios, or evaluating the contours they produce from a medical standpoint. It seems likely that the difficult legislative environment and distance to market limits the number of groups willing to dedicate time and energy to rendering their models suitable for clinics. The regulatory landscape for healthcare is complex and can be a significant obstacle to the implementation of new technologies, which is why research on these issues is important.

5.3.3. How Can Research Practices in Medical Image Segmentation Be Improved?

In addition to the general remarks made under the previous two headlines, we suggest using the following good practices, which often appear to be overlooked, to improve the methodology in individual studies:

- Follow good reporting/documentation guidelines: We found a surprising number of studies lacking critical information needed to reproduce or even implement the methods given in the study. In particular, multiple studies (and abstracts) fail to report details about the patients (e.g., the class balance), the training procedure (e.g., learning rate, data augmentation parameters, and dropout rate), or the validation procedure (e.g., whether the train-test split was random or not). A good place to start is to follow proposed guidelines such as [55] or [56].
- Do cross-validation: Despite being a standard practice in machine learning, a surprising number of studies do not cross-validate their models and instead opt to use a

single train-test split. This severely limits the validity of the conclusions, particularly for smaller datasets, and is strongly discouraged.

- Implement more robust baselines: Implementing a strong baseline is critical in order to adequately assess a new model (particularly due to the lack of open benchmarks). Yet, a number of studies appear to use dated or suboptimally implemented references such as a naïve U-net. A good place to start is models like SegFormer [57] or nn-Unet [58], which are open-source and can be copied directly from their respective repositories.

5.3.4. Do Authors Agree on Conclusions, and Is It Possible to Spot Trends in the Employed Methods?

Authors overwhelmingly agree that deep learning has the potential to greatly help in the process of delineating regions of interest in medical images—not a single paper reviewed in this study specifically concluded that deep learning was actively inferior to traditional approaches. However, very few papers study well-established model architectures on diverse datasets and body regions. Thus, instead of seeing the field converge on very strong models with wide applicability—like the transformer network in natural language processing—we see a continuing trend to propose novel architectures that perform very well on a small, constrained dataset.

6. Limitations

This review contains both objective and subjective analyses and may be considered both systematic and narrative, or neither. To prevent a biased selection and interpretation, we employed an automated selection procedure without hand-picking papers to exclude or include. As a result, some papers from the search results may be less relevant than others. Moreover, due to the large number of papers and queries answered by ChatGPT, we did not check the correctness of all answers. In our quality control of about 660 answers, the model only made one error, where it conflated the sample size and the number of images in the study. Lastly, the model was only presented with the abstracts of the papers.

7. Conclusions

In this review, we have analyzed the current state of research in medical image segmentation by examining 807 studies that make use of deep learning for radiotherapy applications. Our statistical evaluation revealed that 58% of the publications were based on CT, 33% on MRI, and 8% on PET imaging. The three most studied cancer areas were the head and neck, lung, and brain regions, while the three least studied areas were the spleen, pancreas, and kidney. The median number of patients across all studies was 137. Several issues in the field were highlighted, including the lack of benchmark datasets, the need for open-sourcing code, the importance of collecting more high-quality data, and the need to evaluate existing models and training techniques instead of developing new ones. We also suggested good practices to improve methodology in individual studies, such as following good reporting/documentation guidelines, conducting cross-validation, and implementing more robust baselines. Overall, we hope that this provides valuable insights into the challenges and opportunities in medical image segmentation research and that our suggestions can help researchers improve the quality and rigor of their future work.

Supplementary Materials: The following supporting information can be downloaded at: https://www.mdpi.com/article/10.3390/cancers15174389/s1, Table S1: Full List of Studies.

Author Contributions: Conceptualization, G.M.; methodology, L.J.I.; software, L.J.I.; validation, L.J.I.; formal analysis, L.J.I.; investigation, L.J.I.; resources, L.J.I.; data curation, L.J.I.; writing—original draft preparation, L.J.I.; writing—review and editing, P.S., F.M., G.M., F.C., G.C., M.Z. and M.G.V.; visualization, L.J.I.; supervision, G.M., B.A.J.-F., F.C., G.P. and R.O.; project administration, G.M. All authors have read and agreed to the published version of the manuscript.

Funding: This research received no external funding.

Institutional Review Board Statement: Not applicable.

Informed Consent Statement: Not applicable.

Data Availability Statement: Data of the manuscript are available upon reasonable request.

Acknowledgments: IEO: the European Institute of Oncology, is partially supported by the Italian Ministry of Health (with "Ricerca Corrente" and "5 × 1000" funds) and by Institutional grants from Accuray Inc. and Ion Beam Applications (IBA).

Conflicts of Interest: B.A.J.-F. received speaker fees from Roche, Bayer, Janssen, Ipsen, Accuray, Astellas, Elekta, IBA and Astra Zeneca (all outside the current project). The remaining authors declare no conflict of interest. M.G.V. and G.C. received a research fellowship from the Associazione Italiana per la Ricerca sul Cancro (AIRC) entitled "Radioablation ± hormonotherapy for prostate cancer oligorecurrences (RADIOSA trial): potential of imaging and biology" registered at Clinical Trials.gov NCT03940235, approved by the Ethics Committee of IEO and Centro Cardiologico Monzino (IEO-997). The funders had no role in the design of the study; in the collection, analyses, or interpretation of data; in the writing of the manuscript; or in the decision to publish the results.

References

1. Brouwer, C.L.; Steenbakkers, R.J.; van den Heuvel, E.; Duppen, J.C.; Navran, A.; Bijl, H.P.; Chouvalova, O.; Burlage, F.R.; Meertens, H.; Langendijk, J.A.; et al. 3D Variation in Delineation of Head and Neck Organs at Risk. *Radiat. Oncol.* **2012**, *7*, 32. [CrossRef]
2. Veiga-Canuto, D.; Cerdà-Alberich, L.; Sangüesa Nebot, C.; Martínez de las Heras, B.; Pötschger, U.; Gabelloni, M.; Carot Sierra, J.M.; Taschner-Mandl, S.; Düster, V.; Cañete, A.; et al. Comparative Multicentric Evaluation of Inter-Observer Variability in Manual and Automatic Segmentation of Neuroblastic Tumors in Magnetic Resonance Images. *Cancers* **2022**, *14*, 3648. [CrossRef]
3. Van de Steene, J.; Linthout, N.; de Mey, J.; Vinh-Hung, V.; Claassens, C.; Noppen, M.; Bel, A.; Storme, G. Definition of Gross Tumor Volume in Lung Cancer: Inter-Observer Variability. *Radiother. Oncol.* **2002**, *62*, 37–49. [CrossRef]
4. Senan, S.; van Sörnsen de Koste, J.; Samson, M.; Tankink, H.; Jansen, P.; Nowak, P.J.C.M.; Krol, A.D.G.; Schmitz, P.; Lagerwaard, F.J. Evaluation of a Target Contouring Protocol for 3D Conformal Radiotherapy in Non-Small Cell Lung Cancer. *Radiother. Oncol.* **1999**, *53*, 247–255. [CrossRef]
5. Covert, E.C.; Fitzpatrick, K.; Mikell, J.; Kaza, R.K.; Millet, J.D.; Barkmeier, D.; Gemmete, J.; Christensen, J.; Schipper, M.J.; Dewaraja, Y.K. Intra- and Inter-Operator Variability in MRI-Based Manual Segmentation of HCC Lesions and Its Impact on Dosimetry. *EJNMMI Phys.* **2022**, *9*, 90. [CrossRef]
6. Rasch, C.; Eisbruch, A.; Remeijer, P.; Bos, L.; Hoogeman, M.; van Herk, M.; Lebesque, J.V. Irradiation of Paranasal Sinus Tumors, a Delineation and Dose Comparison Study. *Int. J. Radiat. Oncol. *Biol. *Phys.* **2002**, *52*, 120–127. [CrossRef]
7. Becker, A.S.; Chaitanya, K.; Schawkat, K.; Muehlematter, U.J.; Hötker, A.M.; Konukoglu, E.; Donati, O.F. Variability of Manual Segmentation of the Prostate in Axial T2-Weighted MRI: A Multi-Reader Study. *Eur. J. Radiol.* **2019**, *121*, 108716. [CrossRef]
8. Menze, B.H.; Jakab, A.; Bauer, S.; Kalpathy-Cramer, J.; Farahani, K.; Kirby, J.; Burren, Y.; Porz, N.; Slotboom, J.; Wiest, R.; et al. The Multimodal Brain Tumor Image Segmentation Benchmark (BRATS). *IEEE Trans. Med. Imaging* **2015**, *34*, 1993–2024. [CrossRef]
9. Heller, N.; Sathianathen, N.; Kalapara, A.; Walczak, E.; Moore, K.; Kaluzniak, H.; Rosenberg, J.; Blake, P.; Rengel, Z.; Oestreich, M.; et al. The KiTS19 Challenge Data: 300 Kidney Tumor Cases with Clinical Context, CT Semantic Segmentations, and Surgical Outcomes. *arXiv* **2019**, arXiv:1904.00445.
10. Ji, Y.; Bai, H.; Ge, C.; Yang, J.; Zhu, Y.; Zhang, R.; Li, Z.; Zhanng, L.; Ma, W.; Wan, X.; et al. AMOS: A Large-Scale Abdominal Multi-Organ Benchmark for Versatile Medical Image Segmentation. *Adv. Neural Inf. Process. Syst.* **2022**, *35*, 36722–36732.
11. Litjens, G.; Toth, R.; van de Ven, W.; Hoeks, C.; Kerkstra, S.; van Ginneken, B.; Vincent, G.; Guillard, G.; Birbeck, N.; Zhang, J.; et al. Evaluation of Prostate Segmentation Algorithms for MRI: The PROMISE12 Challenge. *Med. Image Anal.* **2014**, *18*, 359–373. [CrossRef]
12. Li, Z.; Kamnitsas, K.; Glocker, B. Overfitting of Neural Nets Under Class Imbalance: Analysis and Improvements for Segmentation. In *Proceedings of the Medical Image Computing and Computer Assisted Intervention—MICCAI 2019*; Shen, D., Liu, T., Peters, T.M., Staib, L.H., Essert, C., Zhou, S., Yap, P.-T., Khan, A., Eds.; Springer International Publishing: Cham, Switzerland, 2019; pp. 402–410.
13. Gu, J.; Zhao, H.; Tresp, V.; Torr, P. Adversarial Examples on Segmentation Models Can Be Easy to Transfer. Available online: https://arxiv.org/abs/2111.11368v1 (accessed on 25 June 2023).
14. Weiss, K.; Khoshgoftaar, T.M.; Wang, D. A Survey of Transfer Learning. *J. Big Data* **2016**, *3*, 9. [CrossRef]
15. Shorten, C.; Khoshgoftaar, T.M. A Survey on Image Data Augmentation for Deep Learning. *J. Big Data* **2019**, *6*, 60. [CrossRef]
16. Sagi, O.; Rokach, L. Ensemble Learning: A Survey. *WIREs Data Min. Knowl. Discov.* **2018**, *8*, e1249. [CrossRef]
17. Yang, C.; Qin, L.; Xie, Y.; Liao, J. Deep Learning in CT Image Segmentation of Cervical Cancer: A Systematic Review and Meta-Analysis. *Radiat. Oncol.* **2022**, *17*, 175. [CrossRef]
18. Kalantar, R.; Lin, G.; Winfield, J.M.; Messiou, C.; Lalondrelle, S.; Blackledge, M.D.; Koh, D.-M. Automatic Segmentation of Pelvic Cancers Using Deep Learning: State-of-the-Art Approaches and Challenges. *Diagnostics* **2021**, *11*, 1964. [CrossRef]
19. Liu, X.; Li, K.-W.; Yang, R.; Geng, L.-S. Review of Deep Learning Based Automatic Segmentation for Lung Cancer Radiotherapy. *Front. Oncol.* **2021**, *11*, 717039. [CrossRef]

20. Fernando, K.R.M.; Tsokos, C.P. Deep and Statistical Learning in Biomedical Imaging: State of the Art in 3D MRI Brain Tumor Segmentation. *Inf. Fusion* **2023**, *92*, 450–465. [CrossRef]
21. Altini, N.; Prencipe, B.; Cascarano, G.D.; Brunetti, A.; Brunetti, G.; Triggiani, V.; Carnimeo, L.; Marino, F.; Guerriero, A.; Villani, L.; et al. Liver, Kidney and Spleen Segmentation from CT Scans and MRI with Deep Learning: A Survey. *Neurocomputing* **2022**, *490*, 30–53. [CrossRef]
22. Badrigilan, S.; Nabavi, S.; Abin, A.A.; Rostampour, N.; Abedi, I.; Shirvani, A.; Ebrahimi Moghaddam, M. Deep Learning Approaches for Automated Classification and Segmentation of Head and Neck Cancers and Brain Tumors in Magnetic Resonance Images: A Meta-Analysis Study. *Int. J. Comput. Assist. Radiol. Surg.* **2021**, *16*, 529–542. [CrossRef]
23. Zöllner, F.G.; Kociński, M.; Hansen, L.; Golla, A.-K.; Trbalić, A.Š.; Lundervold, A.; Materka, A.; Rogelj, P. Kidney Segmentation in Renal Magnetic Resonance Imaging—Current Status and Prospects. *IEEE Access* **2021**, *9*, 71577–71605. [CrossRef]
24. Ali, H.M.; Kaiser, M.S.; Mahmud, M. Application of Convolutional Neural Network in Segmenting Brain Regions from MRI Data. In *Proceedings of the Brain Informatics*; Liang, P., Goel, V., Shan, C., Eds.; Springer International Publishing: Cham, Switzerland, 2019; pp. 136–146.
25. Ranjbarzadeh, R.; Dorosti, S.; Jafarzadeh Ghoushchi, S.; Caputo, A.; Tirkolaee, E.B.; Ali, S.S.; Arshadi, Z.; Bendechache, M. Breast Tumor Localization and Segmentation Using Machine Learning Techniques: Overview of Datasets, Findings, and Methods. *Comput. Biol. Med.* **2023**, *152*, 106443. [CrossRef]
26. Habijan, M.; Babin, D.; Galić, I.; Leventić, H.; Romić, K.; Velicki, L.; Pižurica, A. Overview of the Whole Heart and Heart Chamber Segmentation Methods. *Cardiovasc. Eng. Technol.* **2020**, *11*, 725–747. [CrossRef]
27. Islam, M.Z.; Naqvi, R.A.; Haider, A.; Kim, H.S. Deep Learning for Automatic Tumor Lesions Delineation and Prognostic Assessment in Multi-Modality PET/CT: A Prospective Survey. *Eng. Appl. Artif. Intell.* **2023**, *123*, 106276. [CrossRef]
28. Mohammed, Y.M.A.; El Garouani, S.; Jellouli, I. A Survey of Methods for Brain Tumor Segmentation-Based MRI Images. *J. Comput. Des. Eng.* **2023**, *10*, 266–293. [CrossRef]
29. Punn, N.S.; Agarwal, S. Modality Specific U-Net Variants for Biomedical Image Segmentation: A Survey. *Artif. Intell. Rev.* **2022**, *55*, 5845–5889. [CrossRef]
30. El Jurdi, R.; Petitjean, C.; Honeine, P.; Cheplygina, V.; Abdallah, F. High-Level Prior-Based Loss Functions for Medical Image Segmentation: A Survey. *Comput. Vis. Image Underst.* **2021**, *210*, 103248. [CrossRef]
31. Sharma, N.; Aggarwal, L.M. Automated Medical Image Segmentation Techniques. *J. Med. Phys.* **2010**, *35*, 3–14. [CrossRef]
32. Lin, X.; Li, X. Image Based Brain Segmentation: From Multi-Atlas Fusion to Deep Learning. *Curr. Med. Imaging Rev.* **2019**, *15*, 443–452. [CrossRef]
33. Hesamian, M.H.; Jia, W.; He, X.; Kennedy, P. Deep Learning Techniques for Medical Image Segmentation: Achievements and Challenges. *J. Digit. Imaging* **2019**, *32*, 582–596. [CrossRef]
34. Latif, G.; Alghazo, J.; Sibai, F.N.; Iskandar, D.N.F.A.; Khan, A.H. Recent Advancements in Fuzzy C-Means Based Techniques for Brain MRI Segmentation. *Curr. Med. Imaging* **2021**, *17*, 917–930. [CrossRef]
35. Trimpl, M.J.; Primakov, S.; Lambin, P.; Stride, E.P.J.; Vallis, K.A.; Gooding, M.J. Beyond Automatic Medical Image Segmentation-the Spectrum between Fully Manual and Fully Automatic Delineation. *Phys. Med. Biol.* **2022**, *67*, 12TR01. [CrossRef]
36. Sakshi; Kukreja, V. Image Segmentation Techniques: Statistical, Comprehensive, Semi-Automated Analysis and an Application Perspective Analysis of Mathematical Expressions. *Arch. Comput. Methods Eng.* **2023**, *30*, 457–495. [CrossRef]
37. Shao, J.; Chen, S.; Zhou, J.; Zhu, H.; Wang, Z.; Brown, M. Application of U-Net and Optimized Clustering in Medical Image Segmentation: A Review. *CMES* **2023**, *136*, 2173–2219. [CrossRef]
38. Qureshi, I.; Yan, J.; Abbas, Q.; Shaheed, K.; Riaz, A.B.; Wahid, A.; Khan, M.W.J.; Szczuko, P. Medical Image Segmentation Using Deep Semantic-Based Methods: A Review of Techniques, Applications and Emerging Trends. *Inf. Fusion* **2023**, *90*, 316–352. [CrossRef]
39. Huang, L.; Ruan, S.; Denœux, T. Application of Belief Functions to Medical Image Segmentation: A Review. *Inf. Fusion* **2023**, *91*, 737–756. [CrossRef]
40. Fu, Y.; Lei, Y.; Wang, T.; Curran, W.J.; Liu, T.; Yang, X. A Review of Deep Learning Based Methods for Medical Image Multi-Organ Segmentation. *Phys. Medica* **2021**, *85*, 107–122. [CrossRef]
41. OpenAI Introducing ChatGPT. Available online: https://openai.com/blog/chatgpt (accessed on 25 June 2023).
42. Koss, J.E.; Newman, F.D.; Johnson, T.K.; Kirch, D.L. Abdominal Organ Segmentation Using Texture Transforms and a Hopfield Neural Network. *IEEE Trans. Med. Imaging* **1999**, *18*, 640–648. [CrossRef] [PubMed]
43. Popple, R.A.; Griffith, H.R.; Sawrie, S.M.; Fiveash, J.B.; Brezovich, I.A. Implementation of Talairach Atlas Based Automated Brain Segmentation for Radiation Therapy Dosimetry. *Technol. Cancer Res. Treat.* **2006**, *5*, 15–21. [CrossRef]
44. Sharma, N.; Ray, A.K.; Sharma, S.; Shukla, K.K.; Pradhan, S.; Aggarwal, L.M. Segmentation and Classification of Medical Images Using Texture-Primitive Features: Application of BAM-Type Artificial Neural Network. *J. Med. Phys.* **2008**, *33*, 119–126. [CrossRef]
45. Sharif, M.S.; Abbod, M.; Amira, A.; Zaidi, H. Novel Hybrid Approach Combining ANN and MRA for PET Volume Segmentation. In Proceedings of the 2010 IEEE Asia Pacific Conference on Circuits and Systems, Kuala Lumpur, Malaysia, 6–9 December 2010; pp. 596–599.
46. Sharif, M.S.; Abbod, M.; Amira, A.; Zaidi, H. Artificial Neural Network-Based System for PET Volume Segmentation. *J. Biomed. Imaging* **2010**, *2010*, 105610. [CrossRef]

47. Zeleznik, R.; Weiss, J.; Taron, J.; Guthier, C.; Bitterman, D.S.; Hancox, C.; Kann, B.H.; Kim, D.W.; Punglia, R.S.; Bredfeldt, J.; et al. Deep-Learning System to Improve the Quality and Efficiency of Volumetric Heart Segmentation for Breast Cancer. *NPJ Digit. Med.* **2021**, *4*, 43. [CrossRef]
48. Deng, Y.; Hou, D.; Li, B.; Lv, X.; Ke, L.; Qiang, M.; Li, T.; Jing, B.; Li, C. A Novel Fully Automated MRI-Based Deep-Learning Method for Segmentation of Nasopharyngeal Carcinoma Lymph Nodes. *J. Med. Biol. Eng.* **2022**, *42*, 604–612. [CrossRef]
49. Graffy, P.M.; Liu, J.; O'Connor, S.; Summers, R.M.; Pickhardt, P.J. Automated Segmentation and Quantification of Aortic Calcification at Abdominal CT: Application of a Deep Learning-Based Algorithm to a Longitudinal Screening Cohort. *Abdom. Radiol.* **2019**, *44*, 2921–2928. [CrossRef] [PubMed]
50. Chen, R.J.; Lu, M.Y.; Williamson, D.F.K.; Chen, T.Y.; Lipkova, J.; Noor, Z.; Shaban, M.; Shady, M.; Williams, M.; Joo, B.; et al. Pan-Cancer Integrative Histology-Genomic Analysis via Multimodal Deep Learning. *Cancer Cell* **2022**, *40*, 865–878.e6. [CrossRef] [PubMed]
51. Hager, P.; Menten, M.J.; Rueckert, D. Best of Both Worlds: Multimodal Contrastive Learning with Tabular and Imaging Data. In Proceedings of the IEEE/CVF Conference on Computer Vision and Pattern Recognition, Vancouver, BC, Canada, 17–24 June 2023; pp. 23924–23935.
52. Hong, D.; Gao, L.; Yokoya, N.; Yao, J.; Chanussot, J.; Du, Q.; Zhang, B. More Diverse Means Better: Multimodal Deep Learning Meets Remote-Sensing Imagery Classification. *IEEE Trans. Geosci. Remote Sens.* **2021**, *59*, 4340–4354. [CrossRef]
53. Vale-Silva, L.A.; Rohr, K. Long-Term Cancer Survival Prediction Using Multimodal Deep Learning. *Sci. Rep.* **2021**, *11*, 13505. [CrossRef]
54. Venugopalan, J.; Tong, L.; Hassanzadeh, H.R.; Wang, M.D. Multimodal Deep Learning Models for Early Detection of Alzheimer's Disease Stage. *Sci. Rep.* **2021**, *11*, 3254. [CrossRef]
55. Luo, W.; Phung, D.; Tran, T.; Gupta, S.; Rana, S.; Karmakar, C.; Shilton, A.; Yearwood, J.; Dimitrova, N.; Ho, T.B.; et al. Guidelines for Developing and Reporting Machine Learning Predictive Models in Biomedical Research: A Multidisciplinary View. *J. Med. Internet Res.* **2016**, *18*, e323. [CrossRef]
56. Mongan, J.; Moy, L.; Kahn, C.E. Checklist for Artificial Intelligence in Medical Imaging (CLAIM): A Guide for Authors and Reviewers. *Radiol. Artif. Intell.* **2020**, *2*, e200029. [CrossRef]
57. Xie, E.; Wang, W.; Yu, Z.; Anandkumar, A.; Alvarez, J.M.; Luo, P. SegFormer: Simple and Efficient Design for Semantic Segmentation with Transformers. In Proceedings of the Advances in Neural Information Processing Systems, Virtual, 6–14 December 2021; Curran Associates, Inc.: Red Hook, NY, USA, 2021; Volume 34, pp. 12077–12090.
58. Isensee, F.; Jaeger, P.F.; Kohl, S.A.A.; Petersen, J.; Maier-Hein, K.H. NnU-Net: A Self-Configuring Method for Deep Learning-Based Biomedical Image Segmentation. *Nat. Methods* **2021**, *18*, 203–211. [CrossRef] [PubMed]

cancers

MDPI

Systematic Review

Deep Learning in Thoracic Oncology: Meta-Analytical Insights into Lung Nodule Early-Detection Technologies

Ting-Wei Wang [1,2,3,†], Chih-Keng Wang [2,4,†], Jia-Sheng Hong [1], Heng-Sheng Chao [5], Yuh-Min Chen [2,5] and Yu-Te Wu [1,6,7,*]

1 Institute of Biophotonics, National Yang-Ming Chiao Tung University, Taipei 30010, Taiwan
2 School of Medicine, College of Medicine, National Yang-Ming Chiao Tung University, Taipei 30010, Taiwan
3 Department of Computer Science, Whiting School of Engineering, Johns Hopkins University, Baltimore, MD 21218, USA
4 Department of Otolaryngology-Head and Neck Surgery, Taichung Veterans General Hospital, Taichung 40705, Taiwan
5 Department of Chest Medicine, Taipei Veteran General Hospital, Taipei 112, Taiwan
6 Brain Research Center, National Yang-Ming Chiao Tung University, Taipei 30010, Taiwan
7 College Medical Device Innovation and Translation Center, National Yang-Ming Chiao Tung University, Taipei 30010, Taiwan
* Correspondence: ytwu@nycu.edu.tw; Tel.: +886-2-2826-7000 (ext. 5707)
† These authors contributed equally to this work.

Simple Summary: Detecting lung nodules, which may indicate thoracic cancer, is a critical challenge in medical imaging. Recent advances in artificial intelligence, particularly deep learning, show promise for improving diagnostic accuracy. This study evaluates the effectiveness of deep learning models, such as convolutional neural networks, in identifying lung nodules on computed tomography images. By analyzing results from 48 studies, we aim to highlight the strengths and limitations of these models. Our findings emphasize the potential of artificial intelligence to transform lung cancer diagnosis while addressing the need for more inclusive and diverse studies to ensure these technologies are reliable and applicable across various patient populations. This work could help guide researchers, clinicians, and developers in advancing medical imaging solutions for cancer detection.

Abstract: Background/Objectives: Detecting lung nodules on computed tomography (CT) images is critical for diagnosing thoracic cancers. Deep learning models, particularly convolutional neural networks (CNNs), show promise in automating this process. This systematic review and meta-analysis aim to evaluate the diagnostic accuracy of these models, focusing on lesion-wise sensitivity as the primary metric. **Methods:** A comprehensive literature search was conducted, identifying 48 studies published up to 7 November 2023. The pooled diagnostic performance was assessed using a random-effects model, with lesion-wise sensitivity as the key outcome. Factors influencing model performance, including participant demographics, dataset privacy, and data splitting methods, were analyzed. Methodological rigor was maintained through the Checklist for Artificial Intelligence in Medical Imaging (CLAIM) and Quality Assessment of Diagnostic Accuracy Studies-2 (QUADAS-2) tools. Trial Registration: This review is registered with PROSPERO under CRD42023479887. **Results:** The meta-analysis revealed a pooled sensitivity of 79% (95% CI: 72–86%) for independent datasets and 85% (95% CI: 83–88%) across all datasets. Variability in performance was associated with dataset characteristics and study methodologies. **Conclusions:** While deep learning models demonstrate significant potential in lung nodule detection, the findings highlight the need for more diverse datasets, standardized evaluation protocols, and interventional studies to enhance generalizability and clinical applicability. Further research is necessary to validate these models across broader patient populations.

Keywords: deep learning; lung nodule detection; convolutional neural networks; computed tomography scans; meta-analysis

1. Introduction

Lung carcinoma, a leading cause of cancer-related deaths, results from the uncontrolled proliferation of abnormal cells in pulmonary tissues. Lung cancer is the most frequently diagnosed malignancy worldwide, with approximately 2.38 million new cases and 1.27 million deaths in 2023 [1]. The severe clinical symptoms of lung cancer considerably affect patients' quality of life and place a substantial burden on health-care systems globally [2,3].

Despite advances in treatment strategies, the trend of diagnosing lung cancer at advanced stages remains a major challenge, adversely affecting survival [4]. For non-small-cell lung cancer, the 5-year survival rates are 65%, 37%, and 9% for localized, regional, and distant stages, respectively. By contrast, small-cell lung cancer has 5-year survival rates of 30%, 19%, and 3% for these stages, respectively [5]. Imaging modalities, such as computed tomography (CT), including its low-dose acquisition technique (LDCT), play pivotal roles in the early detection of lung cancer. The National Lung Screening Trial revealed the superiority of low-dose CT (LDCT) over conventional chest radiography, demonstrating a 20% reduction in mortality when LDCT was used for screening [6]. Furthermore, the NELSON trial revealed the efficacy of LDCT, and the results indicated a 26% reduction in mortality among men and an even more pronounced decrease of up to 61% in women compared with those who did not undergo screening [6]. These findings emphasize the importance of early detection for improving patient outcomes.

Despite the proven benefits of these imaging techniques, their integration into lung cancer diagnosis encounters some challenges. A major limitation is the delayed diagnosis of lung cancer, which is often detected only when advanced symptoms become apparent [7]. This delay in detection considerably reduces the effectiveness of early intervention strategies. In addition, these diagnostic methods are prone to high false-positive rates and the risk of overdiagnosis. These problems not only lead to unnecessary medical procedures and increased health-care costs but also cause considerable psychological distress among patients [8]. Thus, the integration of these diagnostic tools into clinical practice requires a careful evaluation of their limitations and their potential impact on patient health and health-care systems.

Substantial advancements have been made in lung cancer imaging in terms of artificial intelligence (AI), particularly in computer-aided detection (CADe) and computer-aided diagnosis (CADx). These developments are primarily reflected in the augmentation of detection capabilities [9], refined characterization of pulmonary nodules [10,11], and enhancement of risk assessment accuracy [12]. Among these advancements, a key development has been the integration of convolutional neural networks (CNNs) into the analysis of CT images. Empirical research has validated the effectiveness of CNNs in increasing the precision of detection and reducing the incidence of false positives [13]. This progress in AI and deep learning technologies represents a pivotal shift in the diagnostic landscape of lung cancer, increasing the accuracy and efficiency of early-detection methods.

Despite the promising role of CNNs, the inherent "black box" nature of these models limits their interpretability and explainability in direct end-to-end applications [14]. To address this problem, an alternative approach is to deconstruct the processes of CADe and CADx and subject them to critical analysis. Previous meta-analyses have primarily focused on the diagnostic accuracy of deep learning models [15–17]. This review examines the detection sensitivity of deep learning models for early lung cancer detection on CT images through CADe. We systematically synthesized and evaluated evidence on the role of AI in enhancing detection sensitivity and reducing the workload of radiologists. This review provides a comprehensive overview of the current state of AI in lung nodule detection and its potential implications for clinical practice, policy-making, and future research. Such an exploration can revolutionize the lung cancer screening process, optimizing early detection and thereby affecting patient outcomes.

2. Materials and Methods

2.1. General Guidelines

This systematic review and meta-analysis adhered to the Preferred Reporting Items for Systematic Reviews and Meta-Analyses (PRISMA) 2020 guidelines [18]. We followed the PRISMA checklist to ensure the highest methodological rigor in the design and reporting of this study. Detailed information regarding our compliance with these guidelines is provided in Supplementary Tables S1 and S2. In addition, this study was registered with PROSPERO under CRD42023479887. Because this systematic review and meta-analysis did not involve direct human participation, ethical approval and informed consent requirements were deemed not applicable.

2.2. Database Search and Identification of Eligible Studies

Two reviewers (T-WW and J-SH) conducted a comprehensive literature review focusing on studies applying deep learning for chest CT images of lung cancer. The literature search was performed in PubMed, Embase, and Web of Science (Supplementary Table S3). The search period was from the inception of each database until 7 November 2023. Our selection process involved an initial screening of titles and abstracts and was supplemented by manual searches to ensure a comprehensive coverage of the relevant literature. Any discrepancies between reviewers during the selection phase were resolved through consultation with a third expert.

We included studies that recruited adults with lung cancer and used chest LDCT and CT images in conjunction with deep learning techniques. To maintain the focus and quality of our review, we excluded various study types and articles, including review articles, posters, conference presentations, and supplements. In addition, we excluded studies focusing on classification or false-positive reduction, articles not written in English, case reports, studies with dataset problems (e.g., incomplete dataset splitting), retracted articles, studies that did not use deep learning methodologies, studies that employed non-CT imaging methods, and those with irrelevant outcomes.

2.3. Data Extraction and Management

T-WW and J-SH conducted data extraction, focusing on various metrics relevant to lung nodule detection. Our investigative scope was expansive, covering various study characteristics, including study design, participants' race, study duration, number of patients, data sources utilized, types and sizes of nodules, size thresholds, series and lesion numbers, lesion sizes, and methods employed for validation.

We evaluated the dimensions and types of algorithms employed in these studies. In addition, we examined various advanced preprocessing techniques, including generative methods, lung segmentation approaches, intensity standardization, resolution adjustments, image cropping, and data augmentation strategies. Furthermore, we analyzed false-positive reduction, multiscale approaches employed, model input dimensions, and specific deep learning models.

We analyzed the performance of deep learning algorithms, focusing on lesion-wise sensitivity. This performance metric was calculated to determine average lesion-wise sensitivity across an extensive range of false-positive thresholds per scan, including 1/8, 1/4, 1/2, 1, 2, 4, and 8. This metric also reflects precision, enabling a comprehensive assessment of the performance of deep learning models in the detection of lung nodules.

2.4. Methodological Quality Appraisal

The methodological quality of each study included in our review was thoroughly evaluated using the Checklist for Artificial Intelligence in Medical Imaging and the Quality Assessment of Diagnostic Accuracy Studies-2 tools [19,20]. T-WW and J-SH independently conducted this rigorous appraisal for the unbiased and comprehensive assessment of the studies. Given the complexities inherent in evaluating AI applications in medical imaging, any discrepancies were resolved through consultation with senior researchers. This step was crucial in harmonizing any conflicting interpretations and maintaining the integrity of the evaluation process.

2.5. Statistical Analysis

Two meta-analyses were performed to evaluate lesion-wise sensitivity, which was reported as a competition performance metric across the selected studies. The first analysis focused on independent datasets. When different studies utilized the same dataset, the highest-performing algorithm was chosen for inclusion. The second analysis included all reported results from all validation datasets. When studies reported multiple algorithms, the highest-performing algorithm was chosen for inclusion. For studies that presented median values and interquartile ranges, we converted them into mean values and standard deviations by using established formulas [21,22]. Given the heterogeneous study populations, we employed a random-effects model with restricted maximum likelihood (REML) [23], which offers more reliable estimates of between-study variance by adjusting for the degrees of freedom used in parameter estimation. The results of this comprehensive analysis are depicted in forest plots.

Subgroup analyses were conducted considering various factors, such as race (Asian vs. Western vs. mixed), nature of the database (open-source vs. private), validation methods (internal vs. external validation), dataset splitting methods (train/test split vs. cross-validation), and specific features of model architectures, including dimensionality (2D vs. 3D), image preprocessing procedures, false-positive reduction techniques, multiscale involvement, and types of algorithms [24]. Additionally, a meta-regression [25] was performed to explore correlations between competition performance metrics and variables such as the size of the training dataset and the number of lesions. The Q test was used to quantify discrepancies or heterogeneity across studies, with the statistical significance threshold set at $p < 0.05$. Heterogeneity was classified into the following categories based on I2 indices: trivial (0–25%), minimal (26–50%), moderate (51–75%), and pronounced (76–100%) [26]. To address potential biases in publication, Egger's test was applied to assess funnel plot asymmetries [27].

3. Results

3.1. Study Identification and Selection

Our systematic literature review, depicted in the PRISMA flowchart (Figure 1), initially yielded 3485 studies. After removing 1255 duplicates, we screened 2330 articles by using

EndNote. Of these, we excluded 2053 articles due to insufficient relevance. Further evaluation of 277 full-text articles led to additional exclusions for various reasons, such as the non-use of deep learning or the use of non-CT methods (Table S4). Finally, we included 48 studies [28–74] in our comprehensive meta-analysis.

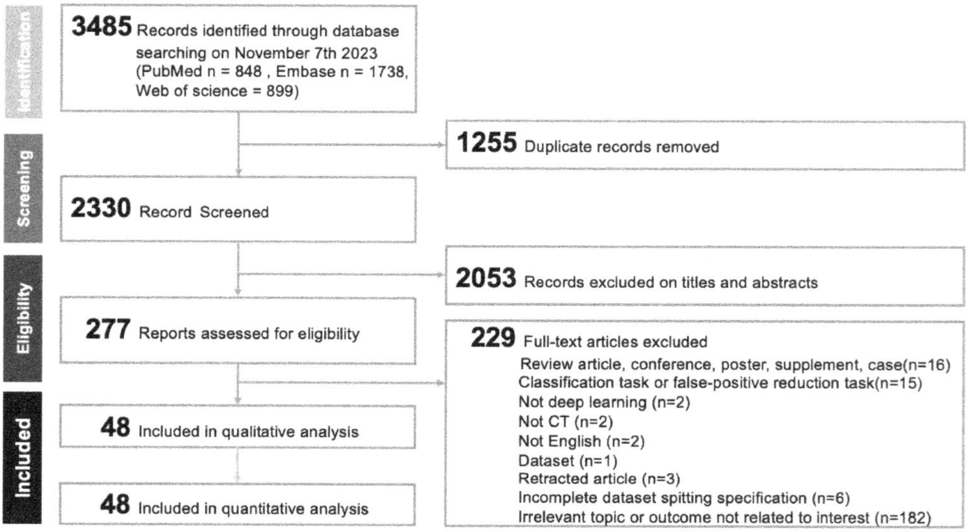

Figure 1. PRISMA flowchart for study selection.

3.2. Basic Characteristics of Included Studies

Table 1 presents a comprehensive summary of patient and study characteristics from these 48 studies on lung cancer that were conducted from 2018 to 2023. These studies involved patient cohorts of varying sizes, with Zhao et al. (2023) [28] having the largest cohort of 4556 patients and Guo et al. (2020) [64] having the smallest cohort of 306 patients. Regarding lung cancer characterization, the studies primarily focused on nodules, often employing size thresholds of >3 mm. However, some studies [31,38,41,49,57,71] used different criteria. The lesion counts and sizes reported in the training and testing sets varied substantially, reflecting the heterogeneity of lung cancer. The validation methods employed in these studies mainly included training and testing frameworks, with several studies opting for cross-validation techniques. This observation highlights the importance of robust model validation in lung cancer research. Moreover, the consistent use of manual referencing across these studies emphasized the vital role of human expertise in ensuring data accuracy and contextual relevance, a key aspect of medical research.

3.3. Characteristics and Performance of Deep Learning Algorithms

Table 2 provides a comprehensive overview of the diverse methods used in lung cancer imaging research, highlighting the integration of various preprocessing techniques and deep learning algorithms. The data indicated a significant trend toward the use of generative algorithms, which were employed by several studies [19,33,57] for data augmentation. Lung segmentation, a crucial preprocessing step, was widely applied in many studies [28–31,33–43,47,49–57,59,64,67,69,71–73] for isolating regions of interest for accurate analysis. Intensity clipping [28–37,39–44,46,47,49,50,52–55,58,59,61,62,65,67,68,70] and normalization [28–36,39–44,46–55,58–62,65,67,68,70] were other critical preprocessing steps that were extensively implemented to ensure the standardization of imaging data across diverse datasets. Resolution adjustment [28–33,35,37–39,42–45,47–54,57–59,62,63,65, 67,72,74] was also prominently used to ensure consistent image quality and details across different imaging modalities. Image augmentation [28–30,32,33,35,37,39–41,43,44,47,49–59, 61–69,71–73] and cropping [28–49,51–69,71–74] were widely used to prevent overfitting and improve algorithmic robustness. Furthermore, false-positive reduction techniques [28,29,31, 37,39–43,45–47,49,53–63,65–68,70,71,74] and multiscale analysis [29,30,34,39–42,46,47,49,51–54,56,58,60,62,63,65–67,70,73] were performed to enhance detection accuracy and reliability.

Different imaging dimensions, including 2D [28,37,55,58,59,67,70,71,74], 3D [29–31,33–36,38–54,56,57,60–65,67–69,73], and combined 2D/3D approaches [32,66], were used for lung nodule detection and characterization. Furthermore, these studies used diverse algorithms, ranging from basic U-net to advanced variants, such as U-net++, nnU-net, YOLOv5, Mask R-CNN, Faster R-CNN, and custom CNNs, reflecting the ongoing innovation and customized solutions for lung cancer detection. In these studies, the clinical performance measure values ranged from 0.39 to 0.96, indicating the different levels of efficacy of these approaches, which can be affected by dataset complexities and algorithmic capabilities. Additionally, Supplementary Table S5 provides details on CT protocols and hardware characteristics, offering further insights into the imaging parameters used across studies.

3.4. *Quality Assessment*

Figure S1 offers a comprehensive summary of the quality assessments for the studies included, utilizing the QUADAS-2 tool. Additionally, a detailed analysis focusing on bias risks and applicability concerns is presented in Supplementary Table S6.

Supplementary Table S7 extensively evaluates 48 studies based on the CLAIM criteria. These studies yielded an average CLAIM score of 25.77, equating to approximately 61.36% of the maximum possible score of 42, with a standard deviation of 2.8 and scores ranging from 20.00 to 38.00. A breakdown of the average scores across CLAIM subsections for these studies is as follows: title/abstract section scored 1.7 out of 2 (85%), introduction 1.96 out of 2 (98%), methods 18.46 out of 28 (65.59%), results 1.38 out of 5 (27.5%), discussion 1.27 out of 2 (63.5%), and other information 1 out of 3 (33.3%). This breakdown highlights the varying levels of quality and thoroughness in different sections of the studies.

3.5. *Efficacy of Deep Learning Model Detection of Lung Cancer on CT Images*

An analysis of independent validation datasets for 16 deep learning algorithms revealed considerable variance in performance metrics, ranging from 39% to 96% (Figure 2). The mean performance metric was 79%, with a 95% confidence interval (CI) of 72% to 86%. These results revealed significant heterogeneity, as indicated by a Q-test value of 2214.72 ($p < 0.01$) and a Higgins I2 index of 99.18%. Sensitivity analysis (Figure S2) revealed markedly lower performance in the study by Xu et al. [60], leading to its exclusion from subsequent subgroup analysis and meta-regression. Egger's test yielded a p value of 0.75, indicating no significant publication bias (Figure S3). Subgroup analyses revealed notable differences in performance for factors such as race, validation methods, resolution adjustment, and image cropping. However, variables such as dataset privacy, splitting methodology, slice thickness, generative approaches, lung segmentation, intensity clipping, intensity normalization, data augmentation, false-positive reduction strategies, multiscale analysis, model dimensions, and algorithm type did not significantly affect the performance of these models (Figure 3). The analysis including Xu et al. is presented in Figure S4. In addition, meta-regression analysis did not reveal a significant correlation between the number of training images or lesion counts and the overall effectiveness of the models.

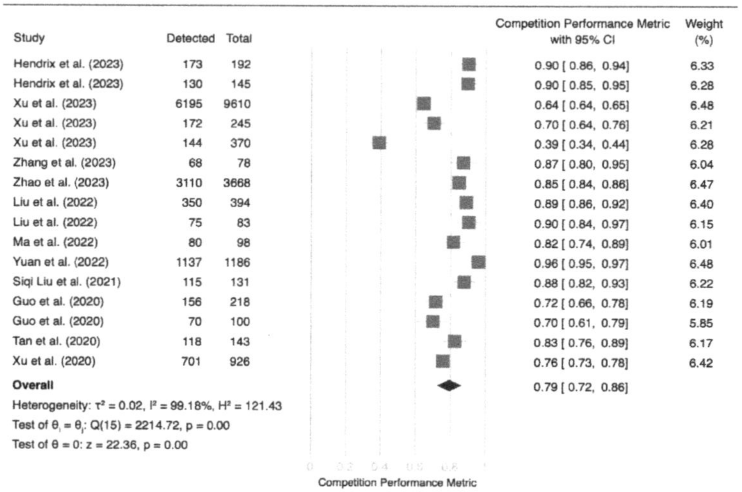

Figure 2. Forest plot of competition performance metrics of deep learning algorithms in independent validation datasets [28,29,31,37,43,44,47,49,52,60,61].

An extensive evaluation of validation datasets for 64 deep learning algorithms revealed substantial variability in performance metrics, ranging from 39% to 96% (Figure 4). The calculated average performance metric was 85%, with a 95% CI ranging from 83% to 88%. This substantial heterogeneity was supported by a Q-test value of 7133.19 ($p < 0.01$) and a Higgins I2 index of 99.23%. Sensitivity analysis (Figure S5) did not reveal a significant difference based on the exclusion of any article. Egger's test yielded a p value of <0.01, indicating the presence of publication bias (Figure S6). However, additional subgroup analysis incorporating conference papers did not reveal significant differences (Figure S7). Subgroup analysis demonstrated significant differences in model performance for race, dataset privacy, and dataset splitting methods. However, no significant differences were observed in model performance for the validation methods, slice thicknesses, generative approaches, lung segmentation, intensity clipping, intensity normalization, resolution adjustment, data augmentation, image cropping, false-positive reduction strategies, multi-scale analysis, model dimensions, or algorithm type (Figure 5). In addition, meta-regression analysis indicated no significant correlations between the number of training images or lesion counts and the overall efficacy of the models.

Table 1. Patient and study characteristics.

First Author	Publication Year	Study Design	Race	Patients	Data Source	Image	Duration	Type	Size Threshold	Series (Train/Test)	Lesion Num (Train/Test)	Size (Train/Test)	Validation
Zhao et al. [28]	2023	Retrospective	I: Western; E: Asian	4556	I: LUNA16, E: Shanghai Chest Hospital	LDCT/CT	2012~2018	I: nodule; E: malignancy	LUNA16 > 3 mm	4556 (888/3668)	4854 (1186/3668)	NR (8.31/15.17)-mean	Train/test
Zhang et al. [29]	2023	Retrospective	Western	888	LUNA 16	LDCT	NR	Nodule	LUNA16 > 3 mm	888 (710/178)	1186 (949/237)	8.31 (NR/NR)-mean	Train/test
Zhang et al. [30]	2023	Retrospective	I: Western E: Asian	928	I: LUNA16, E: Wuhan Hospital	LDCT/CT	NR	Nodule	LUNA16 > 3 mm	928 (800/128)	1264 (1068/196)	NR (8.31/NR)-mean	Train/test
Xu et al. [31]	2023	Retrospective	I1: Western; I2: Asian; I3: Western; I4: Asian	10,848	I1: LUNA16; I2: Tianchi; I3: Russia; I4: PN9	LDCT/CT	2015~2019	Nodule	LUNA16 > 3 mm; Tianchi > 5 mm; Russia > 3 mm	10,848 (8349/2499)	44,719 (34,252/10,467)	NR (8.31/NR/NR/NR)-mean	Train/test
Wang et al. [32]	2023	Retrospective	Western	888	LUNA 16	LDCT	NR	Nodule	LUNA16 > 3 mm	888 (799/89)	1186 (1067/119)	8.31 (NR/NR)-mean	Cross-validation
Shen et al. [33]	2023	Retrospective	Western	888	LUNA 16	LDCT	NR	Nodule	LUNA16 > 3 mm	888 (799/89)	1186 (1067/119)	8.31 (NR/NR)-mean	Cross-validation
Mkindu et al. I [34]	2023	Retrospective	Western	888	LUNA 16	LDCT	NR	Nodule	LUNA16 > 3 mm	888 (799/89)	1186 (1067/119)	8.31 (NR/NR)-mean	Cross-validation
Mkindu et al. II [35]	2023	Retrospective	Western	888	LUNA 16	LDCT	NR	Nodule	LUNA16 > 3 mm	888 (799/89)	1186 (1067/119)	8.31 (NR/NR)-mean	Cross-validation
Lin et al. [36]	2023	Retrospective	Western	888	LUNA 16	LDCT	NR	Nodule	LUNA16 > 3 mm	888 (799/89)	1186 (1067/119)	8.31 (NR/NR)-mean	Cross-validation
Hendrix et al. [37]	2023	Retrospective	Western	1690	LUNA 16, Radboud University Medical Center, Jeroen Bosch Hospital	LDCT/CT	2017~2020	Nodule	LUNA16 > 3 mm	1690 (1490/200)	5107 (4770/337)	NR	Train/test

Table 1. *Cont.*

First Author	Publication Year	Study Design	Race	Patients	Data Source	Image	Duration	Type	Size Threshold	Series (Train/Test)	Lesion Num (Train/Test)	Size (Train/Test)	Validation
Guo et al. [38]	2023	Retrospective	I1: Asian; I2: Asian	184	West China Hospital	LDCT	2008~2017	Nodule	1 mm~30 mm	578 (459/119)	1781 (1314/467)	NR (8.43/7.67)-mean	Train/test
Chen et al. [39]	2023	Retrospective	Western	888	LUNA 16	LDCT	NR	Nodule	LUNA16 > 3 mm	888 (799/89)	1186 (1067/119)	8.31 (NR/NR)-mean	Cross-validation
Zheng et al. [40]	2022	Retrospective	Western	888	LUNA 16	LDCT	NR	Nodule	LUNA16 > 3 mm	888 (799/89)	1186 (1067/119)	8.31 (NR/NR)-mean	Cross-validation
Hui Zhang et al. [41]	2022	Retrospective	Western	1088	I1: LUNA16; I2: Tianchi	LDCT	NR	Nodule	LUNA16 > 3 mm; Tianchi > 5 mm	1088 (799/289)	1432 (1067/365)	NR (8.31/NR)-mean	Train/test
Guanglu Zhang et al. [42]	2022	Retrospective	Western	888	LUNA 16	LDCT	NR	Nodule	LUNA16 > 3 mm	888 (799/89)	1186 (1067/119)	8.31 (NR/NR)-mean	Cross-validation
Yuan et al. [43]	2022	Retrospective	Western	888	LUNA 16	LDCT	NR	Nodule	LUNA16 > 3 mm	888 (799/89)	1186 (1067/119)	8.31 (NR/NR)-mean	Cross-validation
Suzuki et al. [44]	2022	Retrospective	Western	888	LUNA 16	LDCT	NR	Nodule	LUNA16 > 3 mm	888 (799/89)	1186 (1067/119)	8.31 (NR/NR)-mean	Cross-validation
Niu et al. [45]	2022	Retrospective	Western	436	LUNA 16	LDCT	NR	Nodule	LUNA16 > 6 mm	436 (349/87)	684 (548/136)	NR	Train/test
Mei et al. [46]	2022	Retrospective	Asian	8798	PN9	CT	2015~2019	Nodule	NR	8798 (6707/2091)	40,439 (30,828/9611)	NR	Train/test
Ma et al. [47]	2022	Retrospective	Asian	456	First Hospital of China Medical University	CT	NR	GGO	NR	456 (365/91)	486 (388/98)	NR	Cross-validation
Luo et al. [48]	2022	Retrospective	Western	888	LUNA 16	LDCT	NR	Nodule	LUNA16 > 3 mm	888 (799/89)	1186 (1067/119)	8.31 (NR/NR)-mean	Cross-validation

Table 1. *Cont.*

First Author	Publication Year	Study Design	Race	Patients	Data Source	Image	Duration	Type	Size Threshold	Series (Train/Test)	Lesion Num (Train/Test)	Size (Train/Test)	Validation
Liu et al. [49]	2022	Retrospective	I: Western; E1: Western; E2: Western	1118	LUNA 16; SPIE-AAPM; Lung TIME	LDCT/CT	NR	Nodule	LUNA16 > 3 mm, SPIE-AAPM > 10 mm Lung TIME > 2 mm	1118 (799/319)	1663 (1067/596)	NR (8.31/NR/NR)-mean	Train/test
Katase et al. [50]	2022	Retrospective	I: Mixed; E1: Western; E2: Western	2374	Kyorin University Hospital; LUNA 16; SPIE-AAPM; LNDb	LDCT/CT	2013~2018	Nodule	Major axis diameter measured ≥ 3 mm for solid or part-solid nodules and ≥5 mm for ground-glass nodules	2374 (1997/377)	10,924 (10,467/457)	NR (8.3/NR/NR)-mean	Train/test
Huang et al. [51]	2022	Retrospective	Western	888	LUNA 16	LDCT	NR	Nodule	LUNA16 > 3 mm	888 (710/178)	1186 (949/237)	8.31 (NR/NR)-mean	Cross-validation
Guo et al. [52]	2022	Retrospective	Western	888	LUNA 16	LDCT	NR	Nodule	LUNA16 > 3 mm	888 (799/89)	1186 (1067/119)	8.31 (NR/NR)-mean	Cross-validation
Pereira et al. [53]	2021	Retrospective	Western	888	LUNA 16	LDCT	NR	Nodule	LUNA16 > 3 mm	888 (799/89)	1186 (1067/119)	8.31 (NR/NR)-mean	Cross-validation
Peng et al. [54]	2021	Retrospective	Western	888	LUNA 16	LDCT	NR	Nodule	LUNA16 > 3 mm	888 (799/89)	1186 (1067/119)	8.31 (NR/NR)-mean	Cross-validation
Nguyen et al. [55]	2021	Retrospective	Western	961	LUNA 16	LDCT	NR	Nodule	LUNA16 > 3 mm	961 (799/162)	1269 (1068/201)	8.31 (NR/NR)-mean	Cross-validation
Weihua Liu et al. [56]	2021	Retrospective	Western	888	LUNA 16	LDCT	NR	Nodule	LUNA16 > 3 mm	888 (799/89)	1186 (1067/119)	8.31 (NR/NR)-mean	Cross-validation
Siqi Liu et al. [57]	2021	Retrospective	Western	6904	LUNA 16, NLST, in-house	LDCT/CT	NR	Nodule	> 6 mm	6904 (6488/446)	22,450 (22,169/281)	NR	Train/test

Table 1. *Cont.*

First Author	Publication Year	Study Design	Race	Patients	Data Source	Image	Duration	Type	Size Threshold	Series (Train/Test)	Lesion Num (Train/Test)	Size (Train/Test)	Validation
Farhangi et al. [58]	2021	Retrospective	Western	888	LUNA 16	LDCT	NR	Nodule	LUNA16 > 3 mm	888 (799/89)	1186 (1067/119)	8.31 (NR/NR)-mean	Cross-validation
Zheng et al. [59]	2020	Retrospective	Western	888	LUNA 16	LDCT	NR	Nodule	LUNA16 > 3 mm	888 (799/89)	1186 (1067/119)	8.31 (NR/NR)-mean	Cross-validation
Xu et al. [60]	2020	Retrospective	Asian	1109	The First Affiliated Hospital of Nanjing Medical University	CT	2014~2015	Nodule	NR	1109 (998/111)	12,057 (11,131/926)	NR	Train/test
Tan et al.. [61]	2020	Retrospective	I: Western; E: Asian	1003	I: LUNA 16; E: Zhejiang Cancer Hospital,	LDCT/CT	NR	Nodule	LUNA16 > 3 mm	1003 (799/204)	1329 (1067/262)	NR (8.31/NR)-mean	Train/test
Ozdemir et al. [62]	2020	Retrospective	Western	888	LUNA 16	LDCT	NR	Nodule	LUNA16 > 3 mm	888 (799/89)	1186 (1067/119)	8.31 (NR/NR)-mean	Cross-validation
Masood et al. [63]	2020	Retrospective	Western	888	LUNA 16	LDCT	NR	Nodule	LUNA16 > 3 mm	888 (799/89)	1186 (1067/119)	8.31 (NR/NR)-mean	Cross-validation
Guo et al. [64]	2020	Retrospective	Asian	306	West China Hospital	LDCT	NR	Nodule	NR	579 (463/116)	1590 (1272/318)	NR	Train/test
Chenyang et al. [65]	2020	Retrospective	Western	601	LUNA 16	LDCT	NR	Nodule	LUNA16 > 3 mm	888 (799/89)	1186 (1067/119)	8.31 (NR/NR)-mean	Cross-validation
Cao et al. [66]	2020	Retrospective	Western	601	LUNA 16	LDCT	NR	Nodule	LUNA16 > 3 mm	888 (799/89)	1186 (1067/119)	8.31 (NR/NR)-mean	Cross-validation
Xie et al. [67]	2019	Retrospective	Western	601	LUNA 16	LDCT	NR	Nodule	LUNA16 > 3 mm	888 (710/178)	1186 (949/237)	8.31 (NR/NR)-mean	Cross-validation
Winkels et al. [68]	2019	Retrospective	Western	NR	I: NLST, E: LIDC/IDRI	LDCT	NR	Nodule	NR	NR	47,462 (38,889/8582)	NR (NR/8.31)-mean	Train/test

Table 1. *Cont.*

First Author	Publication Year	Study Design	Race	Patients	Data Source	Image	Duration	Type	Size Threshold	Series (Train/Test)	Lesion Num (Train/Test)	Size (Train/Test)	Validation
Nasrullah et al. [69]	2019	Retrospective	Western	601	LUNA 16	LDCT	NR	Nodule	LUNA16 > 3 mm	888 (710/178)	1186 (949/237)	8.31 (NR/NR)-mean	Cross-validation
Xia Huang et al. [70]	2019	Retrospective	Western	601	LUNA 16	LDCT	NR	Nodule	LUNA16 > 3 mm	888 (710/178)	1186 (949/237)	8.31 (NR/NR)-mean	Train/test
Wenkai Huang et al. [71]	2019	Retrospective	Western + Asian	NR	LUNA16, Tianchi	LDCT/CT	NR	Nodule	LUNA16 > 3 mm; Tianchi > 5 mm	1888 (1699/189)	18,125 (16,312/1813)	NR	Cross-validation
Gong et al. [67]	2019	Retrospective	Western	601	LUNA 16	LDCT	NR	Nodule	LUNA16 > 3 mm	888 (799/89)	1186 (1067/119)	8.31 (NR/NR)-mean	Cross-validation
Zhang et al. [72]	2018	Retrospective	Western	601	LUNA 16	LDCT	NR	Nodule	LUNA16 > 3 mm	888 (799/89)	1186 (1067/119)	8.31 (NR/NR)-mean	Cross-validation
Gu et al. [73]	2018	Retrospective	Western	601	LUNA 16	LDCT	NR	Nodule	LUNA16 > 3 mm	888 (799/89)	1186 (1067/119)	8.31 (NR/NR)-mean	Cross-validation
Setio et al. [74]	2018	Retrospective	Western	601	LUNA 16	LDCT	NR	Nodule	LUNA16 > 3 mm	888 (799/89)	1186 (1067/119)	8.31 (NR/NR)-mean	Cross-validation

Table 2. Characteristics and performance of preprocessing techniques and deep learning algorithms.

First Author	Training Size	Lesion Count	Generative	Lung Segmentation	Intensity Clipping	Intensity Normalization	Resolution Adjustment	Image Augmentation	Image Cropping	False-Positive Reduction	Multiscale	Input Dimension	Algorithms	CPM
Zhao et al. [28]	888	1186	Yes	Yes	−1024, 400	−1, 1	1 × 1 × 1	Yes	64 × 64 × 64	Yes	No	2D	UNet++	E: 0.848
Zhang et al. [29]	710	949	No	Yes	−1200, 600	0, 255	1 × 1 × 1	Yes	128 × 128 × 128	Yes	Yes	3D	FPN	0.8934
Zhang et al. [30]	800	1068	No	Yes	−1200, 600	0, 255	Yes	Yes	128 × 128 × 128	No	Yes	3D	SK-ResNet	E: 0.8742

Table 2. *Cont.*

First Author	Training Size	Lesion Count	Generative	Lung Segmentation	Intensity Clipping	Intensity Normalization	Resolution Adjustment	Image Augmentation	Image Cropping	False-Positive Reduction	Multiscale	Input Dimension	Algorithms	CPM
Xu et al. [31]	8349	34252	No	Yes	−1200, 600	0, 255	1 × 1 × 1	No	128 × 128 × 128	Yes	No	3D	NoduleNet+ SGSE	I1: 0.7830; I2: 0.7036; I3:0.3901; I4:0.6446
Wang et al. [32]	799	1067	No	No	−1000, 400	0, 1	Yes	Yes	50 × 50 × 50	No	No	2D/3D	CNN	0.795
Shen et al. [33]	799	1067	Yes	Yes	−1200, 600	0, 255	Yes	Yes	96 × 96 × 96	No	No	3D	CADe	0.8299
Mkindu et al. I [34]	799	1067	No	Yes	−1200, 600	0, 1	No	No	64 × 64 × 64, 16 × 16 × 16, 12 × 12 × 12	No	Yes	3D	MSViT	0.911
Mkindu et al. II [35]	799	1067	No	Yes	−1200, 600	0, 1	1 × 1 × 1	Yes	64 × 64 × 64	No	No	3D	ResECA	0.911
Lin et al. [36]	799	1067	No	Yes	−1200, 600	0, 1	No	No	96 × 96 × 96	No	No	3D	IR-UNet++	0.8741
Hendrix et al. [37]	1490	4770	No	Yes	−1000, 400	No	Yes	Yes	512 × 512	Yes	No	2D	YOLOv5	0.902
Guo et al. [38]	459	1314	No	Yes	No	No	Yes	No	128 × 128 × 20	No	No	3D	CNN	I1: 0.6/ I2:0.6116
Chen et al. [39]	799	1067	No	Yes	−1000, 400	0, 1	1 × 1 × 1	Yes	64 × 64 × 12	Yes	Yes	3D	F-Net, MSS-Net	0.967
Zheng et al. [40]	799	1067	No	Yes	−1200, 600	0, 255	No	Yes	210 × 210 × 210	Yes	Yes	3D	TSND	0.9059
Hui Zhang et al. [41]	799	1067	No	Yes	−1200, 600	0, 255	No	Yes	96 × 96 × 96	Yes	Yes	3D	Faster R-CNN	0.927
Guanglu Zhang et al. [42]	799	1067	No	Yes	−1200, 600	0, 255	1 × 1 × 1	No	128 × 128 × 128	Yes	Yes	3D	FPN+CSA	0.912
Yuan et al. [43]	799	1067	No	Yes	−1200, 600	0, 255	1 × 1 × 1	Yes	48 × 48 × 48	Yes	Yes	3D	3D Residual U-Net model	0.959
Suzuki et al. [44]	799	1067	No	No	−1000, 600	0, 255	1 × 1 × 1	Yes	64 × 96 × 96	No	No	3D	Modified 3D U-net	0.947
Niu et al. [45]	349	548	No	No	No	No	Yes	No	96 × 96 × 96	Yes	No	3D	URCTrans	0.95

Table 2. *Cont.*

First Author	Training Size	Lesion Count	Generative	Lung Segmentation	Intensity Clipping	Intensity Normalization	Resolution Adjustment	Image Augmentation	Image Cropping	False-Positive Reduction	Multiscale	Input Dimension	Algorithms	CPM
Mei et al. [46]	6707	30828	No	No	−1200, 600	0, 255	No	No	128 × 128 × 128	Yes	Yes	3D	SANet	0.6446
Ma et al. [47]	365	388	No	Yes	−300, 1800	Yes	Yes	Yes	64 × 128 × 128	Yes	Yes	3D	Mask RCNN	0.8174
Luo et al. [48]	799	1067	No	No	No	0, 1	1 × 1 × 1	No	96 × 96 × 96	No	No	3D	SCPM-Net	0.892
Liu et al. [49]	799	1067	No	Yes	−1200, 600	0, 255	1 × 1 × 1	Yes	96 × 96 × 96	Yes	Yes	3D	FPN	0.957
Katase et al. [50]	1997	10467	No	Yes	Yes	0–1	1 × 1 × 1	Yes	No	No	No	3D	Faster R-CNN	0.96
Huang et al. [51]	710	949	No	Yes	No	0–1	1 × 1 × 1	Yes	80 × 80 × 80	No	Yes	3D	OSAF-YOLOv3	0.905
Guo et al. [52]	799	1067	No	Yes	−1200, 600	0, 255	No	No	96 × 96 × 96	No	Yes	3D	Multiscale aggregation network	0.92
Pereira et al. [53]	799	1067	No	Yes	−1000, 400	0, 255	Yes	Yes	32 × 32 × 32, 48 × 48 × 48	Yes	Yes	3D	Mask R-CNN	0.9224
Peng et al. [54]	799	1067	No	Yes	−1200, 600	0–1	1 × 1 × 1	No	128 × 128 × 128	Yes	Yes	3D	CEM, SAM, and Res2Net	0.872
Nguyen et al. [55]	799	1068	No	Yes	−1200, 600	0–1	No	Yes	512 × 512	Yes	No	2D	Faster R-CNN	0.882
Weihua Liu et al. [56]	799	1067	No	Yes	No	No	No	Yes	128 × 128 × 128	Yes	Yes	3D	PDCB	0.939
Siqi Liu et al. [57]	6488	22169	Yes	Yes	No	No	Yes	Yes	64 × 64 × 64	Yes	No	3D	Deep Lung	0.9226
Farhangi et al. [58]	799	1067	No	No	−1000, 400	0–1	0.625 × 0.625 × 2	Yes	48 × 48 × 16	Yes	Yes	2D	CNN	0.895
Zheng et al. [59]	799	1067	No	Yes	−1000, 400	0–1	Yes	Yes	512 × 512	Yes	No	2D	DL-CAD	0.922
Xu et al. [60]	998	11131	No	No	No	Yes	No	No	20 × 20 × 6, 30 × 30 × 10, 40 × 40 × 26	Yes	Yes	3D	CNN	0.757

Table 2. *Cont.*

First Author	Training Size	Lesion Count	Generative	Lung Segmentation	Intensity Clipping	Intensity Normalization	Resolution Adjustment	Image Augmentation	Image Cropping	False-Positive Reduction	Multiscale	Input Dimension	Algorithms	CPM
Tan et al.. [61]	799	1067	No	No	−1200, 200	0–1	No	Yes	512 × 512 × 32	Yes	No	3D	CNN	0.956
Ozdemir et al. [62]	799	1067	No	No	−1000, 400	0–1	1 × 1 × 1	Yes	64 × 64 × 64	Yes	Yes	3D	V-net	0.921
Masood et al. [63]	799	1067	No	No	No	No	0.5 × 0.5 × 0.5	Yes	Yes	Yes	Yes	3D	Faster R-CNN	0.946
Guo et al. [64]	463	1272	No	Yes	No	No	No	Yes	128 × 128 × 128	No	No	3D	DeepLN	I1: 0.716/ I2:0.699
Chenyang et al. [65]	799	1067	No	No	−1000, 400	0–1	1 × 1 × 1	Yes	64 × 64 × 64	Yes	Yes	3D	V-Net	0.902
Cao et al. [66]	799	1067	No	No	No	No	No	Yes	64 × 64 × 3	Yes	Yes	2D/3D	TSCNN	0.911
Xie et al. [67]	710	949	No	No	−1000, 4000	0–1	1 × 1 × 1	Yes	512 × 512	Yes	Yes	2D	Faster R-CNN	0.79
Winkels et al. [68]		38889	No	No	−1000, 300	−1, 1	No	Yes	12 × 72 × 72	Yes	No	3D	3D G-CNNs	0.88
Nasrullah et al. [69]	710	949	No	Yes	No	No	No	Yes	96 × 96 × 96	No	No	3D	CMixNet with faster R-CNN	0.9421
Xia Huang et al. [70]	710	949	No	No	−1000, 3000	0, 255	No	No	No	Yes	Yes	2D	Faster R-CNN	0.88
Wenkai Huang et al. [71]	1699	16312	No	Yes	No	No	No	Yes	96 × 96	Yes	Yes	2D	CNN	0.876
Gong et al. [67]	799	1067	No	Yes	−1200, 600	0, 255	1 × 1 × 1	Yes	128 × 128 × 128	Yes	Yes	3D	RPN	0.904
Zhang et al. [72]	799	1067	No	Yes	No	No	1 × 1 × 1	Yes	32 × 32 × 32	No	Yes	3D	DCNN	0.947
Gu et al. [73]	799	1067	No	Yes	No	No	No	Yes	64 × 64 × 64	No	Yes	3D	Deep CNN	0.7967
Setio et al. [74]	799	1067	No	No	No	No	0.5 × 0.5 × 0.5	No	512 × 512	Yes	No	2D	Znet	0.811

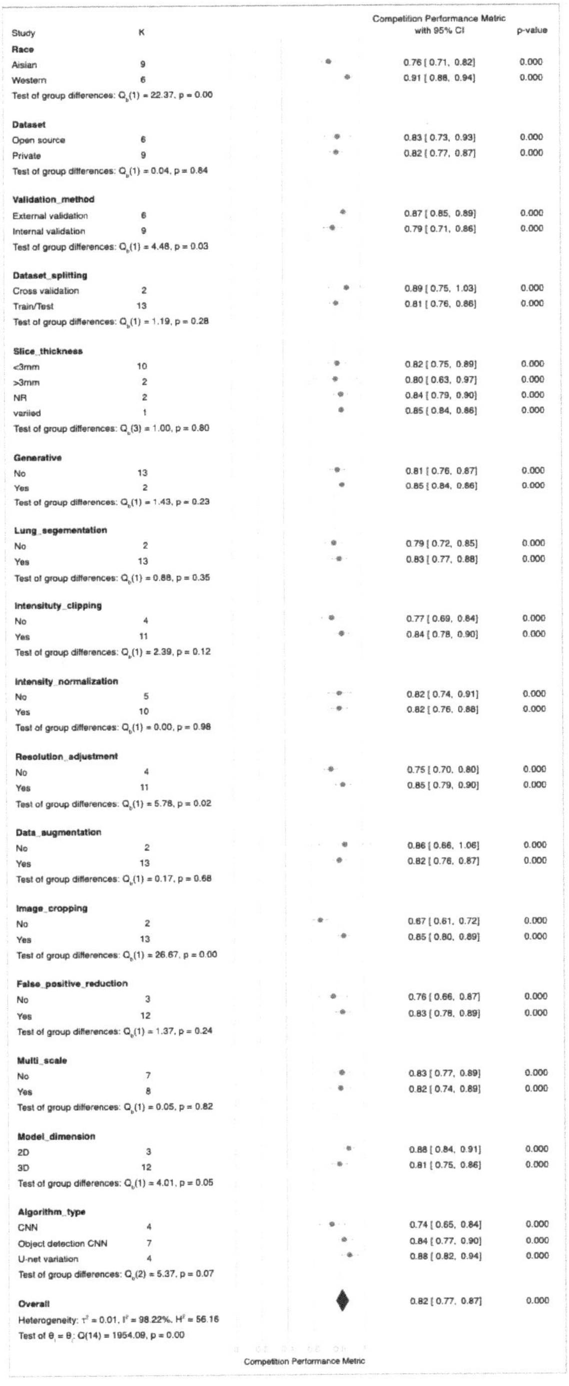

Figure 3. Forest plot of subgroup analysis competition performance metrics of deep learning algorithms in independent datasets.

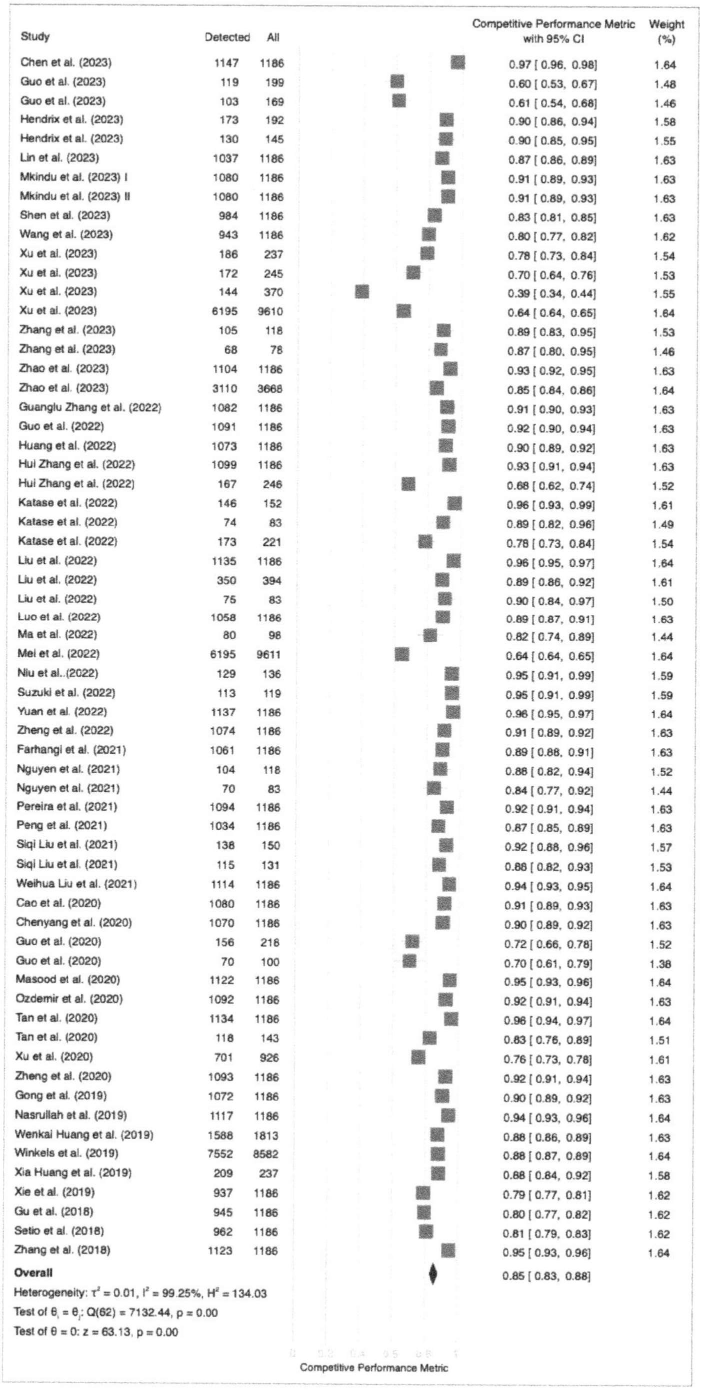

Figure 4. Forest plot of competition performance metrics of deep learning algorithms in all validation datasets [28–39,41–59,61–63,65–74].

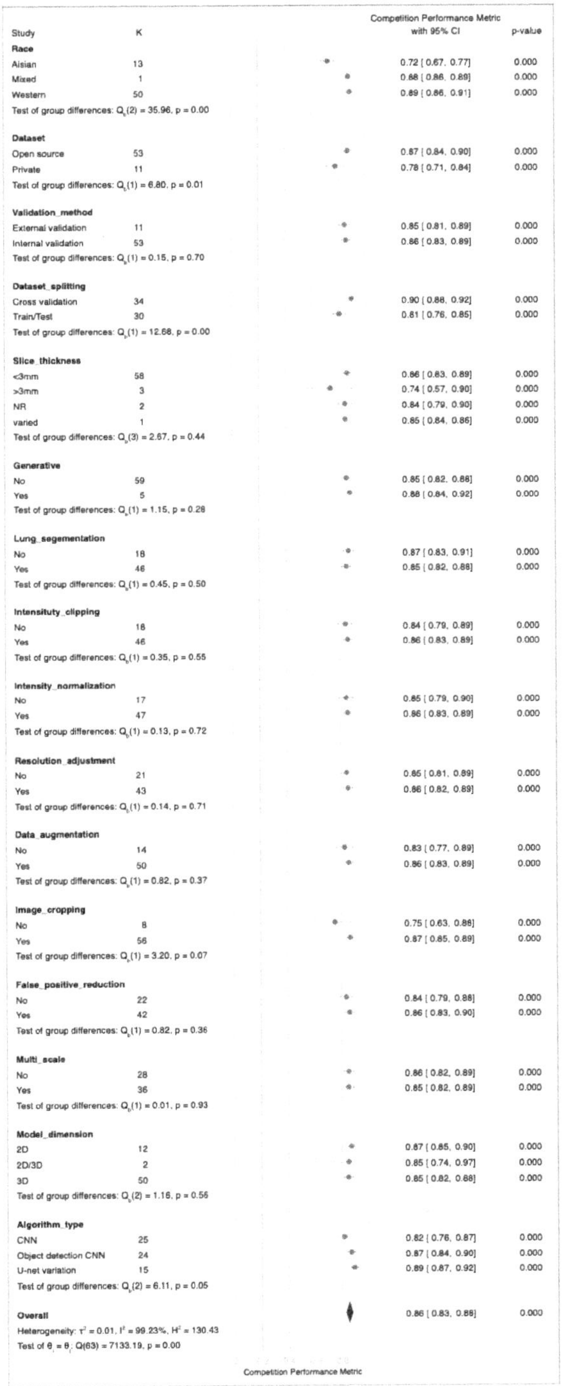

Figure 5. Forest plot of subgroup analysis competition performance metrics of deep learning algorithms in all validation datasets.

4. Discussion

To the best of our knowledge, this is the first systematic review and meta-analysis to evaluate the sensitivity of deep learning models for lung nodule detection using competition performance metrics as a benchmark. Unlike previous studies that primarily focused on diagnostic sensitivity and specificity [75] or segmentation performance using metrics such as the Dice similarity coefficient [76], our study uniquely synthesizes results from 16 deep learning models validated on independent datasets. Through this analysis, we derived a pooled competition performance metric of 79%, with a 95% confidence interval ranging from 72% to 86%, providing a novel perspective on the evaluation of model performance in this domain. Race, validation methods, resolution adjustment, and image cropping significantly affected the performance of these deep learning models. Furthermore, when examining the results for all 64 deep learning algorithms across various validation datasets, the pooled competition performance metric was 85%, with 95% CI values ranging from 83% to 88%. Race, dataset privacy, and dataset splitting methods significantly affected the performance of these deep learning algorithms.

This study revealed the significant effect of race on the performance of deep learning models. Notably, we observed that a higher proportion of individuals of Asian descent exhibited non-solid nodules with a ground-glass opacity appearance [77,78]. This characteristic might have contributed to the decreased performance, either due to the non-solid morphology of nodules or a potential imbalance in distribution within the dataset, leading to reduced sensitivity. Furthermore, we identified that image distortions differentially affected the performance of deep learning models across various subgroups. This suggests the increased sensitivity of these models to variations in input data [79]. Such increased sensitivity might contribute to the substantial effect of race on model performance. A recent study [80] highlighted the importance of fairness and equity in deep learning models, advocating for equitable model performance across different subpopulations in datasets, particularly for variables such as race and gender. Thus, deep learning algorithms that are not only effective but also impartial and inclusive should be developed, considering the diversity of the populations they are intended to serve.

Our analysis of validation methods revealed that external validation exhibited superior performance compared to internal validation, a finding that contrasts with the commonly observed decrease in performance under external validation [81]. One possible explanation is that the external datasets used in this study may have been either more representative of real-world conditions or less heterogeneous, allowing the models to generalize effectively. In addition, robust training procedures, such as appropriate data augmentation and thorough hyperparameter tuning, could have contributed to reducing overfitting and improving model resilience when evaluated on external data. Consequently, this outcome suggests that well-designed deep learning models can maintain high performance across diverse populations, highlighting their potential robustness. However, when the analysis was extended to larger sample sizes across all validation sets, no significant difference was identified between internal and external validation methods. Furthermore, dataset privacy and dataset splitting methods significantly affect model performance. Open-source datasets, such as LUNA16 [74], Tianchi [82], Russia [83], Pn9 [46], SPIE-AAPM Lung CT Challenge [84], Lung Time [85], LNDb [86], and NLST [87], have been extensively utilized for benchmarking various deep learning algorithms. Notably, the LUNA16 dataset consists of low-dose CT (LDCT) scans, whereas several other studies included in this review relied on full-dose CT scans from private datasets. This distinction is important, as LDCT is commonly used for lung cancer screening due to its reduced radiation exposure, but its impact on model performance remains underexplored. Although cross-validation can enhance the representativeness of validation results, it has a risk of overfitting. The findings collectively indicate the significant impact of dataset characteristics on the performance of deep learning models. They highlight the need for further research for validating these models in diverse clinical settings and with varied dataset partitions. Such research would ensure the applicability and reliability of deep learning models across different clinical environments and patient populations, thereby contributing to the development of more robust and universally applicable diagnostic tools in the health-care sector.

In terms of dataset preprocessing, we determined that resolution adjustment and image cropping were significantly correlated with the performance of deep learning models. However, less than five studies focused on this aspect, potentially leading to a lack of statistical power. Further analysis incorporating a broader range of validation datasets did not corroborate these initial findings. Despite the inconclusiveness regarding resolution adjustment and image cropping, the results revealed that preprocessing enhanced model performance. Regarding the algorithms used in deep learning models, segmentation-based U-Net architectures and their variants exhibited higher performance than detection-based CNNs and other customized CNN architectures, aligning with findings from a recent study [28]. A possible explanation is that U-Net's encoder–decoder structure with skip connections may facilitate more precise localization of nodules by preserving spatial information and capturing subtle textural details. In contrast, detection-based CNNs often focus on bounding-box predictions and may therefore miss fine-grained distinctions crucial for small or irregularly shaped nodules. Nonetheless, we did not observe any statistically significant differences in performance across these algorithm types. Furthermore, other model-related factors, such as slice thickness, false-positive reduction strategies, multi-scale analysis, model dimensions, and various preprocessing techniques, did not exhibit significant differences among subgroups.

The study results revealed that the training size and lesion count were not significantly correlated with model performance. This finding is consistent with those of previous studies [79,88,89]. These observations suggest that dataset characteristics exert a more significant effect on the performance of deep learning models than technical factors related to deep learning. This highlights the importance of focusing on dataset characteristics, such as quality, diversity, and representativeness, for enhancing the efficacy of deep learning models in clinical and research applications.

This study demonstrated the potential and inherent challenges of employing deep learning models, especially CNNs, for early lung cancer detection. These models have demonstrated their efficacy in enhancing the precision of pulmonary nodule detection on CT images, improving diagnostic accuracy, and alleviating the workload for radiologists. However, the clinical application of these technologies is more complex. A critical limitation of the included studies is their non-interventional nature, indicating that AI assessments did not affect the diagnostic workflow. Thus, whether the enhanced cancer detection capabilities of these models in research would effectively translate into actual improvements in cancer detection in real-world clinical settings remains to be determined.

Translating deep learning-based lung cancer detection into clinical practice requires a comprehensive, multistep approach. Prospective clinical trials are essential to validate model performance under real-world conditions, ensuring generalizability and robustness across diverse patient populations and workflows. Effective integration into radiology workflows must include training staff, ensuring user-friendly interfaces, and achieving seamless compatibility with existing systems. Adhering to regulatory approvals is crucial to ensure safety and reliability, while implementing robust data privacy and security protocols is necessary to protect patient information and comply with regulations. Furthermore, interpretability and explainability are vital to foster trust and acceptance, enabling clinicians to understand and rely on AI-driven decisions. Lastly, evaluating the cost-effectiveness of these technologies will inform resource allocation and reimbursement strategies. These steps together provide a clear roadmap for bringing deep learning solutions into routine clinical use.

In future work, differentiating between commercially available and non-commercially available AI software could provide valuable insights, as highlighted in the study by Fukumoto et al. [90], which validated the performance of commercially available deep-learning-based lung nodule detection using Synapse Fujifilm. The "black box" nature of many DL models raises concerns regarding their interpretability and reliability in clinical settings. Performance variability based on training dataset characteristics, including racial diversity, can lead to biases. This study revealed performance discrepancies across different datasets, emphasizing the need for extensive validation in varied clinical environments. Future larger-scale prospective or interventional studies should focus on developing practical, fair, inclusive, and interpretable models to integrate DL in thoracic oncology effectively, ensuring their broad applicability across diverse patient populations.

5. Conclusions

This study effectively demonstrated the capability of deep learning models, especially CNNs, in enhancing the detection of lung nodules on CT images. The pooled competition performance metrics of 79% (95% CI: 72% to 86%) on independent datasets and 85% (95%CI: 83% to 88%) on all validation sets indicate the potential of these technologies to substantially improve diagnostic accuracy and reduce the workload of radiologists. However, despite these promising results, several critical challenges exist that must be addressed. These include the non-interventional nature of the studies, the "black box" problem inherent in AI models, and variability in performance based on dataset characteristics. Highlighting the need for extensive, diverse, and interventional research, the study emphasizes developing effective, interpretable, and equitable deep learning models across different patient demographics. This approach is crucial for advancing lung cancer screening and diagnosis in clinical practice.

Supplementary Materials: The following supporting information can be downloaded at: https://www.mdpi.com/article/10.3390/cancers17040621/s1, Figure S1: The results of QUADAS-2 quality assessment for included studies; Figure S2: The results of a sensitivity analysis of deep learning algorithms' competition performance metrics in independent validation dataset using the one-study removal method; Figure S3: Funnel plot of deep learning algorithms' competition performance metrics of the highest-performing results in independent validation dataset; Figure S4: Forest plot of subgroup analysis competition performance metrics of deep learning algorithms in independent datasets; Figure S5: The results of a sensitivity analysis of deep learning algorithms' competition performance metrics in all validation datasets using the one-study removal method; Figure S6: Funnel plot of deep learning algorithms' competition performance metrics of the highest-performing results in independent validation dataset; Figure S7: Forest plot of subgroup analysis competition performance metrics of deep learning algorithms in independent datasets with publication status as moderator (p = 0.82); Table S1: PRISMA-DTA Abstract Checklist [91]; Table S2: PRISMA-DTA Checklist [91]; Table S3: Keywords and search results in different databases; Table S4: Excluded articles and reasons; Table S5: CT protocol and hardware characteristics; Table S6: Quality assessment according to the Quality Assessment of Diagnostic Accuracy Studies 2 (QUADAS-2) criteria; Table S7: The Checklist for Artificial Intelligence in Medical Imaging scores.

Author Contributions: T.-W.W.: Conceptualization, Methodology, Software, Validation, Data Curation, Formal Analysis, Investigation, Writing—Original Draft, and Visualization. C.-K.W.: Conceptualization, Methodology, Validation, Formal Analysis, Writing—Reviewing and Editing, and Investigation. J.-S.H.: Conceptualization, Methodology, Validation, Formal Analysis, Writing—Reviewing and Editing, and Investigation. H.-S.C.: Conceptualization, Formal Analysis, Supervision, Writing—Reviewing and Editing, and Investigation. Y.-M.C.: Conceptualization, Formal Analysis, Supervision, Writing—Reviewing and Editing, and Investigation. Y.-T.W.: Conceptualization, Writing—Reviewing and Editing, Resources, Supervision, Project Administration, and Funding Acquisition. All authors have read and agreed to the published version of the manuscript.

Funding: This research was funded by the Gen. & Mrs. M.C. Peng Fellowship from the School of Medicine, 406 National Yang Ming Chiao Tung University, MD-SY-A3-309-01; Taichung Veterans General Hospital, TCVGH-YMCT1109111, TCVGH-YMCT1119105; the National Science and Technology Council in Taiwan, MOST 110-2634-F-006-022, MOST 110-2221-E-A49A-504-MY3; National Yang Ming Chiao Tung University from the Featured Areas Research Center Program within the framework of the Higher Education Sprout Project by the Ministry of Education (MOE) in Taiwan, 111 W10159; BRC Plan 112W32101; Towards the 2030 Cross-Domain Project for Smart Healthcare and Wellness (2/2)—SMART Plan; NSTC 111-2634-F-A49-014-; NSTC 111-2634-F-006-012; Innovative Translational Center Project 112w94002.

Institutional Review Board Statement: This meta-analysis did not intervene or interact with humans or collect identifiable private information and thus does not require institutional review board approval.

Informed Consent Statement: Not applicable.

Data Availability Statement: Data are contained within the article and Supplementary Materials.

Conflicts of Interest: The authors declare no conflicts of interest.

References

1. Siegel, R.L.; Miller, K.D.; Wagle, N.S.; Jemal, A. Cancer statistics, 2023. *CA A Cancer J. Clin.* **2023**, *73*, 17–48. [CrossRef] [PubMed]
2. Morrison, E.J.; Novotny, P.J.; Sloan, J.A.; Yang, P.; Patten, C.A.; Ruddy, K.J.; Clark, M.M. Emotional Problems, Quality of Life, and Symptom Burden in Patients with Lung Cancer. *Clin. Lung Cancer* **2017**, *18*, 497–503. [CrossRef] [PubMed]
3. McIntyre, A.; Ganti, A.K. Lung cancer—A global perspective. *J. Surg. Oncol.* **2017**, *115*, 550–554. [CrossRef] [PubMed]
4. Hirsch, F.R.; Scagliotti, G.V.; Mulshine, J.L.; Kwon, R.; Curran, W.J., Jr.; Wu, Y.-L.; Paz-Ares, L. Lung cancer: Current therapies and new targeted treatments. *Lancet* **2017**, *389*, 299–311. [CrossRef]
5. SEER*Explorer: An Interactive Website for SEER Cancer Statistics [Internet]. Surveillance Research Program, National Cancer Institute. Available online: https://seer.cancer.gov/explorer/ (accessed on 23 February 2023).
6. De Koning, H.J.; Van Der Aalst, C.M.; De Jong, P.A.; Scholten, E.T.; Nackaerts, K.; Heuvelmans, M.A.; Lammers, J.-W.J.; Weenink, C.; Yousaf-Khan, U.; Horeweg, N.; et al. Reduced Lung-Cancer Mortality with Volume CT Screening in a Randomized Trial. *N. Engl. J. Med.* **2020**, *382*, 503–513. [CrossRef]
7. Duma, N.; Santana-Davila, R.; Molina, J.R. Non-Small Cell Lung Cancer: Epidemiology, Screening, Diagnosis, and Treatment. *Mayo Clin. Proc.* **2019**, *94*, 1623–1640. [CrossRef]
8. Lee, E.; Kazerooni, E.A. Lung Cancer Screening. *Semin. Respir. Crit. Care Med.* **2022**, *43*, 839–850. [CrossRef]
9. Zhang, X.; Liu, B.; Liu, K.; Wang, L. The diagnosis performance of convolutional neural network in the detection of pulmonary nodules: A systematic review and meta-analysis. *Acta Radiol.* **2023**, *64*, 2987–2998. [CrossRef]
10. Ardila, D.; Kiraly, A.P.; Bharadwaj, S.; Choi, B.; Reicher, J.J.; Peng, L.; Tse, D.; Etemadi, M.; Ye, W.; Corrado, G.; et al. End-to-end lung cancer screening with three-dimensional deep learning on low-dose chest computed tomography. *Nat. Med.* **2019**, *25*, 954–961. [CrossRef]
11. Joshua, E.S.N.; Bhattacharyya, D.; Chakkravarthy, M.; Byun, Y.-C. 3D CNN with Visual Insights for Early Detection of Lung Cancer Using Gradient-Weighted Class Activation. *J. Healthc. Eng.* **2021**, *2021*, 6695518. [CrossRef]
12. Mikhael, P.G.; Wohlwend, J.; Yala, A.; Karstens, L.; Xiang, J.; Takigami, A.K.; Bourgouin, P.P.; Chan, P.; Mrah, S.; Amayri, W.; et al. Sybil: A Validated Deep Learning Model to Predict Future Lung Cancer Risk from a Single Low-Dose Chest Computed Tomography. *J. Clin. Oncol.* **2023**, *41*, 2191–2200. [CrossRef] [PubMed]

13. Wankhade, S.; Vigneshwari, S. A novel hybrid deep learning method for early detection of lung cancer using neural networks. *Healthc. Anal.* **2023**, *3*, 100195. [CrossRef]
14. Rudin, C. Why black box machine learning should be avoided for high-stakes decisions, in brief. *Nat. Rev. Methods Prim.* **2022**, *2*, 81. [CrossRef]
15. Liu, M.; Wu, J.; Wang, N.; Zhang, X.; Bai, Y.; Guo, J.; Zhang, L.; Liu, S.; Tao, K. The value of artificial intelligence in the diagnosis of lung cancer: A systematic review and meta-analysis. *PLoS ONE* **2023**, *18*, e0273445. [CrossRef]
16. Forte, G.C.; Altmayer, S.; Silva, R.F.; Stefani, M.T.; Libermann, L.L.; Cavion, C.C.; Youssef, A.; Forghani, R.; King, J.; Mohamed, T.-L.; et al. Deep Learning Algorithms for Diagnosis of Lung Cancer: A Systematic Review and Meta-Analysis. *Cancers* **2022**, *14*, 3856. [CrossRef]
17. Thong, L.T.; Chou, H.S.; Chew, H.S.J.; Lau, Y. Diagnostic test accuracy of artificial intelligence-based imaging for lung cancer screening: A systematic review and meta-analysis. *Lung Cancer* **2023**, *176*, 4–13. [CrossRef]
18. Page, M.J.; McKenzie, J.E.; Bossuyt, P.M.; Boutron, I.; Hoffmann, T.C.; Mulrow, C.D.; Shamseer, L.; Tetzlaff, J.M.; Akl, E.A.; Brennan, S.E.; et al. The PRISMA 2020 statement: An updated guideline for reporting systematic reviews. *BMJ* **2021**, *372*, n71. [CrossRef]
19. Mongan, J.; Moy, L.; Kahn, C.E. Checklist for Artificial Intelligence in Medical Imaging (CLAIM): A Guide for Authors and Reviewers. *Radiol. Artif. Intell.* **2020**, *2*, e200029. [CrossRef]
20. Whiting, P.F.; Rutjes, A.W.S.; Westwood, M.E.; Mallett, S.; Deeks, J.J.; Reitsma, J.B.; Leeflang, M.M.G.; Sterne, J.A.C.; Bossuyt, P.M.M.; QUADAS-2 Group. QUADAS-2: A Revised Tool for the Quality Assessment of Diagnostic Accuracy Studies. *Ann. Intern. Med.* **2011**, *155*, 529–536. [CrossRef]
21. Wan, X.; Wang, W.; Liu, J.; Tong, T. Estimating the sample mean and standard deviation from the sample size, median, range and/or interquartile range. *BMC Med. Res. Methodol.* **2014**, *14*, 135. [CrossRef]
22. Luo, D.; Wan, X.; Liu, J.; Tong, T. Optimally estimating the sample mean from the sample size, median, mid-range, and/or mid-quartile range. *Stat. Methods Med. Res.* **2018**, *27*, 1785–1805. [CrossRef] [PubMed]
23. Borenstein, M.; Hedges, L.V.; Rothstein, H.R. Fixed-Effect versus Random-Effects Models. In *Introduction to Meta-Analysis*; Borenstein, M., Ed.; Wiley: Hoboken, NJ, USA, 2009; pp. 77–86.
24. Borenstein, M.; Higgins, J.P.T. Meta-Analysis and Subgroups. *Prev. Sci.* **2013**, *14*, 134–143. [CrossRef] [PubMed]
25. Morton, S.C.; Adams, J.L.; Suttorp, M.J.; Shekelle, P.G. *Meta-regression Approaches: What, Why, When, and How?* Agency for Healthcare Research and Quality (US): Rockville, MD, USA, 2004; Volume 1. Available online: https://www.ncbi.nlm.nih.gov/books/NBK43897/ (accessed on 7 November 2023).
26. Higgins, J.P.T.; Thompson, S.G.; Deeks, J.J.; Altman, D.G. Measuring inconsistency in meta-analyses. *BMJ* **2003**, *327*, 557–560. [CrossRef]
27. Egger, M.; Smith, G.D.; Schneider, M.; Minder, C. Bias in meta-analysis detected by a simple, graphical test. *BMJ* **1997**, *315*, 629–634. [CrossRef]
28. Zhao, W.; Ma, J.; Zhao, L.; Hou, R.; Qiu, L.; Fu, X.; Zhao, J. PUNDIT: Pulmonary nodule detection with image category transformation. *Med. Phys.* **2023**, *50*, 2914–2927. [CrossRef]
29. Zhang, M.; Kong, Z.; Zhu, W.; Yan, F.; Xie, C. Pulmonary nodule detection based on 3D feature pyramid network with incorporated squeeze-and-excitation-attention mechanism. *Concurr. Comput. Pract. Exp.* **2023**, *35*, e6237. [CrossRef]
30. Zhang, H.; Zhang, H. LungSeek: 3D Selective Kernel residual network for pulmonary nodule diagnosis. *Vis. Comput.* **2023**, *39*, 679–692. [CrossRef]
31. Xu, R.; Liu, Z.; Luo, Y.; Hu, H.; Shen, L.; Du, B.; Kuang, K.; Yang, J. SGDA: Towards 3D Universal Pulmonary Nodule Detection via Slice Grouped Domain Attention. *IEEE/ACM Trans. Comput. Biol. Bioinform.* **2023**, *21*, 1093–1105. [CrossRef]
32. Wang, X.; Su, R.; Xie, W.; Wang, W.; Xu, Y.; Mann, R.; Han, J.; Tan, T. 2.75D: Boosting learning by representing 3D Medical imaging to 2D features for small data. *Biomed. Signal Process. Control* **2023**, *84*, 104858. [CrossRef]
33. Shen, Z.; Cao, P.; Yang, J.; Zaiane, O.R. WS-LungNet: A two-stage weakly-supervised lung cancer detection and diagnosis network. *Comput. Biol. Med.* **2023**, *154*, 106587. [CrossRef]
34. Mkindu, H.; Wu, L.; Zhao, Y. 3D multi-scale vision transformer for lung nodule detection in chest CT images. *Signal Image Video Process.* **2023**, *17*, 2473–2480. [CrossRef]
35. Mkindu, H.; Wu, L.; Zhao, Y. Lung nodule detection of CT images based on combining 3D-CNN and squeeze-and-excitation networks. *Multimed. Tools Appl.* **2023**, *82*, 25747–25760. [CrossRef]
36. Lin, J.; She, Q.; Chen, Y. Pulmonary nodule detection based on IR-UNet++. *Med. Biol. Eng. Comput.* **2023**, *61*, 485–495. [CrossRef]
37. Hendrix, W.; Hendrix, N.; Scholten, E.T.; Mourits, M.; Jong, J.T.-D.; Schalekamp, S.; Korst, M.; van Leuken, M.; van Ginneken, B.; Prokop, M.; et al. Deep learning for the detection of benign and malignant pulmonary nodules in non-screening chest CT scans. *Commun. Med.* **2023**, *3*, 156. [CrossRef]

38. Guo, Q.; Wang, C.; Guo, J.; Bai, H.; Xu, X.; Yang, L.; Wang, J.; Chen, N.; Wang, Z.; Gan, Y.; et al. The Gap in the Thickness: Estimating Effectiveness of Pulmonary Nodule Detection in Thick- and Thin-Section CT Images with 3D Deep Neural Networks. *Comput. Methods Programs Biomed.* **2023**, *229*, 107290. [CrossRef] [PubMed]
39. Chen, Y.; Hou, X.; Yang, Y.; Ge, Q.; Zhou, Y.; Nie, S. A Novel Deep Learning Model Based on Multi-Scale and Multi-View for Detection of Pulmonary Nodules. *J. Digit. Imaging* **2023**, *36*, 688–699. [CrossRef]
40. Zheng, S.; Kong, S.; Huang, Z.; Pan, L.; Zeng, T.; Zheng, B.; Yang, M.; Liu, Z. A Lower False Positive Pulmonary Nodule Detection Approach for Early Lung Cancer Screening. *Diagnostics* **2022**, *12*, 2660. [CrossRef]
41. Zhang, H.; Peng, Y.; Guo, Y. Pulmonary nodules detection based on multi-scale attention networks. *Sci. Rep.* **2022**, *12*, 1466. [CrossRef] [PubMed]
42. Zhang, G.; Zhang, H.; Yao, Y.; Shen, Q. Attention-Guided Feature Extraction and Multiscale Feature Fusion 3D ResNet for Automated Pulmonary Nodule Detection. *IEEE Access* **2022**, *10*, 61530–61543. [CrossRef]
43. Yuan, H.; Wu, Y.; Cheng, J.; Fan, Z.; Zeng, Z. Pulmonary Nodule Detection Using 3-D Residual U-Net Oriented Context-Guided Attention and Multi-Branch Classification Network. *IEEE Access* **2021**, *10*, 82–98. [CrossRef]
44. Suzuki, K.; Otsuka, Y.; Nomura, Y.; Kumamaru, K.K.; Kuwatsuru, R.; Aoki, S. Development and Validation of a Modified Three-Dimensional U-Net Deep-Learning Model for Automated Detection of Lung Nodules on Chest CT Images From the Lung Image Database Consortium and Japanese Datasets. *Acad. Radiol.* **2022**, *29*, S11–S17. [CrossRef]
45. Niu, C.; Wang, G. Unsupervised contrastive learning based transformer for lung nodule detection. *Phys. Med. Biol.* **2022**, *67*, 204001. [CrossRef] [PubMed]
46. Mei, J.; Cheng, M.-M.; Xu, G.; Wan, L.-R.; Zhang, H. SANet: A Slice-Aware Network for Pulmonary Nodule Detection. *IEEE Trans. Pattern Anal. Mach. Intell.* **2022**, *44*, 4374–4387. [CrossRef] [PubMed]
47. Ma, H.; Guo, H.; Zhao, M.; Qi, S.; Li, H.; Tian, Y.; Li, Z.; Zhang, G.; Yao, Y.; Qian, W. Automatic pulmonary ground-glass opacity nodules detection and classification based on 3D neural network. *Med. Phys.* **2022**, *49*, 2555–2569. [CrossRef]
48. Luo, X.; Song, T.; Wang, G.; Chen, J.; Chen, Y.; Li, K.; Metaxas, D.N.; Zhang, S. SCPM-Net: An anchor-free 3D lung nodule detection network using sphere representation and center points matching. *Med. Image Anal.* **2022**, *75*, 102287. [CrossRef]
49. Liu, J.; Cao, L.; Akin, O.; Tian, Y. Robust and accurate pulmonary nodule detection with self-supervised feature learning on domain adaptation. *Front. Radiol.* **2022**, *2*, 1041518. [CrossRef]
50. Katase, S.; Ichinose, A.; Hayashi, M.; Watanabe, M.; Chin, K.; Takeshita, Y.; Shiga, H.; Tateishi, H.; Onozawa, S.; Shirakawa, Y.; et al. Development and performance evaluation of a deep learning lung nodule detection system. *BMC Med. Imaging* **2022**, *22*, 203. [CrossRef]
51. Huang, Y.-S.; Chou, P.-R.; Chen, H.-M.; Chang, Y.-C.; Chang, R.-F. One-stage pulmonary nodule detection using 3-D DCNN with feature fusion and attention mechanism in CT image. *Comput. Methods Programs Biomed.* **2022**, *220*, 106786. [CrossRef]
52. Guo, Z.; Zhao, L.; Yuan, J.; Yu, H. MSANet: Multiscale Aggregation Network Integrating Spatial and Channel Information for Lung Nodule Detection. *IEEE J. Biomed. Health Inform.* **2021**, *26*, 2547–2558. [CrossRef]
53. Pereira, F.R.; De Andrade, J.M.C.; Escuissato, D.L.; De Oliveira, L.F. Classifier Ensemble Based on Computed Tomography Attenuation Patterns for Computer-Aided Detection System. *IEEE Access* **2021**, *9*, 123134–123145. [CrossRef]
54. Peng, H.; Sun, H.; Guo, Y. 3D multi-scale deep convolutional neural networks for pulmonary nodule detection. *PLoS ONE* **2021**, *16*, e0244406. [CrossRef] [PubMed]
55. Nguyen, C.C.; Tran, G.S.; Nguyen, V.T.; Burie, J.-C.; Nghiem, T.P. Pulmonary Nodule Detection Based on Faster R-CNN with Adaptive Anchor Box. *IEEE Access* **2021**, *9*, 154740–154751. [CrossRef]
56. Liu, W.; Liu, X.; Li, H.; Li, M.; Zhao, X.; Zhu, Z. Integrating Lung Parenchyma Segmentation and Nodule Detection with Deep Multi-Task Learning. *IEEE J. Biomed. Health Inform.* **2021**, *25*, 3073–3081. [CrossRef]
57. Liu, S.; Setio, A.A.A.; Ghesu, F.C.; Gibson, E.; Grbic, S.; Georgescu, B.; Comaniciu, D. No Surprises: Training Robust Lung Nodule Detection for Low-Dose CT Scans by Augmenting with Adversarial Attacks. *IEEE Trans. Med. Imaging* **2020**, *40*, 335–345. [CrossRef]
58. Farhangi, M.M.; Sahiner, B.; Petrick, N.; Pezeshk, A. Automatic lung nodule detection in thoracic CT scans using dilated slice-wise convolutions. *Med. Phys.* **2021**, *48*, 3741–3751. [CrossRef]
59. Zheng, S.; Guo, J.; Cui, X.; Veldhuis, R.N.J.; Oudkerk, M.; van Ooijen, P.M.A. Automatic Pulmonary Nodule Detection in CT Scans Using Convolutional Neural Networks Based on Maximum Intensity Projection. *IEEE Trans. Med. Imaging* **2019**, *39*, 797–805. [CrossRef]
60. Xu, Y.-M.; Zhang, T.; Xu, H.; Qi, L.; Zhang, W.; Zhang, Y.-D.; Gao, D.-S.; Yuan, M.; Yu, T.-F. Deep Learning in CT Images: Automated Pulmonary Nodule Detection for Subsequent Management Using Convolutional Neural Network. *Cancer Manag. Res.* **2020**, *12*, 2979–2992. [CrossRef]

61. Tan, M.; Wu, F.; Yang, B.; Ma, J.; Kong, D.; Chen, Z.; Long, D. Pulmonary nodule detection using hybrid two-stage 3D CNNs. *Med. Phys.* **2020**, *47*, 3376–3388. [CrossRef]
62. Ozdemir, O.; Russell, R.L.; Berlin, A.A. A 3D Probabilistic Deep Learning System for Detection and Diagnosis of Lung Cancer Using Low-Dose CT Scans. *IEEE Trans. Med. Imaging* **2019**, *39*, 1419–1429. [CrossRef]
63. Masood, A.; Yang, P.; Sheng, B.; Li, H.; Li, P.; Qin, J.; Lanfranchi, V.; Kim, J.; Feng, D.D. Cloud-Based Automated Clinical Decision Support System for Detection and Diagnosis of Lung Cancer in Chest CT. *IEEE J. Transl. Eng. Health Med.* **2019**, *8*, 4300113. [CrossRef]
64. Guo, J.; Wang, C.; Xu, X.; Shao, J.; Yang, L.; Gan, Y.; Yi, Z.; Li, W. DeepLN: An artificial intelligence-based automated system for lung cancer screening. *Ann. Transl. Med.* **2020**, *8*, 1126. [CrossRef] [PubMed]
65. Chenyang, L.; Chan, S.-C. A Joint Detection and Recognition Approach to Lung Cancer Diagnosis From CT Images with Label Uncertainty. *IEEE Access* **2020**, *8*, 228905–228921. [CrossRef]
66. Cao, H.; Liu, H.; Song, E.; Ma, G.; Jin, R.; Xu, X.; Liu, T.; Hung, C.-C. A Two-Stage Convolutional Neural Networks for Lung Nodule Detection. *IEEE J. Biomed. Health Inform.* **2020**, *24*, 2006–2015. [CrossRef] [PubMed]
67. Gong, L.; Jiang, S.; Yang, Z.; Zhang, G.; Wang, L. Automated pulmonary nodule detection in CT images using 3D deep squeeze-and-excitation networks. *Int. J. Comput. Assist. Radiol. Surg.* **2019**, *14*, 1969–1979. [CrossRef]
68. Winkels, M.; Cohen, T.S. Pulmonary nodule detection in CT scans with equivariant CNNs. *Med. Image Anal.* **2019**, *55*, 15–26. [CrossRef]
69. Nasrullah, N.; Sang, J.; Alam, M.S.; Mateen, M.; Cai, B.; Hu, H. Automated Lung Nodule Detection and Classification Using Deep Learning Combined with Multiple Strategies. *Sensors* **2019**, *19*, 3722. [CrossRef]
70. Huang, X.; Sun, W.; Tseng, T.L.B.; Li, C.; Qian, W. Fast and fully-automated detection and segmentation of pulmonary nodules in thoracic CT scans using deep convolutional neural networks. *Comput. Med. Imaging Graph.* **2019**, *74*, 25–36. [CrossRef]
71. Huang, W.; Xue, Y.; Wu, Y. A CAD system for pulmonary nodule prediction based on deep three-dimensional convolutional neural networks and ensemble learning. *PLoS ONE* **2019**, *14*, e0219369. [CrossRef]
72. Zhang, J.; Xia, Y.; Zeng, H.; Zhang, Y. NODULe: Combining constrained multi-scale LoG filters with densely dilated 3D deep convolutional neural network for pulmonary nodule detection. *Neurocomputing* **2018**, *317*, 159–167. [CrossRef]
73. Gu, Y.; Lu, X.; Yang, L.; Zhang, B.; Yu, D.; Zhao, Y.; Gao, L.; Wu, L.; Zhou, T. Automatic lung nodule detection using a 3D deep convolutional neural network combined with a multi-scale prediction strategy in chest CTs. *Comput. Biol. Med.* **2018**, *103*, 220–231. [CrossRef]
74. Setio, A.A.A.; Traverso, A.; de Bel, T.; Berens, M.S.; Bogaard, C.V.D.; Cerello, P.; Chen, H.; Dou, Q.; Fantacci, M.E.; Geurts, B.; et al. Validation, comparison, and combination of algorithms for automatic detection of pulmonary nodules in computed tomography images: The LUNA16 challenge. *Med. Image Anal.* **2017**, *42*, 1–13. [CrossRef] [PubMed]
75. Wang, T.-W.; Hong, J.-S.; Chiu, H.-Y.; Chao, H.-S.; Chen, Y.-M.; Wu, Y.-T. Standalone deep learning versus experts for diagnosis lung cancer on chest computed tomography: A systematic review. *Eur. Radiol.* **2024**, *34*, 7397–7407. [CrossRef] [PubMed]
76. Wang, T.-W.; Hong, J.-S.; Huang, J.-W.; Liao, C.-Y.; Lu, C.-F.; Wu, Y.-T. Systematic review and meta-analysis of deep learning applications in computed tomography lung cancer segmentation. *Radiother. Oncol.* **2024**, *197*, 110344. [CrossRef]
77. Lui, N.S.; Benson, J.; He, H.; Imielski, B.R.; Kunder, C.A.; Liou, D.Z.; Backhus, L.M.; Berry, M.F.; Shrager, J.B. Sub-solid lung adenocarcinoma in Asian versus Caucasian patients: Different biology but similar outcomes. *J. Thorac. Dis.* **2020**, *12*, 2161–2171. [CrossRef]
78. Bai, C.; Choi, C.-M.; Chu, C.M.; Anantham, D.; Ho, J.C.-M.; Khan, A.Z.; Lee, J.-M.; Li, S.Y.; Saenghirunvattana, S.; Yim, A. Evaluation of Pulmonary Nodules: Clinical Practice Consensus Guidelines for Asia. *Chest* **2016**, *150*, 877–893. [CrossRef]
79. Majumdar, P.; Mittal, S.; Singh, R.; Vatsa, M. Unravelling the Effect of Image Distortions for Biased Prediction of Pre-trained Face Recognition Models. In Proceedings of the 2021 IEEE/CVF International Conference on Computer Vision Workshops (ICCVW), Virtual, 11–17 October 2021; pp. 3779–3788.
80. Krishnakumar, A.; Prabhu, V.; Sudhakar, S.; Hoffman, J. UDIS: Unsupervised Discovery of Bias in Deep Visual Recognition Models. In Proceedings of the BMVC, Online, 22–25 November 2021.
81. Yu, A.C.; Mohajer, B.; Eng, J. External Validation of Deep Learning Algorithms for Radiologic Diagnosis: A Systematic Review. *Radiol. Artif. Intell.* **2022**, *4*, e210064. [CrossRef]
82. Tianchi. Tianchi Medical AI Competition: Intelligent Diagnosis of Pulmonary Nodules. 2017. Available online: https://tianchi.aliyun.com/competition/entrance/231601/introduction (accessed on 7 November 2023).
83. Morosov, S.; Kulberg, N.; Gombolevskiy, V.; Ledikhova, N.; Sokolina, I.; Vladzimirskiy, A.; Bardin, A. Tagged Results of Lung Computed Tomography Scans. RU Patent 2018620500. 2018.
84. Armato, S.G.; Drukker, K.; Li, F.; Hadjiiski, L.; Tourassi, G.D.; Engelmann, R.M.; Giger, M.L.; Redmond, G.; Farahani, K.; Kirby, J.S.; et al. LUNGx Challenge for computerized lung nodule classification. *J. Med. Imaging* **2016**, *3*, 044506. [CrossRef]

85. Dolejsi, M.; Kybic, J.; Polovincák, M.; Tuma, S. The Lung TIME: Annotated lung nodule dataset and nodule detection framework. In Proceedings of the Medical Imaging 2009: Computer-Aided Diagnosis, Lake Buena Vista, FL, USA, 10–12 February 2009; Volume 7260, p. 72601U. [CrossRef]
86. Pedrosa, J.; Aresta, G.; Ferreira, C.; Rodrigues, M.; Leitão, P.; Carvalho, A.S.; Rebelo, J.; Negrão, E.; Ramos, I.; Cunha, A.; et al. LNDb: A lung nodule database on computed tomography. *arXiv* **2019**, arXiv:191108434.
87. National Lung Screening Trial Research Team. The National Lung Screening Trial: Overview and Study Design. *Radiology* **2011**, *258*, 243–253. [CrossRef]
88. Wang, T.-W.; Hsu, M.-S.; Lee, W.-K.; Pan, H.-C.; Yang, H.-C.; Lee, C.-C.; Wu, Y.-T. Brain metastasis tumor segmentation and detection using deep learning algorithms: A systematic review and meta-analysis. *Radiother. Oncol.* **2023**, *190*, 110007. [CrossRef]
89. Wang, T.-W.; Shiao, Y.-C.; Hong, J.-S.; Lee, W.-K.; Hsu, M.-S.; Cheng, H.-M.; Yang, H.-C.; Lee, C.-C.; Pan, H.-C.; You, W.C.; et al. Artificial Intelligence Detection and Segmentation Models: A Systematic Review and Meta-Analysis of Brain Tumors in Magnetic Resonance Imaging. *Mayo Clin. Proc. Digit. Health* **2024**, *2*, 75–91. [CrossRef]
90. Fukumoto, W.; Yamashita, Y.; Kawashita, I.; Higaki, T.; Sakahara, A.; Nakamura, Y.; Awaya, Y.; Awai, K. External validation of the performance of commercially available deep-learning-based lung nodule detection on low-dose CT images for lung cancer screening in Japan. *Jpn. J. Radiol.* **2024**. *online ahead of print*. [CrossRef] [PubMed]
91. McInnes, M.D.; Moher, D.; Thombs, B.D.; McGrath, T.A.; Bossuyt, P.M.; Clifford, T.; Cohen, J.F.; Deeks, J.J.; Gatsonis, C.; Hooft, L.; et al. Preferred Reporting Items for a Systematic Review and Meta-analysis of Diagnostic Test Accuracy Studies: The PRISMA-DTA Statement. *JAMA* **2018**, *319*, 388–396. [CrossRef] [PubMed]

MDPI AG
Grosspeteranlage 5
4052 Basel
Switzerland
Tel.: +41 61 683 77 34

Cancers Editorial Office
E-mail: cancers@mdpi.com
www.mdpi.com/journal/cancers